Linguistics for Teachers Selected Readings

(lĭng gwĭs′tĭks)

Linguistics for Teachers Selected Readings

John F. Savage Boston College

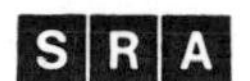

SCIENCE RESEARCH ASSOCIATES, INC.
Chicago, Palo Alto, Toronto, Henley-on-Thames, Sydney, Paris
A Subsidiary of IBM

Printed in the United States of America
Library of Congress Catalog Card No. 72-97928

Contents

Part I—Language and Linguistics

Introduction 2

Linguistics: A Revolution in Retrospect
Albert J. Griffith 16

Linguistics
William G. Moulton 23

Linguistics: A Brief Guide for Principals
Paul C. Burns 33

Language Acquisition: Basic Issues
Stanley F. Wanat 42

Three Processes in the Child's Acquisition of Syntax
Roger Brown and Ursula Bellugi 48

The Nature of Nonstandard Dialect Divergence
Walt Wolfram 67

A Reexamination of Some Assumptions about the Language of the Disadvantaged Child
Susan H. Houston 80

Linguistics in a Relevant Curriculum
Kenneth S. Goodman 92

Postscript 97

Part II—Linguistics and Grammar

Introduction 108

What Grammar?
H. A. Gleason, Jr. 120

Revolution in Grammar
W. Nelson Francis 135

A Concise Structural Grammar
Carl A. Lefevre 152

A Short Introduction to Transformational Grammar
Roderick A. Jacobs 160

John Is Easy to Please
Ved Mehta 165

Linguistics in the Elementary School Classroom
Charles S. Ross and Mary M. Ross 175

Incorporating Transformational Grammar into the English Curriculum
Frank J. Zidonis 187

Snafu, Fubar, or Brave New World?
National Trends in the Teaching of Grammar
James Sledd 194

Postscript 203

Part III—Linguistics and Reading

Introduction 214

Linguistics and Reading
Leonard Bloomfield 225

Linguistics and the Teaching of Reading
Charles C. Fries 237

A Comprehensive Linguistic Approach to Reading
Carl A. Lefevre 243

Reading Comprehension: The Need for a New Perspective
Herbert D. Simons 255

Sociolinguistic Alternatives in Teaching Reading to Nonstandard Speakers
Walt Wolfram 265

Reading the Language of Public Life
Virginia F. Allen 275

Linguistics-Reading Dialogue
Ronald Wardhaugh 281

Implications of Linguistics for the Teaching of Reading
Daisy M. Jones 292

Values of Linguistics in High School Reading
William W. West 302

Postscript 310

Acknowledgments

Sources of the selections contained in this anthology are, in order of appearance:

Albert J. Griffith, "Linguistics: Revolution in Retrospect." *Elementary English* 43 (May 1966): 504–508, 540. Copyright © 1966 by the National Council of Teachers of English. Reprinted by permission of the publisher and Albert J. Griffith.

William G. Moulton, "Linguistics." *Today's Education* 54 (January 1965): 49–53. Copyright 1965, National Education Association. Reprinted by permission of NEA and William G. Moulton.

Paul C. Burns, "Linguistics: A Brief Guide for Principals." *The National Elementary Principal* 40 (September 1965): 37–42. Copyright 1965, National Association of Elementary School Principals, National Education Association. All rights reserved. Reprinted by permission. The quotation on page 34 is from Donald J. Lloyd and Harry R. Warfel, *American English in Its Cultural Setting*. Copyright 1965 Alfred J. Knopf. Reprinted with permission of the publisher.

Stanley F. Wanat, "Language Acquisition: Basic Issues." *The Reading Teacher* 25 (November 1971): 142–147. Reprinted with permission of Stanley F. Wanat and the International Reading Association.

Roger Brown and Ursula Bellugi, "Three Processes in the Child's Acquisition of Syntax." *Harvard Educational Review* 34 (Spring 1964): 133–151. Copyright © 1964 by President and Fellows of Harvard College. The quotation on page 51, from Maclay and Osgood is reprinted with permission from Johnson Reprint Corporation for *Word*.

Walter A. Wolfram, "The Nature of Nonstandard Dialect Divergence." *Elementary English* 47 (May 1970): 739–748. Copyright © by the National Council of Teachers of English for the National Conference on Research in English. Reprinted by permission of the publisher and Dr. Kenneth S. Goodman, President, NCRE.

Susan H. Houston, "A Reexamination of Some Assumptions about the Language of the Disadvantaged Child." *Child Development* 41 (December 1970): 947–963. Copyright 1970 by The Society for Research in Child Development, Inc. All rights reserved. Reprinted with permission of the author and the Society for Research in Child Development.

Kenneth S. Goodman, "Linguistics in a Relevant Curriculum." Reprinted from the April 1969 issue of EDUCATION, Copyright 1969 by the Bobbs-Merrill Company, Inc., Indianapolis, Indiana.

H. A. Gleason, "What Grammar?" *Harvard Educational Review* 34 (Spring 1964): 267–281. Copyright © 1964 by President and Fellows of Harvard College.

W. Nelson Francis, "Revolution in Grammar," *Quarterly Journal of Speech* 40 (October 1954): 299–312. Copyright 1954 by the Speech Communication Association. Reprinted by permission of SCA and the author. The quotation on page 142 by Ralph B. Allen is reprinted with permission of the American Book Company.

Carl A. Lefevre, "A Concise Structural Grammar." Reprinted from the November 1965 issue of EDUCATION. Copyright 1965 by The Bobbs-Merrill Company, Inc., Indianapolis, Indiana.

Roderick A. Jacobs, "A Short Introduction to Transformational Grammar." Reprinted from the November 1965 issue of EDUCATION. Copyright 1965 by The Bobbs-Merrill Company, Inc., Indianapolis, Indiana.

Ved Mehta, "John Is Easy To Please." Reprinted with the permission of Farrar, Straus and Giroux, Inc. from JOHN IS EASY TO PLEASE by Ved Mehta, copyright © 1962, 1963, 1964, 1971 by Ved Mehta. Originally published in *The New Yorker,* May 8, 1971. The quotation on p. 167 is reprinted by permission, from Webster's *New International Dictionary, Second Edition,* © 1959 by G. & C. Merriam Co., Publishers of the Merriam-Webster Dictionaries.

Charles S. Ross and Mary M. Ross, "Linguistics in the Elementary School Classroom." Abridged from *Teacher's Notebook in English,* copyright, 1970, by Harcourt Brace Jovanovich, Inc. and reprinted with their permission.

Frank J. Zidonis, "Incorporating Transformational Grammar into the English Curriculum." *English Journal* 56 (December 1967): 1315–1320. Copyright © 1967 by the National Council of Teachers of English. Reprinted by permission of the publisher and Frank J. Zidonis. Permission to reprint the quotation from Jerome Bruner (page 189) granted by Harvard University Press. Permission to reprint the excerpt by Noam Chomsky, p. 190 "Current Issues in Linguistic Theory" from THE STRUCTURE OF LANGUAGE edited by Jerry A. Fodor and Jerrold J. Katz, © 1964 pp. 50–51 (Prentice-Hall, Inc. Englewood Cliffs, N.J.) granted by the publisher. The quotation on page 193 is from *The Writer and His Craft,* edited by Roy W. Cowden, reprinted with permission of the University of Michigan Press.

James Sledd, "Snafu, Fubar, or Brave New World? National Trends in the Teaching of Grammar." *High School Journal* 49 (January 1966): 162–172. Published by University of North Carolina Press for the School Education, University of North Carolina. Reprinted by permission.

Leonard Bloomfield, "Linguistics and Reading." *Elementary English Review* 19 (April and May 1942): 125–130, 183–186. Copyright © 1942 by the National Council of Teachers of English. Reprinted by permission of the publisher.

Charles C. Fries, "Linguistics and the Teaching of Reading." *The Reading Teacher* 17 (May 1964): 594–598. Reprinted with permission of Mrs. Charles C. Fries and the International Reading Association.

Carl A. Lefevre, "A Comprehensive Linguistic Approach to Reading." *Elementary English* 42 (October 1965): 651–659. Copyright © 1965 by the National Council of Teachers of English. Reprinted by permission of the publisher and Carl A. Lefevre.

Herbert D. Simons, "Reading Comprehension: The Need for a New Perspective." *Reading Research Quarterly* 7 (Spring 1971): 340–341, 354–361. Reprinted with permission of Herbert D. Simons and the International Reading Association. The quotation on page 255 is from E. L. Thorndike, "Reading as Reasoning: A Study of Mistakes in Paragraph Reading." *Journal of Educational Psychology* 8 (1917): 323. Copyright 1917 by the American Psychological Association and reproduced by permission. Permission to quote from George Spache, page 257, granted by Garrard Publishing Co., Champaign, Illinois. The quotation on page 258 is from Thomas S. Kuhn, *The Structure of Scientific Revolutions.* Copyright 1962. Copyright under the International Copyright Union by THE UNIVERSITY OF CHICAGO. All rights reserved. Permission to reprint granted by the University of Chicago Press.

Walt Wolfram, "Sociolinguistic Alternatives in Teaching Reading to Nonstandard Speakers." *Reading Research Quarterly* 6 (Fall 1970): 9–33. Reprinted with permission of Walt Wolfram and the International Reading Association. Permission to reprint excerpts from Goodman (page 268), Shuy (page 269), Wolfram and Fasold (page 270), and Stewart (page 271) granted by the Center for Applied Linguistics, Washington. D.C.

Virginia F. Allen, "Reading the Language of Public Life." An unpublished paper reprinted by permission of Professor Virginia F. Allen.

Ronald Wardhaugh, "Linguistics-Reading Dialogue." *The Reading Teacher* 21 (February 1968): 432–441. Reprinted with permission of Ronald Wardhaugh and the International Reading Association.

Daisy M. Jones, "The Implications of Linguistics for the Teaching of Reading." *Elementary English* 46 (February 1969): 176–183. Copyright © 1969 by the National Council of Teachers of English. Reprinted by permission of the publisher and Daisy M. Jones.

William C. West, "Values of Linguistics in High School Reading." *The New England Reading Association Journal* 4 (Winter 1969): 40–46. Copyright 1969, New England Reading Association. Reprinted by permission. Permission to reprint the excerpt from Emmett Betts (page 303) granted by The Bobbs-Merrill Company, Inc. Permission to reprint the quotation from Charles Kreidler (page 303) granted by the Center for Applied Linguistics, Washington, D.C.

Preface

A Few Words about What Follows

Linguistics has become a magic word in the language instruction of today. Vigorous activity during the past twenty-five years has stretched linguistics beyond the esoteric enclaves of graduate departments of modern languages and brought it cascading down through the high school and elementary grades. High school students are being led to discover the sociological forces that affect language use. Elementary school children are transforming kernel sentences to generate new language combinations. Even some kindergarteners are being taught that the initial phoneme in *Bill*, *ball*, and *boy* is a "lip-popping" sound. We have, indeed, a curriculum and instructional revolution on our hands.

Reactions to this revolution have run the gamut from total confidence to total confusion. At one extreme are the frontiersmen who, spurred on by over-inflated claims by advocates and book salesmen, see linguistics as the panacea to solve all the ills of English teaching. At the other extreme are the skeptics who see linguistics as another fad that will quickly burn itself out in the galaxy of educational innovations.

Many educators in the middle are not absolutely certain of what to think. They aren't quite sure what linguistics has to offer or how practical it is to apply to their work in the classroom. When they try to find out, they are often awed, confused, or driven away by the nature of the materials they have to wade through in an effort to find out. For many teachers in the front line of battle, linguistics is still something veiled in an aura of mystery, a new force that they are either unwilling or unable to cope with in the day-to-day business of classroom teaching.

The collection of articles that follows is an attempt to remove some of the mystery that still surrounds linguistics. It has evolved from a careful review of literally hundreds of articles in a burgeoning collection that has appeared in the professional literature over the past few years and that continues to appear monthly. These articles are mostly for teachers. The selection of articles was made by a teacher for use by other teachers. Most are chosen from educational periodicals. They were selected to help teachers begin to understand what linguistics is all about and how it is affecting elementary language instruction.

There are differences between linguists and teachers. For one thing, the linguist is concerned with languages, a variety of languages. His primary job is the complex task of language analysis. By contrast, the teacher is primarily concerned with only one language, English. His primary job is not one of language analysis but the more practical task of language instruction.

The linguist's approach to language study is scientific. He searches out linguistic data and analyzes it. He is often more interested in the vehicle of communication than with the content of the message that is being communicated (although semantics is one part of the linguistic domain). The teacher's approach to language is different. Society charges teachers with the job of imparting the standard accepted form of language to the young. Teachers are hired to instruct children how to speak and write language "properly." Propriety is not the main concern of the linguist. He is primarily interested in what he observes as the commonly used forms of language. The linguist identifies what the standard form of language is; the teacher instructs children in the use of this form. Teachers are most often concerned with the normative, rather than the descriptive, aspects of language.

There are other differences. The teacher has a major concern with literature, an area of only peripheral concern to the linguist. The concern of the linguist is broader, since he studies all aspects of language and how language relates to culture. While the teacher needs to be well aware of the relationships between language and culture, his major concern is usually more limited to developing his pupils' abilities to know and apply standards of usage. The linguist is a scientist who analyzes language; the teacher is a pedagogue who teaches it. The former searches for information and formulates theories; the latter applies this information and these theories in a functional setting.

These differences notwithstanding, their mutual concern with language creates a bond between the linguist and the language teacher. The abyss that long existed between the linguist and the teacher is closing rapidly. The field of linguistics has a lot to offer teachers. Teachers don't need to be linguists, but they do need to be aware of the linguists' techniques, his discoveries about language, and the latest developments in linguistic science, at least those developments that relate to work in the classroom.

Some of the articles that follow were written by teachers; others by linguists. With only one exception, all were written for an educational audience and were selected on this basis.

The articles in the text were chosen with an eye to practicality. They were selected because they contain ideas and information that language arts teachers can use and apply in their work. Although there is an occasional argument on the side of one theory or another, articles of a polemic nature centering exclusively upon philosophical differences among the various schools of linguistic thought were by-passed. So were many fine articles written specifically for teachers of foreign languages.

Most of the articles are direct and to the point. A couple of the more lengthy ones were edited. The language is not so technical that it requires a background of linguistic training to be understood. Two of the beginning selections were included to familiarize the reader with some of the jargon that linguists use.

The articles that follow represent an attempt to present current linguistic thinking as it is being applied to education. Leonard Bloomfield's "Linguistics and Reading" was published in pre-(linguistic) revolutionary days (1942), and W. Nelson Francis' "Revolution in Grammar" was published in the early years of the revolution (1954). All the other articles were published within the past ten years. *However*, when reading the articles, it is important to keep the date of publication in mind. Linguistics is a fast-moving field and keeping up-to-date requires a full-time effort. New theories are often quickly outdated. By the time many teachers had mastered the "modern theory" contained in Paul Roberts' *Patterns of English* (1956), they discovered his *English Syntax* (1964) that proclaimed and explained an altogether new theory. Similarly, several of the articles included in this book were written in the early and middle 1960s and reflect an orientation toward structural grammar, a theory that was soon afterwards replaced by transformational-generative grammar.

By the time you read this, it is likely that new discoveries will have been made, new theories postulated, other theories modified in the light of new information: old questions will have been answered and new questions will have been raised; new arguments will be raging; new research will have been done; and new linguistically-oriented materials will be available for use in schools. Never mind! This book will at least provide a background that might help you understand these projected developments in the light of what has already gone on in the field of linguistics.

Covering the whole field of linguistics in a single book is at best difficult, at worst impossible (short of a volume that would rival in size the *Encyclopedia of Educational Research*). This collection of articles represents a sample of authoritative thinking, both by linguists who formulate theories about language and by educators who put these theories to work in the classroom. It is by no means encyclopedic. A lot of good material had to be left out. Footnotes and references at the end of each selection are, for the most part, left intact for those who care to follow up.

One final point about the book itself: you're apt to find some repetition from one selection to the other. The writer of an article has to work with severe space limitations. He has to supply a background and make his point in a few pages. Since different articles on the same topic were selected, you will sometimes find the same thing said in a different way about a particular topic. But that's OK. The repetition might help to clarify and/or reinforce material that is important to know.

A Word About Organization

This book, like Gaul, is divided into three parts. Part I, *Linguistics and Language*, is a representative group of readings designed to provide a broad introduction to the linguistic domain. Some articles are of a general descriptive nature to help answer the questions: What is linguistics, anyway? What's it doing in the curriculum? Other articles in part I focus specifically on two areas with tremendous implications for language-arts teachers: namely, language acquisition and the matter of dialect divergence.

Part II, *Linguistics and Grammar,* deals with that part of the language curriculum that linguistics has touched most forcefully. Selections in the second part were chosen to present a rationale for new grammatical models and to present some basic parts of those models known as Structural Grammar and Transformational-Generative Grammar.

Part III, *Linguistics and Reading*, explores the ways linguistic theory is being applied to reading instruction and attempts to shed some light on the question: Just what is a linguistic approach to reading?

The three parts of the book are not mutually exclusive. Some of the articles in part I refer ahead in mentioning the applications of linguistics in teaching reading. Some articles in part III refer back to ideas about grammar presented in part II, and to general linguistic theory included in part I.

Each of the three parts is immediately preceded by an introduction and followed by a postscript and a list of discussion questions and activities. The purpose of the introduction is to explain what follows and to put the ideas presented by the different authors into some perspective. The postscripts are aimed at suggesting some practical applications and implications of linguistics in order to help language arts teachers bridge the gap between linguistic theory and classroom practice. Because of the nature of the selections chosen, practical suggestions are contained in many of the articles as well. The discussion questions and activities are suggested for further learning and general application of the material presented in the articles. The book also contains a basic glossary of linguistic terms used throughout the anthology.

A Final Word

What follows has been designed as an introduction to linguistics for those who need it and a review for those who can use it. It is intended for anyone who is full of questions about linguistics: for teachers who want to get a better grip on that which is so strongly influencing the learning materials and instructional practices of their language curricula; for linguists who want to find out how the results of their studies might be applied in schools; for administrators who want to find out what's going on in classrooms and who want to learn the right kinds of questions to ask when a book salesman tries to sell them "a new linguistic program"; or for anyone who wants to find out something about the force behind the revolution that is going on in language arts today. It is hoped that it will be a particularly useful source of supplementary reading material for courses in language arts and reading, at both the preservice and inservice levels. In short, what follows is intended to provide a useful, consumable, palatable introduction to linguistics as it is being applied in schools.

The editor is deeply indebted to the authors, professional organizations, and publishing companies who have granted permission to reprint the material contained in this book. Sincere thanks are also due Joanne Kenny and Julia Groden whose interest and many hours of work were indispensible in the preparation of the manuscript. Above all, for her encouragement and practical help, I thank my wife Mary Jane, to whom this book is dedicated.

Basic Glossary

The following glossary is basic *in two ways:*

First, it is not exhaustive. It contains only those terms that teachers are apt to encounter in recently published linguistic materials—terms that are used in the selections throughout this book, in other basic linguistics texts, and in linguistically-oriented classroom materials. The number of entries could be expanded at least tenfold to include all the jargon contained in the whole linguistic domain.

Secondly, the definitions themselves are basic. They are concise and therefore sometimes oversimplified. Each definition could be expanded and elaborated upon. Linguists would no doubt differ in defining some of these terms. An attempt has been made here to keep the definitions brief and simple.

A glossary is usually found at the end of a book. In this anthology, it is presented at the beginning, before the terms are used in context. Look over the glossary before you read the selections. Scan those items with which you are already familiar. Carefully read the definitions of the terms that are new to you: it will save you time later on.

Affix. A word element that is attached to a stem or base word. In English, we have prefixes (*un*like) and suffixes (like*ness*).

Allomorph. *See* morpheme.

Allophone. *See* phoneme.

Anglo Saxon. *See* Old English.

Biolinguistics. The study of the relation between the production of language and the biological (or physiological) functions necessary to produce language.

Cant. A special vocabulary of a particular group, containing terms that are designed to conceal meaning from those outside the group.

Comparative linguistics. The branch of linguistics that deals with similarities and differences among language spoken in a particular time period. Also called *synchronic linguistics.*

Decoding. The process in reading of translating printed symbols into speech sounds.

Derivational affixes. Affixes that change words from one part of speech (or *form class*) to another. For example, sail*or*, quick*ly*.

Descriptive linguistics. The branch of linguistic science concerned with making descriptive, verifiable statements about the sound and meaning systems of a particular language.

Deep structure. A concept from transformational grammar, indicating the underlying structural relationships or organization of a sentence; contains information necessary for deriving meaning from sentences.

Determiner. A word that signals that a noun will follow. For example, *the*, *a*, *these*, *many*, *three*.

Dialect. A specific form of a language spoken in a particular geographic region or by a particular social group.

Dialectology. The study of dialects.

Embedding. A process of insertion of one sentence into another sentence. For example, *The boys are smiling* is embedded in *The smiling boys ran home.*

Encoding. Converting a message into a code, particularly into a language code, as from a mental image to spoken language or from spoken to written language code.

Etymology. The derivation of words.

Final contour. *See* Juncture.

Form-class word. A grammatical class to which words belong because of their structural characteristics (the affixes that are added to the words, their position in a sentence, function words that accompany them, and so on). The four form-classes of structural grammar roughly correspond to noun, verb, adjective, and adverb.

Function words. Words with little or no lexical meaning, that do not take inflections and are used to connect form words with syntactical structures in sentences. Function words roughly correspond to such parts of speech as prepositions, conjunctions, pronouns, and other "minor" parts of speech in traditional grammar.

Grammar. The internal structure of language; the rules by which a language operates. See Francis' description of what people mean by grammar, pp. 135–137.

Grapheme. A graphic symbol used in writing; a basic unit of the writing system of a language. Refers to letters of the alphabet, punctuation marks, and so forth.

Historical linguistics. The branch of linguistics that deals with the study of languages through time, how they develop, how they change. Also known as *diachronic linguistics.*

Immediate constituent (IC). The parts of a language construction. For example, the ICs of *The book is on the table* are *the book* and *is on the table*: the ICs of *The book* are *The* and *book.*

Inflectional endings. Suffixes that do not change the part of speech (or form class) of a word when they are added to the base. For example, boy*s*, girl'*s*, larg*er*.

Intonation. The rhythmic pattern or melody of speech. It is also called the *suprasegmental-phoneme system* and consists of *pitch, stress,* and *juncture.*

Jargon. The technical vocabulary commonly understood and used by a particular group, frequently related to vocational or occupational interests.

Juncture. The transition from one speech utterance to another. *Open juncture* distinguishes expressions such as *a name* and *an aim. Sustained juncture* is the pause found after the commas in such expressions as: My friend, George, is not feeling well. *Falling terminal juncture* (or *fade-fall juncture*) is found at the end of a declarative sentence where the voice trails to silence. *Rising terminal juncture* (or *fade-rise juncture*) is found at the end of some interrogative sentences where the pitch level rises.

Kernel sentence. A term from transformational grammar used to describe simple, active, declarative, positive sentences.

Kinesics. The study of how people communicate through body movements, gestures, facial expressions, and the like.

Language. The structured and arbitrary set of vocal symbols that a social group of human beings uses to communicate with one another.

Lexicology. The study of the *lexicon,* the vocabulary of a language.

Linguistics. The scientific study of language.

Middle English. The English language as it was spoken between 1150 and 1500 A.D.

Minimal pairs. Contrasting pairs of utterances that differ in only one sound feature. For example, *pin* and *bin*, *pet* and *pit.*

Modal. A word used with a verb as part of a sentence. There are five modals in English: *may*, *can*, *will*, *shall*, and *must.*

Morpheme. A single, basic, meaning-bearing unit of a language. A morpheme can be a word or part of a word. For example, *cats* consists of two morphemes: *cat,* a *free morpheme* that can stand alone, and *-s*, a *bound morpheme* that must occur with at least one other morpheme. *Allomorphs* are variations within a morpheme class. For example, the vowel change in *men* and the *-en* of *oxen* are allomorphs of the noun-plural morpheme class.

Morphology. The study of the arrangement and interrelationships of morphemes in a language.

Nonstandard language. A form of language that differs from standard language in aspects of sound features, syntax, and/or vocabulary.

Old English. The English language as it was spoken between 450 and 1150 A.D.

Orthography. The spelling system of a language.

Paralanguage. A system of characteristic sound features overlaid on the regular sound system and conveying certain meaning. For example, the emotional cracking of the voice, or talking through a laugh.

Philology. The study of words; a term used especially for historical linguistics.

Phoneme. A basic, indivisible, minimal unit of sound. The smallest usable unit of speech sound in a language. *Allophones* are variations of sounds within a phoneme class. For example, the /p/ in *pot* differs slightly from the /p/ in *spot,* although both belong to the same phoneme class.

Phoneme-grapheme correspondence. The relationship between basic spoken sounds and written symbols (graphemes) used to represent these sounds.

Phonology. The study of the sound system of a language. It includes *phonetics* which is concerned with the production and reception of speech sounds, and *phonemics* which is concerned with identifying and classifying the meaningful speech sounds in a language.

Pitch. The level of speech sounds that is caused by the frequencies used in producing these sounds. In English there are four levels of pitch: /1/ *low*, the level to which the voice normally drops at the end of a declarative sentence; /2/ *normal,* the normal level of the voice in speaking; /3/ *high*, the level to which the voice rises at the end of a question or where the heaviest stress occurs in a sentence; and /4/ *very high*, the level that expresses surprise, shock, or fear.

Psycholinguistics. The study of the relation between psychological and linguistic behavior.

Rhetoric. The art of discourse; the study of the effective use of language.

Semantics. The study of meaning, including the relation between the forms of words and what they signify.

Sentence patterns. Patterns used to characterize or describe the structure of sentences. For example, N + V (Boys run.), N + V + N (Children like candy.).

Slang. Informal language generally containing temporary or fleeting expressions.

Sociolinguistics. The branch of linguistics that deals with the relation between social and linguistic behaviors.

Standard language. The form of language usually spoken by the educated, prestigious, and/or dominant group in a society. The set of language conventions that is accepted for use in education, business, government, and other forms of public life.

Stress. The relative intensity, loudness, or force with which a sound is produced. In English, four degrees of stress are used: /ˊ/ heavy or primary, /^/ secondary, /ˋ/ tertiary, and /˘/ weak stress. Stress is conventionally called *accent* in many school-based reading materials.

Structural grammar. Is a descriptive model of grammar based on the analysis of spoken sentences.

Structural linguistics. The study of the structure of language.

Structure words. *See* Function words.
Surface structure. The *superficial* or observed structural relationships of parts of a sentence. (Compare with Deep structure).
Syntax. The order, patterning, or arrangement of words in meaningful grammatical sentences. Syntax also refers to the study of sentences.
Transformational-generative grammar. A descriptive model of grammar that contains an explicit set of ordered rules that enable us to produce all the possible grammatical sentences of a language and none of the ungrammatical ones. These rules make explicit the relationships that a native speaker perceives intuitively.
Usage. The study of the attitudes that speakers of a language have toward various aspects of that language.

(lĭng

Part I
Language and Linguistics

Introduction

The Study of Language

The study of language has been since ancient times a concern of civilized man. Archaeologists have uncovered sophisticated grammars of Sanskrit that were written centuries before the birth of Christ. At the height of their respective civilizations, ancient Greeks and Romans brought the genius of their great minds to bear on the study of their languages. Grammar and rhetoric persisted as part of the trivium, the curriculum of the Middle Ages. But nobody paid much attention to the study of English prior to the seventeenth century.

English came into being around the year 450 A.D. It evolved from the languages of the Germanic tribes who crossed the Channel and conquered England after the Roman legions left a half a century or so earlier. For the first eleven hundred years of its existence as a language, English developed and changed in what has been designated as three periods of time. Old English (450–1150 A.D.) came directly from the West Germanic dialects and reflected the influence of other languages—notably Celtic, which was spoken before the Teutonic tribes arrived; Latin, which was brought by Christian missionaries; and the North Germanic languages of groups of invading Vikings who eventually settled on the island.

The language was profoundly influenced by the French-speaking Norman invaders who arrived in 1066. During the Middle English period (1150–1500) English underwent the most extensive changes that have ever taken place in the language, and it began to resemble more closely the form of English we speak today.

During the first century of the Modern English period (1500–present) English suffered by comparison with the classical languages, just as it had suffered in the centuries before. Throughout the Middle Ages, Latin had been the subject of language study, since it was the language of the clerics and scholars. In the 1500s the effect of the Renaissance was felt in England and the classical languages continued to be the prestige languages. But by 1600, England had established herself as a major international power and had accumulated a substantial body of literature written in the "vulgar tongue." It was during the 1600s that English began to come into its own as a subject of formal study. In 1640, Ben Jonson produced one of the first grammars dealing with the English language. In the century that followed, linguistic activity in England became intense.

Language study in eighteenth century England centered largely on an obsessive interest in codifying the rules of English, partly in an effort to achieve "correctness" in language and partly in an attempt to protect the language from further "corruption" and change. Language scholars saw themselves as the protectors of the language. Over 200 publications on grammar, rhetoric, and linguistic criticism were produced between 1750 and 1800, more than four times as many as had been produced in the previous 1300-year life of the language.[1] Most of these grammars, as we shall see in the second part of this book, were based on a model of Latin Grammar.

Whereas the eighteenth century had been a period of prescriptivism in language study, nineteenth-century scholars began to develop a scientific spirit in their approach to language. While England was settling back with its new set of grammar rules, language scholars in other parts of Europe were making important discoveries about the history of languages and about the changes in sound systems that came about as languages developed over periods of time. Scholars began to take a more analytical approach to language study. While we can't pinpoint the exact time when the scientific spirit in the study of language arrived, we can say that the linguistic approach was born during the nineteenth century.

During the early part of the twentieth century, language study was closely allied with the developing social science of anthropology. Scholars began to recognize that traditional models and methods of language analysis were inappropriate for studying the languages of non-Western cultures, and so they began to develop the techniques of inquiry that characterize linguistic study today. However, while the awareness and practice of the developing science of linguistics slowly accelerated during the first half of the twentieth century, linguistics still remained the concern of the scholarly few.

Since midcentury, however, linguistics has grown into a more popular discipline that has had a tremendous impact on language teaching in the elementary and secondary schools. During the 1950s, relatively few teachers had occasion to learn or use linguistics. By the early 1960s the need for a background in linguistics was faced by many.

The Scientific Study of Language

Simply defined, linguistics is the scientific study of language. In the selections that follow, linguistics is variously defined in the following ways: "the science of language (that) rests on the simple assumption that language is an observable phenomenon about which empirically verifiable statements can be made" (Griffith); "how language changes through time, how it varies through space, how it differs from one social group to another, and most of

---

[1] For a detailed account of linguistic activity in England during this era, see Sterling A. Leonard, *Doctrine of Correctness in English Usage, 1700–1800*. New York: Russell and Russell, 1962.

all how it *works*" (Moulton); "As a discipline, it is concerned with the scientific study of language" (Goodman). Other more elaborate definitions can be found but all of them come down to the simple definition of linguistics as the scientific study of language.

What sets linguistics apart from traditional language study is the word *scientific,* which is more than a catchword included in the definition to gain prestige or popularity. In his approach to language study, the linguist uses the techniques of scientific inquiry. He is concerned with measurable aspects of language, aspects that are objectively verifiable. He systematically gathers data about language, formulates theories based on this data, and makes his theories subject to revision in the light of new information about the language he is studying. Like any scientist, the linguist does not accept theories about language that are based on authoritarianism, dogmatism, or opinion alone. His study is based on language facts.

We teachers have inherited a rather dogmatic and prescriptive approach to language study (and language teaching) and thus the linquist's approach often bothers us. We get a little uptight when we hear (as Paul Burns points out on page 39) that the linguist might say the expression "I done it" is correct. What the linguist is saying, in this case, goes something like this: "I have gathered data about language as it is used in certain situations and I have found that the expression 'I done it' is used by all native speakers in such-and-such a context." Of course, if the languist's sample is large enough to encompass the language of a broad spectrum of native speakers, he will also discover that other speakers use the expression "I did it" rather than "I done it." It then becomes his job to describe the different standards of language used by native speakers in different contexts and situations. What the linguist doesn't do is immediately condemn "I done it" as bad language.

Linguists generally shun such terms as *good* and *bad,* or *right* and *wrong* in their description of language. Rather, they describe language as being *appropriate* or *inappropriate* to the context and situation in which it is used.

Linguistics is a broad discipline covering many areas, just as language itself touches all aspects of life. The linguist concerns himself with the history and development of language (*historical linguistics*), the similarities and differences among languages spoken at the same time (*comparative linguistics*), the mental activity involved in producing and understanding languages (*psycholinguistics*), the nature and structure of the language being studied (*structural linguistics*), the relation of the language to the culture *(sociolinguistics),* and the function of the physiological organs used in producing language *(biolinguistics).* Within this sprawling domain lies *philology,* the study of written language; *rhetoric,* the study of the effective use of language; *lexicology,* the study of words and their meanings; *etymology,* the study of the origin and derivation of words; *semantics,* the study of meaning in language; *grammar,* the features underlying language and how those features are arranged; *usage,* the attitude of language users toward different aspects of their language; *dialectology,* the study of different varieties of the same language; and other areas. There is no aspect of language that escapes the linguist's attention.

All of these different areas of the linguistic domain should not be thought of as being in separate, distinct, and mutually exclusive cubbyholes. Although there is considerable overlap from one area to another (just as there is considerable overlap of different areas of the natural sciences), each area has a focus unique enough to make it a separate branch of linguistic science.

What the Linguist Sees When He Looks at Language

To the linguist, language is a set of vocal sounds that human beings use to communicate. These sounds arbitrarily symbolize objects, events, and ideas in the human experience. Language is seen by the linguist as being systematic, dynamic, complete, and tied closely to the culture of the people who speak it. Let's look briefly at the characteristics that the linguist identifies in defining or describing language.

Language is human. That is, only humans possess the power of language. Animals can communicate. In fact, some species (such as dolphins) are said to have a fairly sophisticated communication system. But what animals lack is the power to use language symbols to represent their thoughts. Language is an aspect of behavior that only humans can learn. Language vastly expands man's powers of communication and places his civilization a large step above the societies of lower forms of life.

Language is speech. To the linguist, speech is the primary form of language. Because we teachers have dealt so long with reading, composition, spelling, handwriting, and literature—all facets of written language—we have often tended to lose sight of the primacy of speech. But many fully developed languages have existed without any writing system at all. By the time they come to school, most children have already learned to use language to communicate effectively. The adult illiterate is likewise "in command" of his language even though he can neither read nor write. Language, then, is learned and most often practiced in its oral form, and thus speech is seen as the primary form of language. Written language is an imperfect representation of speech.

Because speech is the primary form of language, phonology is the first concern of the linguist. In his analysis, the linguist identifies those basic elements that are part of the sound system of language. He calls these basic minimal units of sound *phonemes.* In American English, there are approximately forty-three phonemes (although some linguists identify as few as thirty-three, depending on their analysis). Linguists identify and describe these phonemes according to the way they are made. *Consonants* are sounds made when the breath stream is blocked, forced through a small opening, redirected or otherwise interfered with at various places in the human vocal tract. *Vowels* are made when the breath escapes with minimal interference; the flow of air through the vocal tract is modified rather than impeded.

As an example of how this analysis is carried on, the linguist hears such pairs of words as *pit* and *bit*, *pit* and *pet*, *pit* and *pig*. (Such pairs of words are called *minimal pairs,* since they differ in only one single sound feature). He notices that these differences, although minimal, are significant enough to make different words. Just looking at the word /pit/ (slanting brackets are used to indicate that the written word represents a transcription of sound), the linguist describes the elements in the following way: /p/ is a voiceless-bilabial stop (the stream of air is stopped with the two lips and the vocal cords do not vibrate as the sound is made); /i/ is a high-front vowel (the tongue is in a relatively high position toward the front of the mouth as the sound is made); /t/ is a voiceless-alveolar stop (the breath is stopped by the front of the tongue touching the alveolar ridge). The linguist continues in this way until he has identified and described all the phonemes of the language.

While identifying these sound elements the linguist is also aware of the intonation features that accompany the production of these sounds—the loudness and softness, the pitch, the pauses in the stream of sound. (Burns describes the intonation system of American English more fully on pages 33–41, and Lefevre writes about its function in the reading on pages 249–251).

As he is studying the language, the linguist also finds that certain sounds and groups of sounds carry meaning. For example, combinations of phonemes that make up words such as cat, desk, book, cup, and so on, have certain meanings. He calls these meaning-bearing elements *morphemes.* When he hears expressions such as three cats, lots of books, many cups, several desks, and so forth, he concludes that the *-s* at the end of these words signals a meaning of "more than one." He calls these elements *morphemes* too, since they carry a certain meaning. (The linguist also finds that this element can be pronounced /z/ as in dogs and pencils; /ɨz/ as in glasses and matches; and that there are variations to the morpheme, as in children, deer, men, alumni, and the like.) Similarly, he finds that elements such as *-s, -ed, -tion, -est, un-, re-,* and others all carry certain meaning in the language and so he calls these units morphemes as well.

As he studies the elements of sound and form in a language, the linguist finds that the arrangement of larger units determines meaning in a language as it is used. In a language such as English, the order in which elements are arranged largely determines the meaning of a message that the language conveys. Consider, for example, these two sentences: John ate the fish. The fish ate John. The words (morphemes) are exactly the same in each sentence, but the meaning of each sentence is very different (especially for John). The study of the arrangement of these larger structural elements in language is called *syntax*.

In the linguist's view, language is seen according to this trilevel structure: phonology, morphology, and syntax. The description and examples used in the previous few pages have been oversimplified. A fuller and more detailed account of these areas can be found in a number of sources.[2]

By the time most children go to school, they possess a significant amount of knowledge about the phonological, morphological, and syntactical systems of their language. They're not consciously aware that they have all this information, of course, but they can, nevertheless, use language to communicate. With occasional exceptions, they can produce all the sounds needed to make words. They have internalized the morphological rules for performing such linguistic functions as making words plural and expressing past tense. In fact, they know these rules so well that they overgeneralize and use expressions such as "I runned and catched the ball." They can arrange words in their proper order to convey the meaning of the message they want to get across. They can follow all the steps that William Moulton describes in his article (page 23).

During the past decade, linguists have devoted a great deal of attention and research to determine how the young child learns so much about his language with little or no formal instruction. The focus of this research has changed from earlier studies of size of vocabulary and elimination of speech "errors" to the mastery of syntactical and morphological rules as indicators of early language acquisition. What the linguists have found is that a child experiences a period of rapid language growth that usually occurs between one-and-a-half and three-and-a-half years of age, and that in the two or three years that follow, he acquires all the basic language rules that he will need to use as an adult. This is not to say that language learning ceases when a child reaches the age of six or seven. Mastery of more complex language structures continues during the school years,[3] vocabulary expands, and the child learns to deal with language in its written form. These stages of growth notwithstanding, most of the language he will ever learn is learned during the first few years of life.

That the child acquires language at an early age is apparant; how he

---

[2] Along with many of the references found at the end of the articles that follow, some good, recent, not-too-technical sources of information about the topics introduced here are: *A Survey of Modern Grammars* by Jeanne Herndon. New York: Holt, Rinehart & Winston, 1970; *Introduction to Linguistics* by Ronald Wardhaugh. New York: McGraw-Hill, 1972; *Language as a Lively Art* by Ray Past. Dubuque, Iowa: William C. Brown Company, 1970; *The New English* by William S. Chisholm. New York: Funk and Wagnalls, 1969.

[3] Carol Chomsky, "Stages of Language Development and Reading Experience." *Harvard Educational Review* 42 (February 1972): 1–33.

acquires it is not so evident. Various theories of language acquisition have been suggested. Stanley Wanat highlights the three major theories of language acquisition—the behaviorist, nativistic, and cognitive theories—in his article "Language Acquisition: Basic Issues." Roger Brown and Ursula Bellugi report on a study that they conducted on the process of language learning during the years of early childhood. And at the conclusion of Ved Mehta's article in part II, Noam Chomsky's theories of language acquisition are quoted. Significant discoveries about how children learn language have been made in the past ten years. More are bound to follow.

Language is symbolic and arbitrary. Language symbols represent concrete objects, activities, experiences, or ideas. Words merely stand for—or symbolize—real things. This symbolic nature of language allows us to abstract ideas and experiences and talk about life in ancient China or a walk on the moon, even though we've never experienced either directly.

The language symbols we use to represent reality are arbitrary; there is no inherent quality in any object or experience that necessitates our attaching a prescribed verbal symbol to it. We call a four-legged canine creature *dog,* for example, because English speakers agree that this word will be used to represent this creature, not because there is any inherent quality in the creature that demands that it be called *dog.* The French call the creature *chien,* the Spanish call it *perro,* the Germans say *hund,* and speakers of other languages attach still different labels. Words are symbols that take on commonly agreed-upon meanings, and the symbol-referent relationship is an arbitrary one.

Language is systematic, dynamic, and complete. Language is not merely a haphazard collection of sounds and symbols but a *systematic set* of sounds and symbols. For example, to form the plural of words or the third person singular of verbs, we chiefly use the sounds /s/, /z/, and /ɨz/ at the end of the base form. (While both of these operations use the same sound elements, they involve different morphemes.) The use of these separate sounds is systematically patterned. We use /s/ when the final sound of the base word is /p, t, k, f, θ/; /z/ when the stem ends with the sounds /b, d, g, v, ð, m, n, η, r, l, y, w/; and /ɨz/ when the stem ends with the sounds /s, z, š, ž, č, ǰ/.*

To use another example, if we take the five words *not, gone, might, he, have* in any random order and arrange them so that they make sense, most mature native speakers would arrange them into the sentence *He might not*

---

* For those to whom some of these symbols may be unfamiliar: θ = the final sound of *bath*; ð = the final sound of *breathe*; η = the final sound of *sing*; š = the final sound of *dish*; ž = the final sound of *mirage*; č = the final sound of *match*; and ǰ = the final sound of *cage.*

have gone (or possibly *Might he not have gone?*) The system of our language dictates the order in which elements must be arranged if our language is to serve our purpose of effective communication. While the system of any language is indeed complex, it is observable and describable and the child learns the system as he learns the language.

Any living language is in a constant state of change. New words are coined and the old ones fall into disuse. Standards of language change too (as evidenced by the departure of *It* is *I* and *to whom* from most school grammar books). If language didn't change, we would still be speaking a dialect similar to the one reflected in the old English epic *Beowulf,* a language completely unintelligible to most modern-English speakers. From generation to generation, changes in language are comparatively slight, but they become very great over a period of time.

Language is also complete; that is, it contains everything we need to communicate all our ideas and experiences to others. Although the ancient Greeks did not have a word for airplane, their language contained elements that would allow them to talk about the imagined entity of "a great metal bird that could fly through the sky at great speeds." Our language has all the elements that speakers need to achieve total communication, even if they have to invent or borrow words to represent that which is completely new to them.

Language is a cultural phenomenon. One cannot separate language and culture, since there is an intimate relation between a language and the people who speak it. Because language develops according to the needs and characteristics of a culture, any language reflects the culture of the people who speak it. It is part of the complex of beliefs, values, and customs that make up a culture. Over the past century, the study of language has closely paralleled the study of culture.

All cultures have conventions—commonly agreed-upon standards of behavior, dress, eating habits, and the like. Since language is a form of human behavior, it too is conventional. It is used according to the accepted standards commonly followed by native speakers of a particular group.

Much of what has already been said about language as a conventional part of a culture can also be said of language as a conventional part of a subculture; that is, that the particular form of language spoken by any group or subgroup in a society is an integral part of the culture and value system of that group. The particular variety of language spoken by a subgroup within the broader language community is called a *dialect.*

Linguists classify dialect according to two general types. A *regional dialect* is the form of language used by speakers living in a certain geographic area (for example, New England or the South). While we use such general labels as New England accent or Southern drawl, it is important to remember that smaller dialect areas with striking language differences can be identified within larger dialect regions. The second type of dialect, *social dialect*, is the form of speech that distinguishes people from different social classes: the affluent educated upper class, for example, as compared with the less affluent and less educated lower social classes.

Dialects differ in three major aspects: *phonology, vocabulary*, and *grammar*. The phonological differences are the most obvious ones. We are all familiar with the differences that mark the speech of someone, let's say, from Georgia (where /i/ and /e/ are both pronounced the same before nasal sounds, causing words like pin and pen, Jim and gem to sound alike) compared to someone from eastern Massachusetts (where /r/ generally disappears in a postvocallic position, making *car* sound like "cah" and *corn* like "cahn"). These rather gross phonological differences are fairly conspicuous to all of us, but the skilled dialectologist can tell which part of town you're from (assuming you come from a large enough town) based on sound features of your speech alone.

Vocabularly also differs from dialect to dialect. Driving for as short a distance as from Boston to New York you will find, in respective dialect areas along the route, roadside lunch stands advertising submarine sandwiches, grinders, hoagies, and heroes—all referring to the same thing (a sandwich on a long roll containing a variety of ingredients). And whether you fry your eggs on a skillet, in a frying pan, a fry pan, or a spider will depend on what part of the country you're from. There are thousands of these vocabulary differences from one dialect area to another.

Grammatical features are more characteristic of social-class dialect. While certain grammatical constructions are unique to some regional dialects (as the well-publicized Pennsylvania Dutch expression, Throw grandfather down the stairs his hat), such language constructions as *we was, he ain't*, and *I don't got no more* are not entirely unique to one geographical region or another. Expressions such as these are more characteristic of a person's educational level or social class.[4]

In recent years linguists have devoted a great deal of attention to the study of dialect divergence in the United States. The results of this research on the topic of subgroup dialects and the thinking that has resulted therefrom has shed a whole new light on the topic and has had enormous implications for teachers.

At any time in any language, dialects exist. One dialect is usually con-

---

[4] The subject of social and regional dialects has been treated here in a very brief and cursory way. Some further valuable and interesting reading on dialectology can be found in three publications of the National Council of Teachers of English: *Dimensions of Dialect*, edited by Eldonna Evertts (1967); *Dialects USA* by Jean Malmstrom and Annabel Ashley (1963); and *Discovering American Dialects* by Roger Shuy, one of the premier dialectologists in the United States today, (1967). Carroll E. Reed's *Dialects of American English*. Cleveland: World Publishing Co., 1967; and *The Linguistic Atlas of the United States and Canada*, a mammoth work many years in the making, are also informative sources.

sidered to be the *standard* dialect. Since the values of the dominant social group in any culture are the most widely held, the language of this group usually emerges as the standard dialect. In Old English where dialect differences were sharply marked from one area to another, West Saxon came to be considered the standard dialect. In Middle English, the standard dialect was East Midland. It was the dialect spoken in the most heavily populated region of England, the one used in London and other centers of learning, and the one that is represented in Chaucer's writing. In modern American English, the standard dialect is the language of the white upper and middle classes.

Standard English, of course, is a statistical abstraction, like the typical American family or the average third-grade class. While it may be labeled and described, it is an abstraction in that no two members in the category are exactly alike. Standard American English is the variety of language habitually used by educated native speakers and might be typified by the language used by network radio and television announcers. Virginia F. Allen, in her article in part II, calls it "the language of public life . . . the set of grammatical conventions governing communications which are beamed at the general public, across ethnic and sociocultural lines."

Side by side with this standard language, literally thousands of subgroup dialects exist. When linguists began to study these subgroup dialects, they made some interesting discoveries. They found, among other things, that all subgroup dialects have the same general language features that mark any language—that the phonological and grammatical systems are just as regular and ordered, that they are complete, that they are totally adequate as communication systems, that they reflect the characteristics of the culture in which they are spoken, that they are capable of logical operations, and that they have a beauty all their own. In short, linguists found that subgroup dialects are effective and perfectly adequate devices for verbal communication (which is the major purpose of language).

We've long been aware of dialect divergence in our language, but how we view these differences has changed dramatically in light of linguistic research. There are two ways of looking at dialect differences: one way sees subgroup dialects as deficient models and the other sees subgroup dialects as different models of language. Walter Wolfram, in "The Nature of Dialect Divergence," sums up the deficient versus different views: "In a *deficit* model, speech differences are viewed and described with reference to a norm. . . The *difference* model considers each language variety to be a self-contained system which is neither inherently superior nor deficient." What are the implications of each of these points of view?

Traditionally, the deficit view prevailed in schools. Dialects were viewed in a hierarchial structure, with standard English at the top of the heap. Standard English was the norm, the yardstick by which all other varieties of language were to be measured (and taught). Subgroup dialects were considered sloppy, careless, awkward, and faulty. The language that the pupil learned as a child, the language of his family and peer group, was considered something to be eradicated and replaced by standard English. Early intervention programs (such as Head Start) and formal school programs tried (and failed) to replace the child's language with one that was all but foreign to him. The language that the child spoke was thought to reflect a cognitive deficiency, and many children were thought to be nonverbal because their language was nonstandard. (In her article Susan Houston examines many of these assumptions in the light of research in this area.) The results of this elitist kind of thinking in schools have fallen somewhere between futility and disaster.

The view that any subgroup dialect has a form and structure all its own—that it is a different rather than a deficient form of language—has changed this hierarchial approach to the matter of dialect divergence. Standard English is no longer the single, universally accepted norm. Since language is seen in light of the context or situation in which it is used, developing dialect versatility in children has become the aim of teachers whose pupils speak a subgroup dialect. In other words, subgroup dialects are not to be scorned and eradicated, but rather the child in school is exposed to standard English so that he will be able to use it when the situation demands. The idea is to make pupils aware of what language to use and when to use it, to make pupils bidialectal (in much the same way that foreign-language teachers try to make pupils bilingual), to enable learners to use an alternate form of language when they encounter situations in which they are likely to profit from using the alternate form.

The distinction between the linguistic versus the social factors of any dialect is an important one. No dialect of any language is intrinsically good or bad, better or worse than any other dialect (including standard dialect). "That one language variety is associated with a socially stigmatized group, and, therefore, socially stigmatized has nothing to do with the actual linguistic capacity of the system." (Wolfram) The problem, then, is not with the subgroup dialect itself but with the attitudes of people toward the status of speakers of the dialect.[5]

No matter how one looks at subgroup dialect differences, most agree that it is advantageous, even necessary, for all children to at least be familiar with (if not in complete control of) standard English. But this need comes from social, economic, and/or academic reasons, not linguistic ones. When and how this exposure should take place are questions that

---

[5] Many fine articles on the topic of dialect divergence as it relates to school can be found in the May 1968 issue of *Elementary English*. The research studies contained in the references following the articles by Wolfram and Houston make additional profitable reading.

have been answered by different people in different ways.

The best time for a formal concentrated program of standard English seems to be the upper elementary and junior high school grades, since younger children are hardly aware of the social forces that suggest the need for mastering a second dialect. Some people, however, make a case for teaching standard English as soon as a child enters school, even before he starts to learn to read.

How best to teach standard English is a question to which there is no easy answer. Language is a skill that is learned by practice and use. Patterned practice (dialogue in which patterns containing grammatical constructions typical of standard English are repeated), role playing, structured discussion, fluency drills and other techniques have been suggested. Two things do need to be present when developing pupils' dialect diversity, however. The first is that pupils ought to be aware of the reason why such learning is advantageous; that is, it is for social reasons, and there is nothing wrong with the language they speak outside of the classroom. Secondly, the teacher needs to be aware of the "conflict points" between standard English and the dialect of pupils; that is, the specific points (mostly grammatical) in which the child's dialect differs from the standard English spoken in the American speech community at large.

This, then, is how the linguist views language: as a human phenomenon, man's greatest invention; as speech, sounds arranged according to an ordered system designed to transmit a message from one speaker to another; as a living, dynamic, changing, evolving entity; as having all the elements we need to share ideas with one another; as being intimately tied to the culture and value system of the people who speak it. When the linguist looks at language, that is what he sees.

But What Is the Linguistic Approach?

The linguistic approach means different things to different people, so it is difficult to state a definition that will suit everybody. Nevertheless, what constitutes the linguistic approach is an important question for teachers. While there is no single approach, a linguistic orientation to language teaching can be said to consist of two components. First, linguistic study has resulted in a new body of knowledge or information about language. This information is part of the curriculum in a linguistically oriented program. Secondly, the linguistic approach is a method of language study that makes it different from the way language was taught before. This second characteristic—call it an attitude toward language study, language teaching, and language itself—is probably the most important characteristic of the linguistic approach.

The content of a linguistic program consists of those facts about language that linguists have uncovered. The history of language, which explains in part how our language got to be the way it is, is part of this content. So are the theories of new grammars. So are the facts about language structure that Burns writes about. In fact, linguistics has been defined by some as a body of knowledge or information about language, and this body of content is taught as part of a linguistics program.

When (and if) a child should learn the terminology and content of linguistics is debatable. On the one hand, people use the you-can-teach-anything-to-any-child-at-any-age-as-long-as-you-do-it-in-an-intellectually-honest-way type of thinking to justify the introduction of linguistic concepts and terminology in the early grades. On the other hand, you have the argument that whether or not a child knows that the phoneme /p/ is a voiceless bilabial stop or that [-'s] is a possessive-forming morpheme, he can still use language effectively, just as a person can drive a car without knowing the principle of the internal combustion engine. Despite this latter argument, one finds content from linguistics increasingly included in recently published materials designed for classroom use.

While the issue of whether children should learn this content is questionable, one issue is more definite: that teachers certainly should know this material. For as Griffith says in his article, "No one would want an English teacher to 'treat' his child's language unless the teacher has a thorough knowledge of the science that underlies the practical arts and skills he exercises and teaches."

The method or attitude with which this content is taught, however, is the prime factor and the best indicator of the linguistic approach. Dull, dogmatic language teaching can still be carried on under the name of linguistics. The linguistic approach is a discovery approach. It starts with the children's language and uses techniques of inquiry in studying that language. "Inquiry and discovery techniques can help him (the child) to examine his own language in relevant ways." (Goodman). The linguistic approach employs an investigative process, not indoctrination. The answers can't be found in the back of the book. Creating an interest in language, not merely teaching facts about it, is of prime importance.

This approach to language study and language teaching requires an open mind regarding language. It recognizes that there are few absolutely unchangeable right or wrong answers on language matters. It is marked by an awareness that language changes, that slang often becomes part of standard language, and that many of the prescriptive rules that were taught in the past are either largely irrelevant or grossly incorrect. It recognizes the legitimacy of the language a child brings to school and requires a certain degree of what has been called *linguistic tolerance.* It requires a change of thinking on the part of the teacher.

These, then, are two benchmarks of the linguistic approach: a new body of content about the structure of language and an inquiry approach to the study of this content. More specific examples of how linguistics can be put to work in the classroom are presented in the postscript following this part of the book.

Another question that is paramount in the minds of teachers is: Will the linguistic approach have any positive results? Will it help pupils speak or write or read any better? Will it help them appreciate literature or love their language any more than they do now? Will there be anything tangible to show (besides gray hair on the teacher's head) after a linguistic approach has been tried?

The twofold purpose of a language program is to teach children *about language* and to help them *learn to use language* effectively. Conventionally, the latter skills-oriented goal was the major one aimed at in language arts classes. In linguistic programs, children learn more about their native tongue. This is the justification for the linguistic approach given by some teachers: that linguistics "puts some teeth" into the language curriculum. People with this point of view eschew practical claims and contend that knowledge about language is its own reason for being in the curriculum.

On practical grounds alone, linguistics can hardly be justified. As Albert Griffith writes, "The real question is not whether scientific linguistics instruction is practical, but whether any language instruction, traditional, linguistic, or otherwise, is practical . . . The experiments recounted from time to time in *College English, The English Journal,* and other periodicals indicate that linguistic instruction is not inferior to, and is probably better than, traditional instruction in effecting improvements in student language skills. But there is still little evidence anywhere to demonstrate that the English teacher, whatever his methods and theories, earns his keep from his practical achievements alone."

One thing is clear, however: linguistics is no miracle drug to cure the ills of English teaching and guarantee instant success for all children. At best, linguistics presents a more accurate picture of our language. At worst, it is no more harmful than what we have been doing for years. This may be reason enough for a linguistic approach.

In his article Albert J. Griffith looks at linguistics in terms that teachers can understand and relate to. He sets out to answer the two oft-asked questions: What is linguistics? and What do we do with it?

In answering the first question, he delightfully disposes of some of the myths surrounding linguistics—that it is a fad, a mystic cult, or a subversive plot—and defines it in brief and practical terms.

In answering the second question, he rejects the need for students' knowledge of linguistics on practical grounds alone. He accepts the possibility of linguistics as part of a student's liberal education. For teachers, however, Griffith contends that a knowledge of linguistics is a practical necessity, essential to those whose profession it is to teach English.

Linguistics: A Revolution in Retrospect

Albert J. Griffith

A third of a century has passed since Leonard Bloomfield brought forth his book *Language*, the great fountainhead of modern American linguistics. It was some twenty-five years ago that the seminal works on the doctrine of usage appeared; the important descriptive studies of Fries, Trager and Smith, and Pike are all a dozen or more years old; even the source book of the supposedly ultra new generative grammars has been around for almost a decade.

Whatever else it may have been, the linguistics "revolution" is now history—recent, of course, but no longer without some perspective in time. It is now something that ought to be capable of fairly dispassionate perusal and evaluation, of the same sort now given to other events contemporaneous with it: the Great Depression, World War II, the launching of Sputnik I.

Yet, well-chronicled as every phase of its progress and regression has been, linguistics is still something of a futuristic phantom to thousands of language arts teachers all over the country who quake in terror when the subject comes up—as it inevitably does nowadays—in the academic homilies of conventions and workshops and in the awesome deliberations of curriculum revision committees. Two questions, the most basic of the myriad questions surrounding the mystery of linguistics, constantly recur: What is it? And what do we do with it?

No perfectly simple or dynamically positive answer, capable of dispelling all the perplexity possible in a teacher's mind, can be given for either of these questions. And yet something approaching an answer can be found negatively: by disposing of some of the myths that have grown up around this unlovely lorelei, linguistics.

What Linguistics Is Not

Linguistics is not, first of all, what the "leave it alone, maybe it'll go away" school would have it be: a progressivist fad, one of those ephemeral fashions which perennially afflict us, but make no permanent impressions upon us. The late Flannery O'Connor once wrote a short story about a Southern school teacher who for "twenty summers when she should have been resting . . . had to take a trunk in the burning heat to the state teachers' college." Her only revenge for this, Miss O'Connor writes, was a "mild" one which didn't satisfy her sense of justice: "when she returned in the fall, she always taught in the exact way she had been taught not to teach." Many English teachers, one might suspect, attempt a similar mute and mild revenge by blithely ignoring in their teaching the linguistic principles forced upon them in summer institutes, professional periodicals, and district workshops. But any hope they may have that linguistics will someday fade away into the nether world where raccoon coats, boogie-woogie, and the hula hoop now repose is likely to be disappointed. We may see McGuffey readers resurrected around us to symbolize the conservative stand against the fickle forces of progressivism, but we are no more likely to see English teaching return to what it was before the linguistics revolution than we are likely to see astronomy turn back to astrology or chemistry to alchemy. Like the physics teacher someone reported who is still teaching the phlogiston theory of fire on the assumption that the oxidation theory is a fad which will one day disappear, those who are "waiting out" the linguistics fad are probably in for a long wait.

If linguistics is not a progressivist fad, neither is it what the "I haven't been initiated, I cannot partake" people try to make it: a mystic cult, whose mysteries are revealed to true believers only. It is true that the average English teacher picking up a copy of one of the new transformational grammars might well think he has a Numerological Society manual or a Rosicrucian tract; and it is true that runic phrases like "constructional homonymity" and "tagmemic representation" and "morphophonemic change" and "immediate constituents" and "terminal strings" and "optional permutations" are almost like passwords by which the members of the current in-groups of the profession can be recognized. But there is nothing to prevent the outsider from learning these shibboleths himself; he needs no formal induction, no baptism, no candlelight ceremonies; he doesn't even have to take a pledge of allegiance or swear a blood oath to begin the Way of the Linguist.

The real opponents of linguistics, however, are not the fad fighters or the cult kidders, but the "it's un-American, I refuse to co-exist" group, who view linguistics as a particularly subtle subversive plot. "What was good enough for grandmother is good enough for me," these people shout. For them, Kosygin, Castro, and Chomsky provide the unholy triumvirate of our day. "We've always taught English the old way," they say; "it's against free enterprise to change." The Linguistic Society of America, they are sure, has secret cells in every school, in conspiratorial alliance with the International Bankers, the UN, the ADA and the NAACP. These Minute Men are ready to face the linguists in an eyeball to eyeball showdown, despite the missile gap that followed on the lexicographic front when the linguists got control of Webster's *Third* (a real fission-fusion device if there ever was one). Linguistics infiltration of the MLA, the CEA, and the NCTE is such that a good old-fashioned "Language, si! Linguistics, no!" is hardly ever found in the pages of the professional journals any more. But the antilinguistics group still finds plenty of champions in the popular press—Dwight Macdonald in the *New Yorker*, Mario Pei in *Saturday Review*, Wilson Follett in *Atlantic*, J. Donald Adams in the *New York Times Book Review*, and (most grandiloquently of all) Lincoln Barnett in *Horizon*—to see that neither capitulation nor coexistence will come easy.

The Science of Language

For most teachers, however, linguistics is neither fad, cult, nor plot, though it may alternately amuse, puzzle, and terrify. Linguistics is simply an unknown quantity, which (perhaps not altogether through their own fault) they have failed to assess. But despite the fuss and furor, linguistics is not all that complicated. It is basically nothing more than the science of language and rests on the simple assumption that language is (among other things) an observable phenomenon about which empirically verifiable statements may be made. Linguistics has its practical drawbacks: it is incomplete, constantly subject to revision and modification, sometimes incredibly picayunish and technical, sometimes daringly broad and conjectural, perennially on the verge of total illumination but never quite out of the dark. It is often confusing as well, as independent observers with different data, different methods, different tools reach different conclusions, coin different terms, make different applications. But these are the drawbacks of any science—drawbacks inherent in the empirical approach, not drawbacks peculiar to linguistics alone. No one would demand that the physicist once and for all explain matter or the biologist life; why should the linguist be expected to produce full-blown an immediate overview of language?

Perhaps it is only the teacher's patience wearing thin. Too long English teachers have been told that their job is to teach composition, literature, and language—without ever knowing precisely what they were supposed to teach about these, especially about language. Most teachers who like to teach language arts like it because they love literature, not because they love to correct themes or conduct drills on grammar. Someday, perhaps, curricular reconstruction will allow some to be solely and simply the literary esthetes they have always wished to be, and other specialists will be assigned to teach the skills of composition and the scientific facts of language research. For the present, unfortunately, English teachers are doomed to the three fold task laid down by the Basic Issues conferences and other official interpreters of the profession, and this task includes the teaching of language.

The Necessary Task

Language must be taught, then, and it is. Or something that vaguely passes for it is taught. Somewhere, in between the chapters on library use and movie selection and telephone etiquette, our textbooks contain amorphous little sections on grammar and vocabulary and mechanics and spelling, which seem somehow to be related to the language teaching task. Exactly what the goal of these chapters and the teaching of them should be, few would be willing to say. Most students are native speakers of English whose linguistic habits have not been significantly altered since their preschool days. Basically all they have traditionally been given are several systems of interlocking and sometimes overlapping classifications of language features and some arbitrary admonitions about what to do with these language features.

There is nothing wrong, of course, in telling students that sentences can be classified as declarative, interrogative, imperative, or exclamatory, for, sure enough, they can be so classified, just as the physical elements can, sure enough, be classified as earth, air, fire, and water. There is nothing wrong with telling students that parts of speech include words that name things, words which modify other words, words which show relationships, and so forth, but it is a little like listing the ingredients of a cake as one egg, several hundred calories, some protein, oxygen, icing, and a cylindrical surface.

There may be nothing wrong, either, with telling students that English has three moods, six tenses, three persons, two numbers, and three genders on the analogy with Latin; but just for variety could one not stretch his imagination a little more and teach them that English has five moods like Menomini, two tenses like Slavic, four persons like Algonquian, three numbers like Sanskrit, or twenty genders like Bantu? If we are going to force English to fit the categories of a language other than itself, we might as well be eclectic about it.

Unquestionably, students are given as much misinformation as information in their English classes. Few could fail to be aware of this fact today, with the propaganda barrage the linguists and the linguistic popularizers have launched. And yet how few have acted to correct the situation. Even discounting the "no, never!" people as unconvertible, there are still too many of the "yes, but not yet" people, and the "yes, more or less" people, those who are hearers but not doers of the word.

The Pragmatic Question

Inevitably, these proscrastinating and temporizing brethren raise the crucial questions: What good will it do to switch to linguistics? What will be the practical results? As in so many other areas of American life, the utilitarian test seems here, too, to be the final criterion. If linguistics can be shown to produce a measurable improvement in the oral and written communication of students, the benevolent pragmatist will be satisfied. But if there is no practical advantage . . .

The real question is not whether scientific linguistics instruction is practical, but whether any language instruction, traditional, linguistic, or otherwise, is practical. This is a question teachers do not always like to contemplate, for the wrong answer might endanger their jobs. Paul Roberts, in an article in *College English*, 22 (October 1960): 1–9, says all teachers must envy the first-grade teacher: "She receives in September youngsters who are largely illiterate and dismisses them largely literate in June." Nowhere else in the English curriculum, Roberts says, can we see such "obvious and consistent progress" or such a "clear connection between the instruction and the improvement." The experiments from time to time recounted in *College English, The English Journal*, and other periodicals indicate that linguistic instruction is not inferior to, and possibly better than, traditional instruction in effecting improvements in student language skills. But there is still little evidence anywhere to demonstrate that the English teacher, whatever his methods and theories, earns his keep from his practical achievements alone.

Perhaps, however, practical results are not the primary goal. Children do somehow learn to speak their native language before they even come to school. A significantly large majority do learn, either because of or in spite of their instruction, to manipulate the written records of their language with some ease. John Keats and F. Scott Fitzgerald never learned to spell but managed to get by passably well by virtue of their other communication skills. Synthetic ability, the talent for creation, is not the same as, nor necessarily dependent on, analytic ability.

As the transformationists put it, a native speaker is a grammar of his language—a machine, as it were, for producing the output recognizable as grammatical utterances of that language. He does not therefore have to *learn* a grammar in school in order to speak; he gained the essential input long before the school marm ever got hold of him. (The activity usually called teaching grammar, incidentally, is usually not teaching the system, the interior logic of the language, which the child already knows and overextends, but the exceptions to the system, the logical absurdities inherent in the language, such as irregular verbs and plural pronouns with singular form, and so forth.) In short, Johnny won't be reduced to grunts and groans, even if he never sets foot in an English classroom.

The Liberal Pursuit

Why, then, do we have these classrooms at all? Because Johnny has more needs than the merely practical. Because Johnny should know more than just how to earn his bread. Because Johnny needs a liberal as well as a vocational education. Because, as Newman says, knowledge is its own end.

In the old days, grammar had its place right there in the ancient trivium, the basis of the liberal education. It was one of the liberal arts, something studied because it was good to know, not necessarily because it was good to use. Linguistics is the descendant of the medieval trivium's old grammar: the liberal pursuit of language knowledge. It is thus comparable to the new math which has gripped the schools. Most people, for practical purposes, need no more math than is necessary to tell time, make change, and figure their income tax; the old math was certainly good enough for this. Why then is set theory introduced to kindergartners today? Because of the belief that it is good for them to know it, that the knowledge is its own end. Uses for analytic grammar are probably even more restricted than uses for analytic mathematics; yet it is good for men to know it, for again the knowledge is its own end.

Linguistics can be taught, then, because it is true or tries to be true, which is perhaps the same thing. No one need become partisan, waxing polemical over each new thesis or discovery. We still recognize that science may need more than one model to represent the reality of a given phenomenon, and, just as the physicist needs both the wave theory and the quantum theory to explain the phenomenon of light, so the linguist may need more than one model to explain the reality of a language. Until we have the single model grammar that is complete, simple, and consistent, we will have to make do with the preliminary models—the current structural grammars, generative grammars, glossematic grammars, and so on—which organize the facts we at this stage possess.

Yet, one other point needs to be made. Even if it is true that linguistics instruction from the first grade to the first year of college is primarily liberal rather than practical, it does not necessarily follow that linguistics instruction remains impractical even on advanced levels. Analytical knowledge of their language may be an academic luxury to students, but it is a practical necessity for their teachers. Teachers do not so much need this linguistic knowledge because they must impart it to others (though they may and should do this to a degree even at the lowest levels), but because they must teach skills (reading, composition, explication) which depend on language. To read, write, and interpret well themselves, teachers, like their students, may get by with intuitive linguistic knowledge, but to teach others these three skills they may have to understand in a more conscious way the processes of language. Thus one may keep himself fairly healthy without any knowledge of anatomy, physiology, hygiene, or medicine; to be a professional healer of others, however, one may find these sciences indispensable.

Professional Competence at Issue

There is not much certainty as to how much linguistic knowledge a third grader or a high school junior or a college freshman needs to possess. But it is certain that an English teacher—at any of these levels—can benefit very practically from an extensive knowledge of linguistic science. Here, though, a little learning is truly a dangerous thing: the absurd errors in "phonics" instruction, the simplistic misconceptions about "usage" categories, the naive misapplications of "sentence pattern" and "transformation" drills are examples enough. No one wants a physician to treat him unless the physician has as thorough a knowledge of the basic sciences of his profession as his times will permit; no one should want an English teacher to "treat" his child's language unless the teacher too has a thorough knowledge of the science which underlies the practical arts and skills he exercises and teaches.

This is a demand which many English teachers may well resent. Many schoolroom veterans do not want to start over learning their subjects anew. It is possible, of course, that other professionals feel the same way: perhaps many physicists resented Einstein and Teller and Oppenheimer and others for complicating their subject and forcing them to reorientate themselves in their own field. It is doubtful, though, that such resentment has led many physicists to ignore relativity or nuclear energy or thermodynamics on the basis that their subject was simpler without these concepts. It may be hoped resentment will not lead English teachers to such a course either.

Teachers may, like Flannery O'Connor's character, have to "take a trunk in the burning heat to the state teacher's college" next summer, or attend an institute here and a workshop there, or perhaps just buy a few books and read a few periodicals, but if they wish to be professionals they must somehow develop the necessary linguistic competence. Once they fully realize the issues, they undoubtedly will.

William G. Moulton sees the main job of the linguist as one of studying how two people are able to talk together. Taking a close look at the act of communication, Moulton clearly delineates eleven steps in the communication process. The first three steps involve *encoding:* semantic, grammatical, and phonological. The next five involve the process of *transmission:* sending the message from the brain to the speech organs, the movements of the speech organs, the vibrations of the air molecules to produce sound, the reception of sound in the hearer's ear, and the path of the message from the ear to the brain. The final three steps involve *decoding:* phonological, grammatical, and semantic. As he describes these eleven steps, Moulton introduces both terminology and concepts basic to linguistic study.

Moulton, a professor of linguistics at Princeton University, has also written *Linguistic Guide to Language Learning.* New York: Modern Language Association, 1970.

Linguistics

William G. Moulton

How language changes through time, how it varies through space, how it differs from one social group to another, and most of all how it works—these things are studied in linguistics. Because modern linguistics has roots which go back to the early nineteenth century and beyond, many people are familiar with some of the things which interested linguists then and still interest them today.

They find it understandable that a linguist should try to find the line which separates those areas in New England where *barn* is "barrn" (with *r*) from those areas where it is "bahn" (without *r*); and they may even envy him a bit when he goes to an Indian reservation or South America or Africa to investigate some hitherto undescribed tongue and thus add his little bit to our meager knowledge of the world's 2,000 to 4,000 languages. (No one knows how many there are.)

But when a linguist says that he is doing some research which he hopes will help us understand a little better how it is that "two people are able to talk together," most people shake their heads in puzzlement.

Yet how two people are able to talk together is, of course, the central problem. During the 1930s and 1940s, most American linguists attacked it by trying to work out better techniques of discovering the structure of language—any language—and of analyzing and classifying what they found. Then, in the late 1950s there came a rather dramatic swing in another direction: away from mere classification of data toward a search for universals and a broad, inclusive theory of language.

In a sense this has been merely a return to some of the prime interests of our nineteenth-century predecessors—Wilhelm von Humboldt, for example. It has also brought American linguistics out of the scholarly isolation from which it suffered for a time, and into closer contact with such related disciplines as psychology and philosophy. (The contact with anthropology has always been close.)

How *are* two people able to talk together? Since most of us never ask this question, but take the matter for granted, it is useful to consider just what goes on. Let us assume that we have a speaker A and a hearer B, that A says something to B, and that B understands him without difficulty. Here an act of communication by means of language, has taken place. But *how* did it take place? What went on inside A? How did the communication move from A to B? And what went on inside B? The process seems to consist of at least eleven different steps. (See the diagram that follows.)

1. Semantic Encoding

We assume that A has some sort of "meaning" (or whatever we want to call it) which he wishes to convey to B. His first step is to get this meaning into proper shape for transmission in the language he is using. (English, we shall say.) Since this is like putting a message in shape to fit the code in which it is to be sent, we can call the process *semantic encoding.*

If A wants to talk to B about some sort of time-piece, his encoding will depend on whether he means the kind that hangs on the wall or stands on a table (a *clock*), or the kind that is carried in the pocket or worn on the wrist (a *watch*). In German the single semantic unit *Uhr* includes both types. If he wants to ask whether B "knows" something, he can use the single semantic unit *know.* Spanish would force him to choose between *conocer* (for a person, place or thing) and *saber* (for a fact).

As these examples show, each language "slices the pie of reality" in its own capricious way. In English, we group a host of different objects, of many types, colors, sizes, and shapes, into the semantic unit *stool.* If to a stool we add a back, however, it suddenly becomes the semantic unit *chair.* If we widen it so that two or more people can sit ont it, it is a *bench.* If to a chair we add upholstery, it is still a *chair.* But if to a bench we add upholstery, it suddenly becomes a *sofa.*

Using a bold and imprecise metaphor, we can think of every language as a vast sieve with thousands of semantic slots in it. Any idea which we want to express in that language first has to be put through this sieve. And every language has a special sieve of its own. The discipline which studies such metaphorical sieves is semantics. (A semanticist would

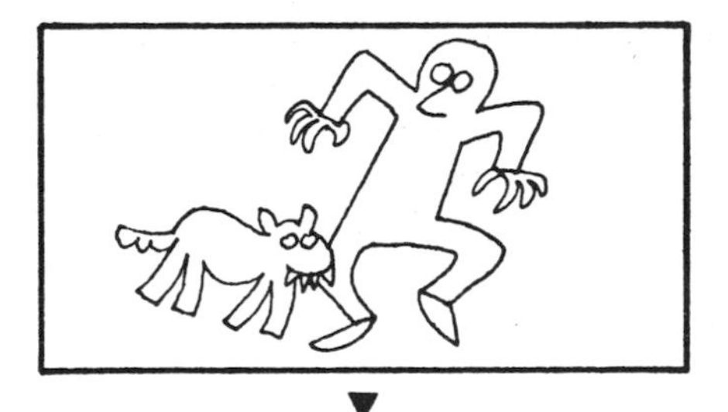

Encoding the message

1 Semantic encoding

2 Grammatical encoding

3 Phonological encoding

Transmission

4 From the brain

5 Speech organs

6 Sound waves

7 The ear

8 To the brain

Decoding the message

9 Phonological decoding

10 Grammatical decoding

11 Semantic decoding

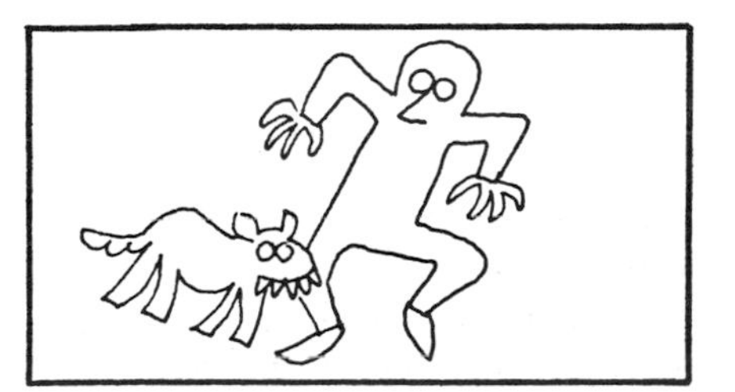

The speaker and his "code"

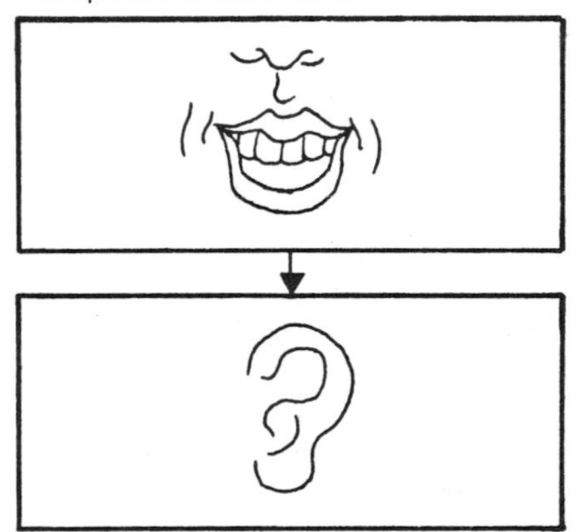

The hearer and his "code"

describe his valuable and difficult work more elegantly, but this a reasonable approximation to part of what he does.)

2. Grammatical Encoding

Once speaker A has found the proper semantic units for his message, he must next arrange them in the particular way the grammar of his language requires. If in English he wants to get across the idea of "dog," "man," and "bite"—with the dog and not the man doing the biting—he has to encode it in the order *dog bites man*: the order *man bites dog* gives quite a different message.

The grammatical code of Latin employs totally different devices. For the meaning "dog bites man" it marks the unit "dog" as nominative (*canis*), the unit "man" as accusative (virum), and it can then combine these words with mordet "bites" in any order whatever. For the opposite message it would mark "dog" as accusative (canem), "man" as nominative (vir), and it could then again combine these with mordet in any order at all.

English grammar signals the difference between subject and object by means of word order; Latin grammar signals it by means of inflectional endings; other languages use still other devices.

The basic units used in grammatical encoding are called morphemes (from Greek morphē "form"). Morphemes may be either words: *dog*, *bite*, *man*, or parts of words; the *-s* of *bites*, the *-ing* of *biting*, and so forth. Some clearly correspond to semantic units: *dog*, *bite*, *man*; with others, however, the semantic connection is less clear, for example, *-s*, *ing*. Still others seem to have no semantic connection at all, the *to* of *try to come*, for example, or the *-ly* of *quickly*.

Morphemes are then arranged grammatically into such higher level units as words; *bites*, *biting*, *quickly* (some morphemes are of course already words: *dog*, *bite*, *man*, *quick*); then phrases of various sorts, for example, *the dog* (which can function, among other ways, as a "subject"); then clauses of various sorts (in English, such constructions contain a subject and predicate); and finally sentences, which are marked in some way as not being parts of still larger constructions.

Recent interest in grammar has focused on the following familiar and yet astonishing (and somehow disturbing) fact—any speaker can say, and any hearer can understand, an infinite number of sentences; and, indeed, many of the sentences we say and hear have never been said before.

How does our grammar provide for this enormous variety and flexibility? If we merely want to reach infinity quickly, we need only allow ourselves to use the word *and* over and over again. There are, however, two far more elegant devices. One is that of *embedding*; putting a construction inside a construction inside a construction, and so on, like a Chinese puzzle. A classic example is the old nursery tale; "This is the cat that killed the rat that ate the malt (and so on and on and on) . . . that lay in the house that Jack built."

Still more elegant is *transformation*, whereby a basic sentence type may be transformed into a large variety of derived constructions. Thus *the dog bites the man* can be transformed into: The dog bit (has bitten, had bitten, is biting, was biting, has been biting, can bite, and so on) the man; the man is bitten (was bitten, has been bitten, and so on) by the dog; (the dog) that bites (and so on) the man; (the man) that the dog bites; (the man) that is bitten by the dog; (the dog) that the man is bitten by; and so on.

3. Phonological Encoding

When grammatical encoding has been completed, the message enters the phonological component of the code as a string of morphemes, and these must now be encoded for sound. This is accomplished by encoding each morpheme into one or more basic phonological units or phonemes (from Greek phōnē̇ "sound"). The morpheme *-s* of *bites* is converted to the phoneme */s/*, *check* to */čĕk/*, *stone to /stōn/*, *thrift* to */θrift/*, and so on.

(Written symbols for phonemes are customarily placed between slant lines to distinguish them from the letters of regular spelling and from the symbols used in phonetic transcription. Just what symbols are used for phonemes is unimportant; one must merely have a different symbol for each phoneme in the language.)

This device of encoding morphemes into *one or more* phonemes each is an extraordinarily powerful one, and in terms of sheer economy it is hard to overestimate its importance. If a language used only one phoneme per morpheme, it could have only as many morphemes as it has phonemes. But if a language uses from one to five phonemes per morpheme (as in the above English examples), the number of possible morpheme shapes soon becomes astronomical.

For a stock of twenty phonemes the figure is 3,368,420; for thirty phonemes it is 25,137,930; and for forty phonemes (English has between thirty and forty, depending on just how you figure them) it reaches the fantastic total of 105,025,640 possible morpheme shapes.

We have given these figures to show what an enormous economy is achieved by having in human language this "duality principle," as it has been called; first an encoding into morphemes, and then a separate encoding of morphemes into *one or more* phonemes each.

There is, however, a very bad flaw in our figure: We have assumed that it is possible for phonemes to occur in any mathematically possible sequence, such as (for English) /ppppp/, /fstgk/, and so forth. But English of course does not do this; like every language, it places very strict limitations on possible sequences of phonemes. Nevertheless, even with the strictest sorts of limits, the duality principle permits every language to form far more morpheme shapes than it will ever use.

If we take English to be a thirty-phoneme language (it has more than thirty, no matter how you figure them), permit no morpheme shapes of more than five phonemes (*glimpse* /glimps/ actually has six), and assume that only one out of every 1,000 possible sequences can be used, we still end up with a total of 25,137 possible morpheme shapes (the above 25,137,930 divided by 1,000)—enough to take care of any language.

If we remind ourselves that English words can easily consist of three or more morphemes (for example, *un-friend-li-ness*), it is clear that we are also provided with an overabundance of possible word shapes—more than enough for Lewis Carroll to invent "slithy toves did gyre and gimble in the wabe," using a few of the thousands of available word shapes which had not previously been claimed.

In the preceding paragraphs, we have assumed, for purposes of presentation, that a message is neatly encoded first semantically, then grammatically, and then phonologically. But since normal speech is full of false starts, hesitations, grammatical slips, and the like, it seems clear that we behave a good deal more like the young lady who when told that she should "think before she spoke," replied with rare honesty: "But I can't do that! How do I know what I'm going to say until I start talking?"

If we do *not* normally plan out our entire message before we start sending it, then we must possess some sort of feedback device which permits us to monitor the message as it is sent and to make necessary adjustments as we proceed—adjusting a present tense verb to agree with its singular subject, for example.

4. From Brain to Speech Organs

When phonological encoding has been completed, the message has been changed from a string of morphemes to a string of phonemes. Speaker A must now somehow program and send on down to his speech organs a set of instructions telling them what movements to make so as to turn each phoneme into sound. We can compare this with the way paper tapes are punched to provide instructions to automatic typewriters, telegraph transmitters, computers, and the like. Programmed in this way, the message is sent sequentially from the brain to the speech organs.

5. Movements of the Speech Organs

Triggered by successive innervations, the speech organs (vocal cords, tongue, lips, and so forth) now perform the proper series of movements. As they do so, an interesting and rather disturbing thing happens. We have assumed that, when the message is sent to the speech organs, it is transmitted in the form of a string of separate instructions, one for each phoneme.

If the message is the word pin /pin/, for example, there are first instructions for producing a /p/, then for producing an /i/, and then for producing an /n/. This seems, at least, to be the most reasonable assumption. If the speech organs responded ideally to these instructions, they would first assume the position for /p/, then move jerkily and instantaneously to the position for /i/, then jerkily and instantaneously to the position for /n/.

Common sense tells us that they cannot do this, and x-ray moving pictures of the speech organs in action prove it beyond a doubt. Instead of moving instantaneously from one position to the next, the speech organs bobble back and forth in a constant flow of motion which does not seem to consist of any specific number of segments at all.

A remarkable transformation has taken place. Where the message previously consisted of a string of discrete segments—three, we assume, in the case of /pin/—it has now been "smeared" into a continuum. As the speech organs move into position to produce the /p/, they already anticipate part of the position for the following /i/. (The reader can test this by whispering the *p*'s of *peer, par, poor;* the sound of each *p* shows clearly which vowel would follow if he went on with the rest of the word.)

As the speech organs then move into the /i/ they carry over part of the position of the /p/ and anticipate part of the position for the following /n/. (We normally "nasalize" such a vowel slightly.) And when the speech organs get to the /n/, they still have part of the position of the preceeding /i/. This drastic change in the shape of the message may seem quite harmless now, but it means that later on this "smeared continuum" of sound will have to be turned back into a string of discrete segments if the message is to be recovered. This is what must take place at stage nine, "phonological decoding."

When the speech organs interact so as to produce a speech sound, they are said to articulate the sound. The study of this aspect of the speech event, *articulatory phonetics,* has long been a highly developed research field.

6. Vibrations of the Air Molecules

As the speech organs articulate, they set the air molecules into vibration and produce audible sound. The study of this aspect of the speech event is *acoustic phonetics.* Here again a great deal of research has been done, and some remarkable advances have been achieved, especially since World War II.

7. Vibrations of the Ear

When the vibrations of the air molecules reach hearer B's eardrum, they produce corresponding vibrations which are then transmitted by means of the three bones of the middle ear to the cochlear fluid of the inner ear. The study of this aspect of the speech event is *auditory phonetics.* It is usually combined with study of the ear in general, and with the study of auditory perception (which of course involves also the activity of the brain farther up the line.)

8. From Ear to Brain

Though this stage is in a sense the mirror image of stage four, "From brain to speech organs," there are two important differences.

First, when the message went from A's brain to his speech organs, it was transmitted as a string of discrete segments; but since it was then turned into a smeared continuum by A's speech organs, this is the shape in which it now reaches B's brain.

Second, speaker A was able to send the message only because, somewhere inside his head, he possessed the proper code; hearer B, however, can receive all the energy in the message whether he knows the code or not —though of course he can do nothing further with it unless he *does* know the same code. We can "hear" all there is to hear in a foreign language message; we can "understand" the message only if we also know the foreign language code.

9, 10, 11. Phonological, Grammatical, and Semantic Decoding

Though we surely use these three different types of decoding when we hear and understand a message, the evidence suggests that we do not use them in a step-by-step procedure but rather race back and forth from one to the other, picking up all the information we can get.

Suppose, for example, that we receive a message which we tentatively decode phonologically as "I hope this'll suture plans." A quick check with the grammatical component of the code reveals that there is indeed a morpheme *suture* marked "transitive verb" (that is to say, we know that one can suture something), so all is well for the moment. But a check farther up the line in the semantic component tells us that one just does not "suture plans" so something must be wrong.

Back we race to the phonological component. Again the message (held in the meantime by some sort of storage device) is decoded as having the phonemic structure "I hope this'll suture plans." But a second check in the grammatical component now reveals that the phoneme sequence "suture plans" can be grammatically either one or two different things; *suture plans* or *suit your plans.* So we check this second possibility in the semantic component of the code. This now makes sense, and we accept it.

Our brain can function so swiftly that all of this happens in a flash. Only rarely does this searching process take so long that it interferes with our understanding of the speaker's next sentence.

In addition to the message itself, our decoding brings us information of three other types. First, there is information about the identity of the speaker (the quality of his voice tells us that it is Jones and not Smith who is speaking), his state of health (hoarse voice, stuffed up nose), and the like. Such things are presumably the same in all languages and hence not part of any code.

Second, there is the kind of information we often refer to as "it wasn't what he said but how he said it"—things indicating that the speaker is angry, excited, sarcastic, unctuous, and so forth. Since such matters are different in English from what they are in French or Vietnamese, they are clearly part of the English language in the wider sense of the term. (They also make a fascinating subject for linguistic study.)

Third, there is information as to where the speaker comes from and what social and educational class he belongs to. If he uses the phonological encoding "thoity-thoid," this will suggest that he comes from Brooklyn or thereabouts; if he says "thihty-thihd" we may suspect that he comes from the vicinity of Boston.

If he uses the grammatical encoding "I seen him when he done it", we will place him at a relatively low social and educational level, even though (and this is an interesting point) the message comes through just as clearly as if he had said "I saw him when he did it." Matters of this third sort are also part of the English language in the wider sense of the term.

In the above description of a speech event, the part which is of most fundamental interest to the linguist is of course the code itself: its phonological component (here great progress was made in the 1930s and 1940s), its grammatical component (again great progress at that time, and a whole new approach opening up since the late 1950s), and its semantic component (long neglected by American linguists, though there has been a recent revival of interest).

When one looks back upon it all, one is perhaps inclined to say: What is it good for? Is it just a game? To the linguist it is more than a game. It is a thing of beauty and wonder, and it needs no more justification than this. At the same time, with a bit of a sigh, he will say that (like such long "useless" fields as astronomy) it *can* be of practical value. It has obvious applications to foreign language teaching and—with great help from the teachers themselves—these applications are now being exploited.

If presented clearly and simply (and this has in general not been the case—nor is it easy) it seems likely that it could also be applied usefully to the teaching of reading and writing, and to the teaching of the English language at all levels. Tentative applications of this sort have already been made; with cooperation on all sides, perhaps they can lead to truly useful results.

Suggested Readings

Carroll, John B. *The Study of Language: A Survey of Linguistics and Related Disciplines in America.* Cambridge: Harvard University Press, 1953.
Hall, Robert A., Jr. *Linguistics and Your Language.* New York: Doubleday (paperback: Anchor Books A–201), 1960.
Gleason, H. A., Jr. *Introduction to Descriptive Linguistics* (rev. ed.). New York: Holt, Rinehart & Winston, 1961. (College text)
Hockett, Charles F. *A Course in Modern Linguistics.* New York: Macmillan, 1958. (More advanced)
Waterman, John T. *Perspectives in Linguistics.* Chicago: University of Chicago Press (paperback: Phoenix Books). 1963. (History of linguistics)
Fries, Charles C. *Linguistics and Reading.* New York: Holt, Rinehart & Winston, 1963. (Applications)

Paul C. Burns is an educator who has written on many aspects of language-arts instruction. His article condenses much information useful to the school practitioner and includes references that both teachers and students will find useful.

The original article opened with quotations from two great linguists: Leonard Bloomfield's lament of teachers' ignorance of linguistics, thus wasting "years of every child's life and reach(ing) a poor result"; and Charles Fries' statement on the need for bringing linguistics to bear on educational problems.

Burns presents some of the basic features of language identified by linguists, introduces concepts about language structure and terminology that linguists use, and suggests how other aspects of linguistic study can be applied in the classroom. His treatment of language structure is based largely on the model of structural grammar (he touches only briefly on transformational grammar) but his description reflects the state of the art in 1965 when the article was originally published.

Linguistics: A Brief Guide for Principals

Paul C. Burns

The growing interest in linguistics among educators and the efforts of linguists to understand the problems of teaching children have resulted in the gradual development of "that kind of communication and that kind of cooperation" between linguists and educators. This drawing together of those who understand the teaching-learning process best and those who know most about the language to be taught provides a logical basis for improving instruction.

Communication between educators and linguists has been directed toward identifying the linguistic concepts which appear applicable to elementary education and to determining when and how they should be introduced into language-arts instruction. The result has been a growing body of literature—in books, professional journals, and commercially published materials for children—interpreting the principles of linguistics, suggesting practical applications of linguistic concepts for classroom use, and describing "linguistically oriented" language programs.

What is meant by "linguistics" or a "linguistically oriented" approach to the language arts? What are some of the major concepts from linguistics which may help us to strengthen instruction in the language arts?

Basic Concepts

The linguistic point of view emphasizes the primacy of speech over writing. The linguist hopes that such characteristics of language as the following can be examined by elementary school pupils:

1. Language is a set or system of sounds (not symbols on a page), and the connection between the sounds and the objects they represent is purely arbitrary. For example, the animal called "the dog" in English is called "le chien" in French. There are many opportunities to develop this concept with pupils in the study of social studies and of a foreign language.

2. Language changes, yet remains durable. Old words may be given new meanings and new uses, and new words may be coined or adapted. "Change is an aspect of human language as regular and relentless as the birth and death of men. It asks no man's permission and waits on no man's approval."[1] Some examples of the ways language changes include:

Meanings change: *nice* once meant foolish but today means *pleasing*.

Makeup of words changes: words are made into compounds, as *beforehand*: neologisms develop, as *edit* from *editor*; portmanteau words are devised, as *smog* from *smoke and fog*.

New words are added: as *blitzkrieg, commando*.

3. There are many social variations in language, such as slang *(scram)*, jargon *(knowing the ropes)*, and cant *(sawbuck)*.

To the linguist, creating interest in language among pupils is of urgent importance. One way to accomplish this in the elementary school language arts program is to develop an understanding of the heritage of language. A number of trade books about language are available for children, teachers, and principals.[2]

Language Structure

Years ago, grammarians superimposed the Latin-grammar system on the English language, and the incompatibility of the two has caused teachers and their pupils unending problems. Modern linguists, recognizing the differences between the Latin and English languages, have devel-

---

[1] Donald J. Lloyd, and Harry R. Warfel, *American English in Its Cultural Setting*. New York: Alfred A. Knopf, 1965. p. 7.

[2] One reference for children is Helene Laird and Charlton Laird, *Tree of Language*. Cleveland, Ohio: World Publishing Company, 1957. And for teachers, Charlton Laird, *The Miracle of Language*. New York: Fawcett World Library, 1957.

oped new ways of looking at language, of sorting out the data, and of classifying the findings.

In brief, linguists state that a language is made up of basic units of sound called *phonemes,* such as *s* in *sing.* Phonemes are the smallest usable units of speech sound.

Phonemes are built into *morphemes* which consist of phonemes used in sequence to form larger working units. Morphemes are indivisible language elements and are the basic meaning-bearing units of language. A free morpheme is a morpheme which can be used by itself. For example, *sing.* A bound-form morpheme, such as *er,* must always be bound to another morpheme. For example, sing*er.*

Morphemes, in turn, are put together into patterns of *syntax.* Syntax refers to the patterning of morphemes into larger structural units.

In analyzing English structure, linguists emphasize *form class, intonation,* and *sentence pattern.*

A *form class* consists of all the words which are interchangeable in a construction. For example since *works* and *sings* can be interchanged in "The boy works" and "The boy sings," the two words—*works* and *sings* —are said, in this instance, to belong to the same form class. There are four form classes in English: noun, verb, adjective, adverb.

Modern linguists do not define these form classes with the old, traditional definitions for the part of speech. They have developed an entirely new and more accurate way of describing language structure. For example, when a verb is defined as "a word that expresses action," such words as *arrival* and *operation* could well be classified as verbs. But since no one says, "He will arrival," *arrival* is not considered to be a verb—not because it does not somehow express action but because it does not occur in what is recognized as a verb structure.

Similarly, while the word *sings* in our previous example, The boy sings, is a "word that expresses action," it may also be used in such a pattern as "Our family used to have Sunday evening sings." In this latter construction, the word *sings* is not considered to be a verb because it is not used in a verb structure.

Linguists suggest more functional definitions and tangible signals to distinguish one major class from another. Thus in rejecting the statement that "a noun is the name of a person, place, or thing; if it is not a name, it is not a noun," they propose a definition such as "A word is a noun because it is used in a particular way in a particular sentence frame." Thus, a noun is a word that can fill the blank in "The ____ was lost"; or a noun is a word like *oogle* in such a statement as, "The oogle was lost." Or a noun can take in inflectional suffix as *s* (more than oneness) or *'s.* Or a noun, by position, comes after such signals *(determiners)* as *the, an, a;* possessive pronouns such as *his, her, my;* or demonstratives such as *this, that.*

Some linguists refer to *structure words*—words that mark structural sentence elements—in the following sense:

> Noun markers: *a, an, the, their, this, my, some*
> Verb markers: *am, are, is, was, have, has, has been, done, did*
> Phrase markers: *up, down, in, out, out of, below, above*
> Clause markers: *if, because, although, even though, that, which*
> Question markers: *who, why, how, when, where, what.*

In brief, words that pattern alike belong to the same word group or class.

It is true, of course, that definitions based solely on morphology (inflectional endings and the like) can lead to confusion. That is, if a noun were defined simply as "a word that forms a plural," then *chaos* could not be classified as a noun. A single signal in the structure, while helpful, is not infallible in our nonperfect language. The signals in our language are generally multiple—position, form (inflectional and derivational endings), and function, and probably in that order of importance.

Intonation is an important structural feature of our language. Intonation involves *stress, pitch,* and *juncture.*

Stress is a matter of the loudness or softness with which syllables are uttered. As an example, consider the word *anticipate.* There are four syllables to the word: an-tic-i-pate. They are not uttered with equal loudness. The second syllable *tic* is the loudest of the four. The weakest is the syllable *i.* Conventionally marked for stress, using the marks / ∧ \ ∪ which indicate descending degrees of loudness, the word would appear àn tíc ĭ pâte.

Stress can help clear up ambiguity, as *the orderly room* (a room that is neat) and *the orderly room* (a room for orderlies). And note the different types of question when any one of the component words is pitched higher and given more stress: Where is he going? (casual) *Where* is he going? Where *is* he going? Where is *he* going? Where is he *going?*

Pitch refers to the idea that if air is made to vibrate rapidly, we have a high pitch; if slowly, we have a low pitch. Various levels of pitch can be detected. For example, if the statement is made, "I am going," the listener will know that the utterance is finished; but if the statement, "I am going . . . . " is made, the listener waits for the speaker to continue. The reason for the feeling of incompletion is not that less has been said, but that the two utterances have different characteristics. Sometimes numerals (1, very low; 2, normal; 3, high; and 4, very high) are assigned to mark pitch. Notice the changing of the statement to a question in the following:

2 3 1
The people who were here went away.
(Declarative sentence)
2 3 3
The people who were here went away?
(Interrogative sentence)

Children's attention can be called to the way in which the voice signals a question or a statement. "When are you going home?" ends with a rising intonation, while the answer, "In a short time," ends with a falling intonation. The word *now* may be either a statement or a question, depending upon the pitch employed. Excitement can be indicated in such a situation as:

4 1
He needs some money!

The need for punctuation is often revealed in the indicated pitch:

3 1
Knowing what he had to do Bill didn't take a moment.

At times pitch or the comma is the only signal which can give meaning to a sentence, as in the following:

3 3
The boys without coats were very cold.
or
The boys, without coats, were very cold.

Attention to such rhythmic patterns of speech will reduce problems of misplaced modifiers and questions about punctuation of nonrestrictive modifiers.

Juncture is the breaking off or interrupting of the speech according to the structure of the sentence—the breaks in the succession of sounds. These gaps are of specific types and come in specific places. One type of juncture enables the listener to distinguish between *announce* and *an ounce.* In *announce,* all the sounds are linked together without a break. But in *an ounce*, there is a break between the second and third sounds. The same phenomenon (called *open juncture*) occurs in such pairs of words as *nitrates* and *night rates* and *I scream* and *ice cream.*

There are other kinds of juncture. *Level* juncture—so called because the voice usually resumes speech, after the gap, at the same level of pitch at which it broke off—can be illustrated: "Bill is waiting without, Paul" and "Bill is waiting, without Paul." The shift of juncture restructures the entire statement. Rising juncture, characterized by rising pitch, is commonly an end signal in an interrogation; falling juncture, characterized by falling pitch, is most commonly the end signal of a declarative sentence. Rising juncture inside an utterance usually separates the elements of a series as "Bill, Tom, Mary, and Jim . . . "

To summarize, an open or plus juncture (+) roughly indicates a word division, as *an + ounce;* single bar juncture (/) roughly indicates word group or phrase divisions, as "The man / in the car / was laughing." The double bar juncture (//) marks a more pronounced interruption and is usually thought of as a comma juncture, as "My brother // who lives in Boston // came to see me." The double cross juncture (#) marks a more pronounced interruption and is associated with terminal pitch patterns at the ends of sentences. "I am going home. # Are you going with me?" #

In brief, the punctuation of writing symbolizes, though imperfectly, the intonation of speech.

Sentence order and pattern refers to the systematic, recurring patterns of words, put together in characteristic designs and composed of a great variety of appropriate fillers. Pupils are tuned to sentence order or patterns that are typical of the English language. "He brought his father a tie" would be accepted as a proper statement. If the sequence were "His father he a tie brought," pupils would instantly recognize it as not typical of the language pattern.

Basic intonation units called sentences tend to pattern themselves in recurring structures called *basic patterns* or types:

1. Father laughed. (Noun—verb or subject—verb)
2. The dog chased the cat. (Noun—verb—noun or subject —verb—object)
3. His dog is a monster. (Noun—linking verb—noun or subject—linking verb—predicate noun)
4. His dog is black. (Noun—linking verb—adjective or subject—linking verb—predicate adjective)
5. The boy laughed loudly. Mother is away. (Noun—verb—adverb or subject—verb—adverb)

Pupils can be asked to write sentences based on these patterns and to experiment with expanding these basic patterns through *elements of expansion* denoting object, time, and place. They can thus discover how meaning and emphasis are influenced by the position of these parts in the sentence. (For example, "The black dog chased the white cat down the street yesterday.") Without getting technical about prepositional phrases, infinitives, or participles, pupils can detect open points in the basic patterns where subordinate units can be inserted; where modifiers can be inserted before the subject, after the subject, before and after the verb.

Another way to show how sentences structure is through *transformations* such as:

The cat was chased by the dog. (passive)
Do dogs chase cats? (question—active)
Dogs do chase cats. (emphatic)
Dogs do not chase cats. (negative)
Don't dogs chase cats? (negative question)

Finally, pupils can learn to say things in different ways by substitutions and style, largely coordination and subordination, as, "The dog chased the cat and father laughed."

Such an interest in manipulating words and sentences can be drawn upon to teach the process of constructing a compound or complex sentence from a series of simple ones. When confusion arises in the pupil's writing of a compound or complex sentence, he has at his command the ability to return to the basics of sentence pattern in order to clarify his thinking and reorganize the structure of the questionable sentence.[3]

Usage and the Dictionary

The linguist might say that "I done it" is correct in the sense that it is correct in relation to the dialect, but that it is perhaps incorrect from a sociological point of view. This does not mean that teachers should neglect attempts to encourage pupils to use "I did it," for pupils who continue to say "I done it" will be handicapped in their relationships with many people with whom they come in contact. In other words, the issue is not to be decided by *Webster's* but by people and situations. The linguist says, "This is what users of English do when they speak and write." The prescriptionist says, "Here is your rule. Obey it." The descriptive linguist's purpose is to supply data, not ethical judgements. *Right* to the linguist means that the element is clear, appropriate to context, and in accordance with contemporary practice of able speakers and writers. *Wrong* means just the opposite.[4]

When it comes to lexicography, the question is whether the dictionary makers should record English as it is actually used by educated people in both their writing and speech (that is, should it be *descriptive*) or whether they should record it as some people think the language should be used (that is, should it be *prescriptive*).

To the linguist, the dictionary is a scientific, unbiased, objective record

---

[3] An excellent reference for principals is Ruth G. Strickland, "The Contribution of Structural Linguistics to the Teaching of Reading, Writing, and Grammar in the Elementary School," *Bulletin of the School of Education, Indiana University* 40, No. 1 (January, 1964).

[4] Two fine references for principals are Robert A. Hall, Jr., *Linguistics and Your Language*. Garden City, N.Y.: Doubleday and Co., 1960; and Margaret M. Bryant, *Current American Usage*. New York: Funk and Wagnalls Co., 1962.

of the English language as it has been in the past and is at the moment of preparing the dictionary. In elementary schools, the comparative study of dictionary status labels (slang, colloquial, dialect, substandard, nonstandard, and so on) will lead into the question of how dictionaries are developed. The linguistic approach views the dictionary as a guidebook, not as a rule book. It does not tell us how words *should* be used, but rather how they *are* used by educated people. It indicates not how words should be spelled, but how writers spell them. It suggests not what compilers think words ought to mean, but what speakers and writers of the language use them to mean. It tells us not which expressions are elegant and which are inelegant, but which are used in elegant circles and which are not.

The urgings of the linguistic scholars for more knowledge about the language can be partly met through the dictionary. For example, through the study of the pronunciation key the pupil learns of the stability of the consonants and the variances of the vowels. He gains insight into the way the language grows and changes by detecting different spellings (as *taboos, tabus*); different pronunciation(as *tomato, either, economic*) acceptable in different parts of the country; different meanings of words (as *track*) depending upon context; and differences in parts of speech depending upon function in a sentence (as *spring*). There is no better source for study of such ideas than the dictionary itself.

Semantics

The linguist is interested in the choice of words (in the responsible and humane use of words) as well as in increasing the number of words in a child's vocabulary.[5] Here attention would be given to words employed to convey attitudes and feelings even though these conditions are not in the words themselves at all. Students of semantics have sharpened and reinforced concern with meaning in a number of crucial ways—by stressing the need for identifying and limiting the referents that our words symbolize; by emphasizing the difficulties inherent in words at a high level of abstraction; by warning of sweeping general terms; and by pointing out how verbal labels prejudge responses.

Attention to responsible use of language will benefit the pupil in many ways. It will help him become a more perceptive listener and reader. It will teach him the art of reading between the lines and the elementary distinction between what is said and what is meant. It will prepare him to look for the precise shade that a word has in its context, the subtle hint conveyed by a metaphor or a simile. It will help to protect him from

---

[5] Stuart Chase, *Power of Words.* New York: Harcourt, Brace, and World, 1954.

the manipulators of language whose emotive language and connotative terms are found everywhere.

Spelling and Reading

To the linguist, a large number of English words are spelled in a regular manner; that is, the grapheme-phoneme correspondence is reliable.

To learn the symbol-sound correspondences rapidly and efficiently, linguists recommend that the pupil's first experiences with written words be with words which are regular in spelling (as *stop*). There should be one letter for one sound until it is learned. Semi-regularly spelled words (as *pay*) would come later; and highly irregular words (as *come*) would be encountered last. It is proposed that instead of controlling the words themselves, there should be control of introduction of sound and the graphic symbols for these sounds.

Such an approach would mean that pupils would turn from learning the spelling of each separate word. Instead, once a second grade child has learned to spell *all,* he would be encouraged to discover that he can now spell many words—*ball, call, fall, hall, tall, halls, calling, called, taller, tallest.* Other patterns would serve to group words for instruction: for example, the short sounds of vowels (*met*); the long vowel-consonant-silent *e* pattern (*mete*); and the long sounds of the vowels. The regular consonants and the consonant blends and digraphs would be systematically and sequentially developed. Spellers who are linguistically oriented present words in groups to show similar features of spelling, emphasizing different ways of spelling the same sound (as the *f* sound spelled with *f, ph, gh*) and in different sounds of the same letter (as in *add, dollar,* and *May*).[6]

Also the recognition in reading of many words built on the same pattern is advocated. Attention to similar word patterns has the advantage of giving extensive experience with a single pattern in order to establish the sound and spelling of each pattern. For further ideas, application, and an understanding of linguistic impact upon reading, principals are referred to two recent books of value.[7]

---

[6] An important reference for principals is Robert A. Hall, Jr., *Sound and Spelling in English*. Philadelphia: Chilton, 1961.

[7] Charles C. Fries, *Linguistics and Reading*. New York: Holt, Rinehart & Winston, 1963; and Carl A. Lefevre, *Linguistics and the Teaching of Reading*. New York: McGraw-Hill, 1964.

Stanley F. Wanat examines the question: how do children learn language? While focusing his attention specifically on reading (the author is research director of the International Reading Association), Wanat presents a comprehensive and concise review of current theories of language acquisition. He classifies these theories as:
1. *Behavoristic,* based on an imitation of models of adult language. (A report of one research project based on this model is presented in the selection following Wanat's article.)
2. *Nativistic,* that language development is related to growth of the brain, and maturation in language parallels maturation in motor and thinking skills. Noam Chomsky's own words on this theory of language acquisition are quoted in the editor's note following Ved Mehta's "John Is Easy to Please," page 174.
3. *Cognitive,* which holds that the child takes an active role in language learning. The author presents this concept in the context of Piaget's theories of cognitive growth.

Wanat concludes that no theory gives an adequate explanation of how a child learns his language. Each, however, has something to offer in piecing together the puzzle of language acquisition.

For further reading, another fine review on this topic is the NCTE/ERIC Report "Language Acquisition and Development: Some Implications for the Classroom" by Carole M. Kirkton. *Elementary English* 48 (March 1971:406–412).

Language Acquisition: Basic Issues

Stanley F. Wanat

The way a child acquires his language is a "natural process" in the sense that we don't have to teach it to him in the same way we have to teach him mathematics. When he enters school, the child can already understand and use a wide range of grammatical structures. How is the child able to do this? And how is his language development related to reading?

Literature Search

Answers to these questions were sought by a team of scholars who were part of the U.S. Office of Education's Literature Search in Reading. Twenty-five researchers drawn from fourteen universities worked the past year examining (1) studies of the reading process; (2) studies of learning to read; and (3) studies of language development related to reading. Martin Kling of Rutgers held overall responsibility for the project, along with John J. Geyer (also of Rutgers), and Frederick B. Davis (University of Pennsylvania).

Recent major efforts. Among earlier but still rather recent major efforts in the study of reading has been the establishment of the Educational Resources Information Center/Clearinghouse on Retrieval of Information and Evaluation of Reading (ERIC/CRIER), a joint project of IRA, Indiana University, and the U.S. Office of Education's Bureau of Research. Its purpose is to make available research reports, materials, and information on reading. Another important effort has been the First-Grade Studies, in which the effectiveness of different methods for teaching reading was considered. A third important thrust in reading research was Project Literacy, directed by Harry Levin at Cornell. This was an interdisciplinary study of some of the basic psychological and linguistic processes which underlie the nature of reading. Project Literacy researchers and teachers made observations, did experiments, and tried out innovations in materials and techniques.

The Literature Search is the latest milestone in reading research, because it has picked out important studies, analyzed them, and has moved forward in trying to fit together some of the pieces of the enormously complex puzzle we call reading. What follows is a presentation and discussion of some of the issues raised in four sections of the Literature Search's *Final Report:* "Background and Development of the Literature Search: Targeted Research and Development Program in Reading," by Martin Kling; "Language Models and Reading," by Irene J. Athey; "Implications of Language Socialization for Reading Models and for Learning to Read," by Doris R. Entwisle; and "Theories of Language Acquisition in Relation to Beginning Reading Instruction," by Ronald Wardhaugh. These four articles can be found in the Fall 1971 issue of the *Reading Research Quarterly.*

Language Development

What is language development and why bother about it? The study of language development (also referred to as developmental psycholinguistics or developmental linguistics or the study of language acquisition) tries to account for how the meaningless cooing, gurgling, and babbling sounds made by the infant turn into the meaningful language spoken by the adult. This field is important to reading specialists because some theorists (notably Eleanor J. Gibson) maintain that competence in the spoken language is an essential first step in learning how to read. The steps in Gibson's theory are: learning to use spoken language, learning to discriminate between graphic symbols, learning spelling-sound correspondences, and learning to handle larger units of structure.

Noam Chomsky of M.I.T. claims that language acquisition is a process in which the child formulates a theory (description) of the structure of his language. It is as if the child were a linguist writing a new grammar, but Chomsky qualifies his claim by saying that the child's grammar-formulation is intuitive, and that the child is probably not even conscious of the rules he formulates. Some of the skills which underlie language development are: the mental ability to deal with the world, the ability to remember things, the ability to break down the language one hears into units of sound and units of meaning and recombine these units, and the ability to generalize.

How do the child's linguistic skills develop? Some theorists stress the child's own active role in the acquisition of language. Other researchers emphasize the innate aspects of language development while a third group concentrates on the rewarding or reinforcement of certain kinds of behavior as the determining factor in language acquisition. These three viewpoints can be labelled Behavioristic, Nativistic, and Cognitive, respectively.

Behavioristic Theory

Following B. F. Skinner's views, the acquisition of language is based on rewarding the child when he imitates or tries to imitate models of adult language. There has been much discussion about the nature of the reward or reinforcement and about the stimulus—the thing which brings about a response from the learner. Techniques based on behavioristic theory have been successful in the classroom. Rewards such as food, use of play equipment, and teacher approval brought about changes in the speech of children in experiments. Two questions posed to behaviorists are: Is reinforcement the most important factor? If imitation is so central, why is it that a response learned in one way is also used in many other ways by the speaker?

The imitation of models that the child hears and the frequency with which he hears these models are key concepts in behavioristic theory. Studies of language acquisition have indicated that although children do imitate what they hear, they also produce many variations of the model. Research has also shown that the child may ignore the model, as in the case where the adult speaker repeatedly presents a correct model, but the child continues to make the same error. Yet, imitation clearly is an important factor in language development, for children raised in an English-speaking environment learn English, and not some other language. The role of frequency of hearing the model is also at issue, since "telegraphic" speech leaves out high-frequency words, and researchers note that language acquisition includes a period of telegraphic speech. Concern with the frequency of items is reflected in basal readers, but such strict vocabulary control may be stifling the curiosity of young readers.

Given the research findings that techniques involving imitation, frequency, and reinforcement do affect the child's acquisition of language, how do we best help the development along? The next theory of language development stresses the innate aspects of language.

Nativistic Theory

Very briefly, the nativistic position holds that language development is related to the growth of the human brain, and that maturation in language parallels maturation in motor and thinking skills. While the behaviorists emphasize outside events, nativistic theory concentrates on what is "inside" the child. Chomsky has been particularly critical of Skinner for ignoring what the child himself brings to the task of language learning. Eric Lenneberg's nativistic theory is based on the notion that language development is biologically determined, and that no other creature besides man has language.

Lenneberg's theory is based upon evidence from the study of language development in normal children, and of children with abnormal language development resulting from congenital and environmental factors. As evidence of the innate biological basis of language, Lenneberg cites the universal properties of language—the characteristics which all languages share. Major issues concerning nativistic models include whether or not language is unique to man, and the nature of language universals. Chomsky's transformational-generative grammar is based on the existence of universals in the mind. Some people have argued that universals across different languages occur because there are universals in the subjects people think about and want to talk about. A problem with nativistic theory is that it does not explain how we get from the child's innate knowledge to his actual language performance.

One aspect of nativistic theory has potentially important implications for the teaching of reading. Lenneberg maintains that there is a "critical" period for language acquisition which is biologically determined. Since, as has already been mentioned, some reading theorists hold that reading is dependent on language development, there may be some optimal relation between stages in language development and stages in learning to read. Current language intervention programs are not directed at children during the time they experience maximum growth in language development, which is before they are four years old.

The nativistic position stresses the internal mechanism—the innate language learning capacity—which the child brings to the task of language acquisition. But trying to account for *all* aspects of language learning in terms of its biological basis is no more informative than trying to account for all aspects of learning how to drive a car in terms of its biological basis. The nativists also fail to take into account the possibility that there may be differences in the innate cognitive and language structure of different children.

Chomsky claims that the child's acquisition of language is relatively independent of intelligence or the particular experiences that the child has had. On the other hand, Basil Bernstein, a British sociologist, holds that social settings bring about particular forms of communication which determine the intellectual orientation of the child. Chomsky maintains that his theory of language holds for the "ideal" speaker in an environment where all the other people speak pretty much alike. Some critics strongly argue that the linguists' assumption of an "ideal" speaker is a basic error, and that all children do not possess the same skills in thinking. As linguists start to analyze actual language behavior, rather than deal with fictionalized ideal speakers, they will move closer to the concerns of psychologists, and linguistic and psychological theories may begin to merge. One of the problems with describing language development is that the goal towards which the child is progressing—the fluency of the mature speaker—has not been adequately described by linguists.

Cognitive Theory

A third theory of language development, cognitive theory, holds that the child takes an active role in learning. The child's cognitive, or thinking, activity is a kind of information processing. Major theories of the ways in which thinking develops in the child take the form of language for granted. Jean Piaget, the Swiss psychologist, states that transformational grammar is close to some of his views. Piaget's concept of "stages" in cognitive growth has implications for reading. If, for example, a child is still at the stage where his perception is "centered," then he can only attend to one part of a situation. He will thus have problems discriminating between a figure and its background. This has obvious implications for the perception of letters. Also, the child whose perception is at this stage will have trouble dealing with the sound of a letter while he is dealing with its visual form, since "centration" is characterized by the inability to deal with more than one thing at a time.

The Dialect Speaker

The language of the dialect speaker—a relatively recent concern in language development—also has implications for the teaching of reading. The child who does not have a good grasp of the language to be read must either be taught that language before reading instruction begins, or else the reading materials must be put into the language or dialect that he speaks. The middle-class child has an advantage because the language he hears and speaks at home is very close to the language he must read in school. Consequently, he has a better chance of success in using context cues to the form and meaning of the sentence.

In teaching dialect speakers how to read, one must try to minimize differences between how they speak most naturally and their reading materials. The establishment of a program to teach reading in the home dialects of American children would necessitate preparing materials in at least seven dialects. Since programs for teaching reading through the use of materials in dialect have not been evaluated, success with this approach is not assured. If, for example, a child does not pronounce the plural marker on words when reading aloud, this does not mean that he cannot read. It may be that his home language is French and that he is transferring language habits from French to English. The same may be true of dialect speakers who can't read past tense forms. Black Americans who talk so-called nonstandard Negro English may not pronounce the past tense marker of verbs when they converse. Therefore, it is not necessarily the case that they "can't read" because they transfer language habits from their home dialect when they read the variety of English we expect to hear in the classroom.

The following implications for teaching are associated with dialect differences. First, the student's task of having to learn a second dialect should be explicitly taken into account. Second, the decoding process should take place within one dialect, and not between dialects. Third, a great deal of attention must be paid to the social context in which learning to read takes place, since there are strong pressures from peer groups against reading in some ghetto settings. For many children, the home situation is so chaotic that instead of developing strategies for attending to information, the children are forced into strategies of tuning out information.

Needed Research

Research has generally ignored differences between and within groups. Consider the relation between sex differences and reading problems: 90 percent of the referrals to reading clinics in the U.S. are boys, whereas in some countries there may be a higher rate of referrals for girls than for boys.

In summary, group differences have generally been ignored in research on language development. Thus, dialect differences, possible ethnic differences in capacities and strategies for processing information, differences in thinking-style, and emotionally-related factors are not adequately taken under consideration. None of the theories reviewed give an adequate explanation of the way a child acquires his language. Each of the theories is wrong in that each unjustifiably claims to provide a complete explanation. Yet, each of these theories is valuable in that each provides part of the information we need to understand language development.

Roger Brown and Ursula Bellugi are leading experts on the theory of language acquisition, and their article on the topic is one of the most authoritative and widely quoted available.

It is a detailed account of a longitudinal study based on the observation of two children who are learning language. The theory of language acquisition here presented highlights both the role of imitation and the role of induction in discovering the basic rules by which our language works. The three processes identified by Brown and Bellugi are: (1) Imitation and Reduction, (2) Imitation with Expansion, and (3) Induction of Latent Structure. Throughout the article the authors take into account the effects of a child's interaction with adults as he is learning language.

The Processes in the Child's Acquisition of Syntax

Roger Brown and Ursula Bellugi

Sometime in the second six months of life most children say a first intelligible word. A few months later most children are saying many words and some children go about the house all day long naming things (table, doggie, ball, and so on) and actions (play, see, drop, and so on) and an occasional quality (blue, broke, bad, and so on). At about eighteen months children are likely to begin constructing two-word utterances; such a one, for instance, as *Push car*.

A construction such as Push car is not just two single-word utterances spoken in a certain order. As single word utterances (they are sometimes called holophrases) both *push* and *car* would have primary stresses and terminal intonation contours. When they are two words programmed as a single utterance the primary stress would fall on *car* and so would the highest level of pitch. *Push* would be subordinated to *car* by a lesser stress and a lower pitch; the unity of the whole would appear in the absence of a terminal contour between words and the presence of such a contour at the end of the full sequence.

By the age of thirty-six months some children are so advanced in the construction process as to produce all of the major varieties of English simple sentences up to a length of ten or eleven words. For several years we have been studying the development of English syntax, of the sentence-constructing process, in children between eighteen and thirty-six months of age. Most recently we have made a longitudinal study of a boy and girl whom we shall call Adam and Eve. We began work with Adam and Eve in October of 1962 when Adam was twenty-seven months old and Eve eighteen months old. The two children were selected from some thirty whom we considered. They were selected primarily because their speech was exceptionally intelligible and because they talked a lot. We wanted to make it as easy as possible to transcribe accurately large quantities of child speech. Adam and Eve are the children of highly-educated parents, the fathers were graduate students at Harvard and the mothers college graduates. Both Adam and Eve were single children when we began the study. These facts must be remembered in generalizing the outcomes of the research.

While Adam is nine months older than Eve, his speech was only a little more advanced in October of 1962. The best single index of the level of speech development is the average length of utterance and in October 1962, Adam's average was 1.84 morphemes and Eve's was 1.40 morphemes. The two children stayed fairly close together in the year that followed; in the records for the thirty-eighth week Adam's average was 3.55 and Eve's, 3.27. The processes we shall describe appeared in both children.

Every second week we visited each child for at least two hours and made a tape recording of everything said by the child as well as of everything said to the child. The mother was always present and most of the speech to the child is hers. Both mother and child became accustomed to our presence and learned to continue their usual routine with us as the observers.

One of us always made a written transcription, on the scene, of the speech of mother and child with notes about important actions and objects of attention. From this transcription and the tape a final transcription was made and these transcriptions constitute the primary data of the study. For many purposes we require a "distributional analysis" of the speech of the child. To this end the child's utterances in a given transcription were cross classified and relisted under such headings as: A + noun; Noun + verb; Verbs in the past; Utterances containing the pronoun *it*, and so on. The categorized utterances expose the syntactic regularities of the child's speech.

Each week we met as a research seminar, with students of the psychology of language,[1] to discuss the state of the construction process in one of the two children as of that date. In these discussions small experiments were often suggested, experiments that had to be done within a few days if they were to be informative. At one time, for instance, we were uncertain whether Adam understood the semantic difference between putting a noun in subject position and putting it in object position. Consequently one of us paid an extra visit to Adam, equipped with some toys. "Adam," we said, "show us the duck pushing the boat." And, when he had done so: "Now show us the boat pushing the duck."

[1] We are grateful for intellectual stimulation and lighthearted companionship to Jean Berko Gleason, Samuel Anderson, Colin Fraser, David McNeill, and Daniel Slobin.

Another week we noticed that Adam would sometimes pluralize nouns when they should have been pluralized and sometimes would not. We wondered if he could make grammatical judgments about the plural; if he could distinguish a correct form from an incorrect form. "Adam," we asked, "which is right, two shoes or two shoe?" His answer on that occasion, produced with explosive enthusiasm, was "Pop goes the weasel!" The two year old child does not make a perfectly docile experimental subject.

The dialogue between mother and child does not read like a transcribed dialogue between two adults. Table 1 offers a sample section from an early transcribed record. It has some interesting properties. The conversation is, in the first place, very much in the here and now. From the child there is no speech of the sort that Bloomfield called "displaced," speech about other times and other places. Adam's utterances in the early months were largely a coding of contemporaneous events and impulses. The mother's speech differs from the speech that adults use to one another in many ways. Her sentences are short and simple; for the most part they are the kinds of sentences that Adam will produce a year later.

TABLE 1

A Section from Adam's First Record

Adam	Mother
See truck, Mommy.	
See truck.	
	Did you see the truck?
No I see truck.	
	No, you didn't see it?
	There goes one.
There go one.	
	Yes, there goes one.
See a truck	
See truck, Mommy.	
See truck.	
Truck.	
Put truck, Mommy.	
	Put the truck where?
Put truck window.	
	I think that one's too large to go in the window.

Perhaps because they are short, the sentences of the mother are perfectly grammatical. The sentences adults use to one another, perhaps because they are longer and more complex, are very often not grammatical, not well formed. Here for instance is a rather representative example produced at a conference of psychologists and linguists: "As far as I know, no one yet has done the in a way obvious now and interesting problem of doing a in a sense a structural frequency study of the alternative syntactical in a given language, say, like English, the alternative possible structures, and how what their hierarchical probability of occurrence structure is."[2] It seems unlikely that a child could learn the patterns of English syntax from such speech. His introduction to English ordinarily comes in the form of a simplified, repetitive, and idealized dialect. It may be that such an introduction is necessary for the acquisition of syntax to be possible but we do not know that.

In the course of the brief interchange of table 1 Adam imitates his mother in saying: "There go one" immediately after she says "There goes one." The imitation is not perfect; Adam omits the inflection on the verb. His imitation is a reduction in that it omits something from the original. This kind of imitation with reduction is extremely common in the records of Adam and Eve and it is the first process we shall discuss.

Imitation and Reduction

Table 2 presents some model sentences spoken by the mothers and the imitations produced by Adam and Eve. These were selected from hundreds in the records in order to illustrate some general propositions. The first thing to notice is that the imitations preserve the word order of the model sentences. To be sure, words in the model are often missing from the imitation but the words preserved are in the order of the original. This is a fact that is so familiar and somehow reasonable that we did not at once recognize it as an empirical outcome rather than as a natural necessity. But of course it is not a necessity, the outcome could have been otherwise. For example, words could have been said back in the reverse of their original order, the most recent first. The preservation of order suggests that the model sentence is pocessed by the child as a total construction rather than as a list of words.

In English the order of words in a sentence is an important grammatical signal. Order is used to distinguish among subject, direct object, and indirect object, and it is one of the marks of imperative and interrogative constructions. The fact that the child's first sentences preserve the word order of their models partially accounts for the ability of an adult to understand these sentences and so to feel that he is in communication with the child. It is conceivable that the child intends the meanings coded by

---

[2] H. Maclay and C. E. Osgood, "Hesitation phenomena in spontaneous English speech." *Word* XV (1959): 19–44.

TABLE 2

Some Imitations Produced by Adam and Eve

Model Utterance	Child's Imitation
Tank car	Tank car
Wait a minute	Wait a minute
Daddy's brief case	Daddy brief case
Fraser will be unhappy	Fraser unhappy
He's going out	He go out
That's an old time train	Old time train
It's not the same dog as Pepper	Dog Pepper
No, you can't write on Mr. Cromer's shoe	Write Cromer shoe

his word orders and that, when he preserves the order of an adult sentence, he does so because he wants to say what the order says. It is also possible that he preserves word order just because his brain works that way and that he has no comprehension of the semantic contrasts involved. In some languages word order is not an important grammatical signal. In Latin, for instance, Agricola amat puellam has the same meaning as Puellam amat agricola and subject-object relations are signalled by case endings. We would be interested to know whether children who are exposed to languages that do not utilize word order as a major syntactic signal, preserve order as reliably as do children exposed to English.

The second thing to notice in table 2 is the fact that when the models increase in length there is not a corresponding increase in the imitation. The imitations stay in the range of two to four morphemes which was the range characteristic of the children at this time. The children were operating under some constraint of length or span. This is not a limitation of vocabulary; the children knew hundreds of words. Neither is it a constraint of immediate memory. We infer this from the fact that the average length of utterances produced spontaneously, where immediate memory is not involved, is about the same as the average length of utterances produced as immediate imitations. The constraint is a limitation on the length of utterance the children are able to program or plan.[3] This kind of narrow span limitation in children is characteristic of most or all of their intellectual operations. The limitation grows less restrictive with age as a consequence, probably, of both neurological growth and of practice, but of course it is never lifted altogether.

---

[3] Additional evidence of the constraint on sentence length may be found in R. Brown and C. Fraser, "The acquisition of syntax." *Verbal Behavior and Learning*, C. N. Cofer and Barbara Musgrave, eds. New York: McGraw-Hill, 1963.

A constraint on length compels the imitating child to omit some words or morphemes from the mother's longer sentences. Which forms are retained and which omitted? The selection is not random but highly systematic. Forms retained in the examples of table 2 include: Daddy, Fraser, Pepper, and Cromer; tank car, minute, briefcase, train, dog, and shoe; wait, go, and write; unhappy and old time. For the most part they are nouns, verbs, and adjectives, though there are exceptions, as witness the initial pronoun *He* and the preposition *out* and the indefinite article *a*. Forms omitted in the samples of table 2 include: the possessive inflection *-s*, the modal auxiliary *will*, the contraction of the auxiliary verb *is*, the progressive inflection *-ing*, the preposition *on*, the articles *the* and *an*, and the modal auxiliary *can*. It is possible to make a general characterization of the forms likely to be retained that distinguishes them as a total class from the forms likely to be omitted.

Forms likely to be retained are nouns and verbs and, less often, adjectives, and these are the three large and "open" parts-of-speech in English. The number of forms in any one of these parts-of-speech is extremely large and always growing. Words belonging to these classes are sometimes called *contentives* because they have semantic content. Forms likely to be omitted are inflections, auxiliary verbs, articles, prepositions, and conjunctions. These forms belong to syntactic classes that are small and closed. Any one class has few members and new members are not readily added. The omitted forms are the ones that linguists sometimes call *functors*, their grammatical functions being more obvious than their semantic content.

Why should young children omit functors and retain contentives? There is more than one plausable answer. Nouns, verbs, and adjectives are words that make reference. One can conceive of teaching the meanings of these words by speaking them, one at a time, and pointing at things or actions or qualities. And of course parents do exactly that. These are the kinds of words that children have been encouraged to practice speaking one at a time. The child arrives at the age of sentence construction with a stock of well-practiced nouns, verbs, and adjectives. Is it not likely then that this prior practice causes him to retain the contentives from model sentences too long to be reproduced in full, that the child imitates those forms in the speech he hears which are already well developed in him as individual habits? There is probably some truth in this explanation but it is not the only determinant since children will often select for retention contentives that are relatively unfamiliar to them.

We adults sometimes operate under a constraint on length and the curious fact is that the English we produce in these circumstances bears a formal resemblance to the English produced by two-year-old children. When words cost money there is a premium on brevity or to put it otherwise, a constraint on length. The result is "telegraphic" English and telegraphic English is an English of nouns, verbs, and adjectives. One does not send a cable reading: "My car has broken down and I have lost my wallet; send money to me at the American Express in Paris" but rather "Car broken down; wallet lost; send money American Express Paris." The telegram omits: my, has, and, I, have, my, to, me, at, the, in. All of these are functors. We make the same kind of telegraphic reduction when time or fatigue constrain us to be brief, as witness any set of notes taken at a fast-moving lecture.

A telegraphic transformation of English generally communicates very well. It does so because it retains the high-information words and drops the low-information words. We are here using "information" in the sense of the mathematical theory of communication. The information carried by a word is inversely related to the chances of guessing it from context. From a given string of content words, missing functors can often be guessed but the message "my has and I have my to me at the in" will not serve to get money to Paris. Perhaps children are able to make a communication analysis of adult speech and so adapt in an optimal way to their limitation of span. There is, however, another way in which the adaptive outcome might be achieved.

If you say aloud the model sentences of table 2 you will find that you place the heavier stresses, the primary and secondary stresses in the sentences, on contentives rather than on functors. In fact the heavier stresses fall, for the most part, on the words the child retains. We first realized that this was the case when we found that in transcribing tapes, the words of the mother that we could hear most clearly were usually the words that the child reproduced. We had trouble hearing the weakly stressed functors and, of course, the child usually failed to reproduce them. Differential stress may then be the cause of the child's differential retention. The outcome is a maximally informative reduction but the cause of this outcome need not be the making of an informative analysis. The outcome may be an incidental consequence of the fact that English is a well-designed language that places its heavier stresses where they are needed, on contentives that cannot easily be guessed from context.

We are fairly sure that differential stress is one of the determinants of the child's telegraphic productions. For one thing, stress will also account for the way in which children reproduce polysyllabic words when the total is too much for them. Adam, for instance, gave us 'pression for expression and Eve gave us 'raff for giraffe; the more heavily-stressed syllables were the ones retained. In addition we have tried the effect of placing heavy stresses on functors which do not ordinarily receive such stresses. To Adam we said: "You say what I say" and then, speaking in a normal way at first: "The doggie will bite." Adam gave back: "Doggie bite." Then we stressed the auxiliary: "The doggie *will* bite" and, after a few trials, Adam made attempts at reproducing that auxiliary. A science fiction experiment comes to mind. If there were parents who stressed functors rather than contentives would they have children whose speech was a kind of reciprocal telegraphic made up of articles, prepositions, conjunctions, auxiliaries, and the like? Such children would be out of touch with the community as real children are not.

It may be that all the factors we have mentioned play some part in determining the child's selective imitations; the reference-making functions of contentives, the fact that they are practiced as single words, the fact that they cannot be guessed from context, and the heavy stresses they receive. There are also other possible factors: for example, the left-to-right, earlier-to-later position of words in a sentence, but these make too long a story to tell here.[4] Whatever the causes, the first utterances produced as imitations of adult sentences are highly systematic reductions of their models. Furthermore, the telegraphic properties of these imitations appear also in the child's spontaneously produced utterances. When his speech is not modeled on an immediately prior adult sentence, it observes the same limitation on length and the same predilection for contentives as when it is modeled on an immediately prior sentence.

Imitation with Expansion

In the course of the brief conversation set down in table 1, Adam's mother at one point imitates Adam. The boy says: "There go one" and mother responds: "Yes, there goes one." She does not exactly reproduce the model sentence of the child but instead adds something to it or expands it. What she adds is a functor, the inflection for third-person on the verb, the very form that Adam had omitted when he imitated his mother.

One of the first things we noticed when we began to study child speech several years ago was the frequency with which adults imitated children. Indeed they seemed to imitate more often than did the children themselves. We later came to realize that adult imitations are seldom exact reproductions; they are usually expansions. The mothers of Adam and Eve responded to the speech of their children with expansions about 30 percent of the time. We did it ourselves when we talked with the children. Indeed we found it very difficult to withhold expansions. A reduced or incomplete English sentence seems to constrain the English-speaking adult to expand it into the nearest properly formed complete sentence. Table 3 lists a few sample expansions from the hundreds in the records.

The first thing worthy of attention in the expansions of table 3 is the fact that the words spoken by the mother preserve the order of the words in the child's sentence. To be sure, words and inflections are added

[4] Brown and Fraser, ibid.

but they are fitted in—before, and after and between the words the child used; they are not generally permitted to disturb the order of the child's words. It is as if these latter were taken as constants by the mother, constants to which some sentence had to be fitted. She acts as if she were assuming that the child means everything he says, all the words and also their order, but as if he might also mean more than he says. From the mother's point of view an expansion is a kind of communication check; it says in effect: Is this what you mean?

TABLE 3

Expansions of Child Speech Produced by Mothers

Child	Mother
Baby highchair	Baby is in the highchair
Mommy eggnog	Mommy had her eggnog
Eve lunch	Eve is having lunch
Mommy sandwich	Mommy'll have a sandwich
Sat wall	He sat on the wall
Throw Daddy	Throw it to Daddy
Pick glove	Pick the glove up

The second thing to notice about table 3 is the character of the forms added to the child's utterances. They include the auxiliaries *is* and *will*; the prepositions *in*, *on*, *to*, and *up*; the verb forms *is*, *have*, *had*, and *having*; the articles *a* and *the*; the pronouns *her*, *he*, and *it*. For the most part, the words added are functors and functors are, of course, the words that the child omits in his reductions.

The interaction between mother and child is, much of the time, a cycle of reductions and expansions. There are two transformations involved. The reduction transformation has an almost completely specifiable and so mechanical character. One could program a machine to do it with the following instructions: Retain contentives (or stressed forms) in the order given up to some limit of length. The expansion accomplished by Adam's mother when she added the third-person inflection to the verb and said "There goes one" is also a completely specifiable transformation. The instructions would read: Retain the forms given in the order given and supply obligatory grammatical forms. To be sure this mother-machine would have to be supplied with the obligatory rules of English grammar but that could be done. However, the sentence "there goes one" is atypical in that it only adds a compulsory and redundant inflection. The expansions of table 3 all add forms that are not grammatically compulsory or redundant and these expansions cannot be mechanically generated by grammatical rules alone.

In table 3 the topmost four utterances produced by the child are all of the same grammatical type; all four consist of a proper noun followed by a common noun. However, the four are expanded in quite different ways. In particular the form of the verb changes: it is in the first case in the simple present tense; in the second case the simple past; in the third case the present progressive; in the last case the simple future. All of these are perfectly grammatical but they are different. The second set of child utterances is formally uniform in that each one consists of a verb followed by a noun. The expansions are again all grammatical but quite unlike, especially with regard to the preposition supplied. In general, then, there are radical changes in the mother's expansions when there are no changes in the formal character of the utterances expanded. It follows that the expansions cannot be produced simply by making grammatically compulsory additions to the child's utterances.

How does a mother decide on the correct expansion of one of her child's utterances? Consider the utterance "Eve lunch." So far as grammar is concerned this utterance could be appropriately expanded in any of a number of ways: "Eve is having lunch"; "Eve had lunch"; "Eve will have lunch"; "Eve's lunch," and so on. On the occasion when Eve produced the utterance, however, one expansion seemed more appropriate than any other. It was then the noon hour, Eve was sitting at the table with a plate of food before her, and her spoon and fingers were busy. In these circumstances "Eve lunch" had to mean "Eve is having lunch." A little later when the plate had been stacked in the sink and Eve was getting down from her chair the utterance "Eve lunch" would have suggested the expansion "Eve has had her lunch." Most expansions are not only responsive to the child's words but also the circumstances attending their utterance.

What kind of instructions will generate the mother's expansions? The following are approximately correct: Retain the words given in the order given and add those functors that will result in a well-formed simple sentence that is appropriate to the circumstances. These are not instructions that any machine could follow. A machine could act on the instructions only if it were provided with detailed specifications for judging appropriateness and no such specifications can, at present, be written. They exist, however, in implicit form in the brains of mothers and in the brains of all English-speaking adults and so judgments of appropriateness can be made by such adults.

The expansion encodes aspects of reality that are not coded by the child's telegraphic utterance. Functors have meaning but it is meaning that accrues to them in context rather than in isolation. The meanings that are added by functors seem to be nothing less than the basic terms in which we construe reality: the time of an action, whether it is ongoing or completed, whether it is presently relevant or not; the concept of possession and such relational concepts as are coded by in, on, up, down—and the like; the difference between a particular instance of a class (Has anybody seen *the* paper?) and any instance of a class (Has anybody seen *a* paper?); the difference between extended substances given shape and size by an "accidental" container (sand, water, syrup, and so forth) and countable "things" having a characteristic fixed shape and size (a cup, a man, a tree). It seems to us that a mother in expanding speech may be teaching more than grammar; she may be teaching something like a world-view.

As yet it has not been demonstrated that expansions are *necessary* for learning either grammar or a construction of reality. It has not even been demonstrated that expansions contribute to such learning. All we know is that some parents do expand and their children do learn. It is perfectly possible, however, that children can and do learn simply from hearing their parents or others make well-formed sentences in connection with various nonverbal circumstances. It may not be necessary or even helpful for these sentences to be expansions of utterances of the child. Only experiments contrasting expansion training with simple exposure to English will settle the matter. We hope to do such experiments.

There are, of course, reasons for expecting the expansion transformation to be an effective tutorial technique. By adding something to the words the child has just produced one confirms his response insofar as it is appropriate. In addition one takes him somewhat beyond that response but not greatly beyond it. One encodes additional meanings at a moment when he is most likely to be attending to the cues that can teach that meaning.

Induction of the Latent Structure

Adam, in the course of the conversation with his mother set down in table 1, produced one utterance for which no adult is likely ever to have provided an exact model: "No I see truck." His mother elects to expand it as "No, you didn't see it" and this expansion suggests that the child might have created the utterance by reducing an adult model containing the form *didn't*. However, the mother's expansion in this case does some violence to Adam's original version. He did not say *no* as his mother said it, with primary stress and final contour; Adam's *no* had secondary stress and no final contour. It is not easy to imagine an adult model for this utterance. It seems more likely that the utterance was created by Adam as part of a continuing effort to discover the general rules for constructing English negatives.

In table 4 we have listed some utterances produced by Adam or Eve for which it is difficult to imagine any adult model. It is unlikely that any adult said any of these to Adam or Eve since they are very simple utterances and yet definitely ungrammatical. In addition it is difficult, by adding functors alone, to build any of them up to simple grammatical

TABLE 4

Utterances Not Likely to Be Imitations

My Cromer suitcase	You naughty are
Two foot	Why it can't turn off?
A bags	Put on it
A scissor	Cowboy did fighting me
A this truck	Put a gas in

sentences. Consequently it does not seem likely that these utterances are reductions of adult originals. It is more likely that they are mistakes which externalize the child's search for the regularities of English syntax.

We have long realized that the occurrence of certain kinds of errors on the level of morphology (or word construction) reveals the child's efforts to induce regularities from speech. So long as a child speaks correctly, or at any rate so long as he speaks as correctly as the adults he hears, there is no way to tell whether he is simply repeating what he has heard or whether he is actually constructing. However, when he says something like "I digged a hole" we can often be sure that he is constructing. We can be sure because it is unlikely that he would have heard *digged* from anyone and because we can see how, in processing words he has heard, he might have come by *digged*. It looks like an overgeneralization of the regular past inflection. The inductive operations of the child's mind are externalized in such a creation. Overgeneralizations on the level of syntax (or sentence construction) are more difficult to identify because there are so many ways of adding functors so as to build up conceivable models. But this is difficult to do for the examples of table 4 and for several hundred other utterances in our records.

The processes of imitation and expansion are not sufficient to account for the degree of linguistic competence that children regularly acquire. These processes alone cannot teach more than the sum total of sentences that speakers of English have either modeled for a child to imitate or built up from a child's reductions. However, a child's linguistic competence extends far beyond this sum total of sentences. All children are able to understand and construct sentences they have never heard but which are nevertheless well-formed, well-formed in terms of general rules that are implicit in the sentence the child has heard. Somehow, then, every child processes the speech to which he is exposed so as to induce from it a latent structure. This latent-rule structure is so general that a child can spin out its implications all his life long. It is both semantic and syntactic. The discovery of latent structure is the greatest of the processes involved in language acquisition and the most difficult to understand. We will provide an example of how the analysis can proceed by discussing the evolution in child speech of noun phrases.

A noun phrase in adult English includes a noun but also more than a noun. One variety consists of a noun with assorted modifiers: *the girl*; *the pretty girl*; *that pretty girl*; *my girl*, and so on. All of these are constructions which have the same syntactic privileges as do nouns alone. One can use a noun phrase in isolation to name or request something: one can use it in sentences, in subject position or in object position or in predicate nominative position. All of these are slots that nouns alone can also fill. A larger construction having the same syntactic privileges as its "head" word is called in linguistics an *endocentric* construction and noun phrases are endocentric constructions.

For both Adam and Eve, in the early records, noun phrases usually occur as total independent utterances rather than as components of sentences. Table 5 presents an assortment of such utterances at time 1. They consist in each case of some sort of modifier, just one, preceding a noun. The modifiers, or as they are sometimes called the *pivot* words, are a much smaller class than the noun class. Three students of child speech have independently discovered that this kind of construction is extremely common when children first begin to combine words.[5,6,7]

It is possible to generalize the cases of table 5 into a simple implicit rule. The rule symbolized in table 5 reads: In order to form a noun phrase of this type, select first one word from the small class of modifiers and select, second, one word from the large class of nouns. This is a *generative* rule by which we mean it is a program that would actually serve to build constructions of the type in question. It is offered as a model of the mental mechanism by which Adam and Eve generated such utterances. Furthermore, judging from our work with other children and from the reports of Braine and of Miller and Ervin, the model describes a mechanism present in many children when their average utterance is approximately two morphemes long.

---

[5] M. D. S. Braine, "The ontogeny of English phrase structure: the first phrase." *Language* XXXIX (1963): 1–13.

[6] W. Miller and Susan Ervin, "The development of grammar in child language." U. Bellugi and R. Brown, eds., *The Acquisition of Language, Child Development Monograph* (1964).

[7] Brown and Fraser, op. cit.

TABLE 5

Noun Phrases in Isolation and Rule for Generating Noun Phrases at Time I

A coat	More coffee
A celery*	More nut*
A Becky*	Two sock*
A hands*	Two shoes
The top	Two tinker-toy*
My Mommy	Big boot
That Adam	Poor man
My stool	Little top
That knee	Dirty knee

NP → M + N

M → *a, big, dirty, little, more, my, poor, that, the, two.*

N → *Adam, Becky, boot, coat, coffee, knee, man, Mommy, nut, sock, stool, tinker-toy, top,* and very many others.

* Ungrammatical for an adult.

We have found that even in our earliest records the M+N construction is sometimes used as a component of larger constructions. For instance, Eve said: "Fix a Lassie" and "Turn the page" and "A horsie stuck" and Adam even said: "Adam wear a shirt." There are, at first, only a handful of these larger constructions but there are very many constructions in which single nouns occur in subject or in object position.

Let us look again at the utterances of table 5 and the rule generalizing them. The class M does not correspond with any syntactic class of adult English. In the class M are articles, a possessive pronoun, a cardinal number, a demonstrative adjective or pronoun, a quantifier, and some descriptive adjectives, a mixed bag indeed. For adult English these words cannot belong to the same syntactic class because they have very different privileges of occurrence in sentences. For the children the words do seem to function as one class having the common privilege of occurrence before nouns.

If the initial words of the utterances in table 5 are treated as one class M then many utterances are generated which an adult speaker would judge to be ungrammatical. Consider the indefinite article *a.* Adults use it only to modify common count nouns in the singlar such as coat, dog, cup. We could not say *a celery* or *a dirt*; celery and dirt are mass nouns. We would not say *a Becky* or *a Jimmy*; Becky and Jimmy are proper nouns. We would not say *a hands* or *a shoes*; hands and shoes are plural nouns. Adam and Eve, at first, did form ungrammatical combinations such as these.

The numeral *two* we use only with count nouns in the plural. We would not say *two sock* since sock is singular, nor *two water* since water is a mass noun. The word *more* we use before count nouns in the plural (more nuts) or mass nouns in the singular (more coffee). Adam and Eve made a number of combinations involving *two* or *more* that we would not make.

Given the initial very undiscriminating use of words in the class M it follows that one dimension of development must be a progressive differentiation of privileges, which means the division of M into smaller classes. There must also be subdivision of the noun class (N) for the reason that the privileges of occurrence of various kinds of modifiers must be described in terms of such subvarieties of N as the common noun and proper noun, the count noun and mass noun. There must eventually emerge a distinction between nouns singular and nouns plural since this distinction figures in the privileges of occurrence of the several sorts of modifiers.

Sixteen weeks after our first records from Adam and Eve (time 2), the differentiation process had begun. By this time there were distributional reasons for separating out articles (a, the) from demonstrative pronouns (this, that) and both of these from the residual class of modifiers. Some of the evidence for this conclusion appears in table 6. In general one syntactic class is distinguished from another when the members of one class have combinational privileges not enjoyed by the members of the other. Consider, for example, the reasons for distinguishing articles (Art) from modifiers in general (M). Both articles and modifiers appeared in front of nouns in two-word utterances. However, in three-word utterances that were made up from the total pool of words and that had a noun in final position, the privileges of *a* and *the* were different from the privileges of all other modifiers. The articles occurred in initial position followed by a member of class M other than an article. No other modifier occurred in this first position; notice the "Not obtained" examples of table 6A. If the children had produced utterances like those (for example, blue a flower, your a car) there would have been no difference in the privileges of occurrence of articles and modifiers and therefore no reason to separate out articles.

The record of Adam is especially instructive. He created such notably ungrammatical combinations as "a your car" and "a my pencil." It is very unlikely that adults provided models for these. They argue strongly that Adam regarded all the words in the residual M class as syntactic equivalents and so generated these very odd utterances in which possessive pronouns appear where descriptive adjectives would be more acceptable.

Table 6 also presents some of the evidence for distinguishing demonstrative pronouns (Dem) from articles and modifiers. (Table 6B.) The pronouns occurred first and ahead of articles in three-and-four-word

TABLE 6 (A and B)

Subdivision of the Modifier Class

A. Privileges Peculiar to Articles

Obtained	Not Obtained
A blue flower	Blue a flower
A nice nap	Nice a nap
A your car	Your a car
A my pencil	My a pencil

B. Privileges Peculiar to Demonstrative Pronouns

Obtained	Not Obtained
That my cup	My that cup
That a horse	A that horse
That a blue flower	A that blue flower
	Blue a that flower

utterances—a position that neither articles nor modifiers ever filled. The sentences with demonstrative pronouns are recognizable as reductions which omit the copular verb *is*. Such sentences are not noun phrases in adult English and ultimately they will not function as noun phrases in the speech of the children, but for the present they are not distinguishable distributionally from noun phrases.

TABLE 7

Rules for Generating Noun Phrases at Time 2

$NP_1 \rightarrow Dem + Art + M + N$	$NP \rightarrow (Dem) + (Art) + (M) + N$
$NP_2 \rightarrow Art + M + N$	
$NP_3 \rightarrow Dem + M + N$	( ) means class within parentheses is optional
$NP_4 \rightarrow Art + N$	
$NP_5 \rightarrow M + N$	
$NP_6 \rightarrow Dem + N$	
$NP_7 \rightarrow Dem + Art + N$	

Recall now the generative formula of table 5 which constructs noun phrases by simply placing a modifier (M) before a noun (N). The differentiation of privileges illustrated in table 6, and the syntactic classes this evidence motivates us to create, complicate the formula for generating noun phrases. In table 7 we have written a single general formula for producing all noun phrases at time 2 [NP→ (Dem) + (Art) + (M) + N] and also the numerous more specific rules which are summarized by the general formula.

By the time of the thirteenth transcription, twenty-six weeks after we began our study, privileges of occurrence were much more finely differentiated and syntactic classes were consequently more numerous. From the distributional evidence we judged that Adam had made five classes of his original class M: articles, descriptive adjectives, possessive pronouns, demonstrative pronouns, and a residual class of modifiers. The generative rules of table 7 had become inadequate; there were no longer, for instance, any combinations like "A your car." Eve had the same set except that she used two residual classes of modifiers. In addition nouns had begun to subdivide for both children. The usage of proper nouns had become clearly distinct from the usage of count nouns. For Eve the evidence justified separating count nouns from mass nouns, but for Adam it still did not. Both children by this time were frequently pluralizing nouns but as yet their syntactic control of the singular-plural distinction was imperfect.

In summary, one major aspect of the development of general structure in child speech is a progressive differentiation in the usage of words and therefore a progressive differentiation of syntactic classes. At the same time, however, there is an integrative process at work. From the first, an occasional noun phrase occurred as a component of some larger construction. At first these noun phrases were just two words long and the range of positions in which they could occur was small. With time the noun phrases grew longer, were more frequently used, and were used in a greater range of positions. The noun phrase structure as a whole, in all the permissible combinations of modifiers and nouns, was assuming the combinational privileges enjoyed by nouns in isolation.

In table 8 we have set down some of the sentence positions in which both nouns and noun phrases occurred in the speech of Adam and Eve. It is the close match between the positions of nouns alone and of nouns with modifiers in the speech of Adam and Eve that justifies us in calling the longer constructions noun phrases. These longer constructions are, as they should be, endocentric; the head word alone has the same syntactic privileges as the head word with its modifiers. The continuing failure to find in noun phrase positions whole constructions of the type, "That a blue flower" signals the fact that these constructions are telegraphic versions of predicate nominative sentences omitting the verb form *is*. Examples of the kind of construction not obtained are: That (that a blue flower); Where (that a blue flower)?

For adults the noun phrase is a subwhole of the sentence, what linguists call an *immediate constituent*. The noun phrase has a kind of psychological unity. There are signs that the noun phrase was also an immediate

TABLE 8

Some Privileges of the Noun Phrase

Noun Positions	Noun Phrase Positions
That (flower)	That (a blue flower)
Where (ball) go?	Where (the puzzle) go?
Adam write (penguin)	Doggie eat (the breakfast)
(Horsie) stop	(A horsie) crying
Put (hat) on	Put (the red hat) on

constituent for Adam and Eve. Consider the sentence using the separable verb *put on.* The noun phrase in "Put the red hat on" is, as a whole, fitted in between the verb and the particle even as is the noun alone in "Put hat on." What is more, however, the location of pauses in the longer sentence, on several occasions, suggested the psychological organization: "Put . . . the red hat . . . on" rather than "Put the red . . . hat on" or "Put the . . . red hat on." In addition to this evidence the use of pronouns suggests that the noun phrase is a psychological unit.

The unity of noun phrases in adult English is evidenced, in the first place, by the syntactic equivalence between such phrases and nouns alone. It is evidenced, in the second place, by the fact that pronouns are able to substitute for total noun phrases. In our immediately preceding sentence the pronoun *It* stands for the rather involved construction from the first sentence of this pharagraph: The unity of noun phrases in adult English. The words called pronouns in English would more aptly be called "pro-noun-phrases" since it is the phrase rather than the noun which they usually replace. One does not replace "unity" with "it" and say The *it* of noun phrases in adult English. In the speech of Adam and Eve, too, the pronoun came to function as a replacement for the noun phrase. Some of the clearer cases appear in table 9.

Adam characteristically externalizes more of his learning than does Eve and his record is especially instructive in connection with the learning of pronouns. In his first eight records, the first sixteen weeks of the study, Adam quite often produced sentences containing both the pronoun and the noun or noun phrase that the pronoun should have replaced. One can see here the equivalence in the process of establishment. First the substitute is produced and then, as if in explication, the form or forms that will eventually be replaced by the substitute. Adam spoke out his pronoun antecedents as chronological consequents. This is additional evidence of the unity of the noun phrase since the noun phrases *my ladder* and *cowboy boot* are linked with *it* in Adam's speech in just the same way as the nouns *ladder* and *ball.*

TABLE 9

Pronouns Replacing Nouns or Noun Phrases and Pronouns Produced Together with Nouns or Noun Phrases

Noun Phrases Replaced by Pronouns	Pronouns and Noun Phrases in Same Utterances
Hit ball	Mommy get it ladder
Get it	Mommy get it my ladder
Ball go?	Saw it ball
Go get it	Miss it garage
Made it	I miss it cowboy boot
Made a ship	I Adam drive that
Fix a tricycle	I Adam drive
Fix it	I Adam don't

We have described three processes involved in the child's acquisition of syntax. It is clear that the last of these, the induction of latent structure, is by far the most complex. It looks as if this last process will put a serious strain on any learning theory thus far conceived by psychology. The very intricate simultaneous differentiation and integration that constitutes the evolution of the noun phrase is more reminiscent of the biological development of an embryo than it is of the acquisition of a conditional reflex.

While Walter A. Wolfrom's article is dated (it includes only ERIC documents processed prior to 1969), nevertheless it examines an issue that is still relevant—that is, whether nonstandard dialects are deficient or merely different models of standard English.

Wolfram reviews studies of nonstandard dialects by those who see them as deficient or inferior to the language in which school work is usually carried on. In his treatment of nonstandard dialects as deficient, the author does not include reference to the work of Basil Bernstein, a British sociolinguist whose writing has strongly influenced thinking along these lines. Houston, however, discusses Bernstein's thinking in the selection following Wolfram's.

Wolfram then reviews the work of those who see nonstandard dialect as a language model different from (and not inferior to) standard English. In this area, the work of Courtney B. Cazden is particularly worthy of note.

Those who would read further in an effort to understand the deficient versus different views are urged to read in their entirety the references that Wolfrom reviews. Another excellent review of certain materials in this area is Anna Maria Malkoc's "Bi-Dialectism: A Special Report from CAL/ERIC." English Journal 60 (February 1971) 279–288.

The Nature of Nonstandard Dialect Divergence

Walt Wolfram

Within the last decade, we have witnessed an expanding interest in the study of nonstandard dialects from a number of different vantage points. Various aspects of nonstandard dialects and their relation to standard dialects have now been investigated. With the increasing number of perspectives on a theme, it has become correspondingly more difficult to keep abreast of all the developments in the field. The various approaches to the problem may keep one rightly perplexed, for the conclusions drawn from similar data may differ dramatically. With the proliferation of papers on a general theme, it also has become increasingly difficult to select a subtopic from a larger area which may be of concern to the potential reader. Finally, the limited and delayed availability of papers through the normal channels of publication may keep one in a constant state of frustration. (Because of this problem, the reader should keep in mind that this description includes only ERIC documents that were processed prior to the fall of 1969.)

The development of ERIC has certainly helped alleviate the problem of limited and delayed availability, but the relevance of various papers to a specific issue and the relative merit of these papers is outside the scope of ERIC. Yet, it is apparent that such evaluative judgments might be of great service to the reader who has neither the time nor interest to survey the many divergent aspects of nonstandard dialects for himself.

The primary purpose of this paper is therefore evaluative. It is designed to investigate a specific issue in this area of nonstandard dialects and to evaluate ERIC documents dealing with this issue. Obviously, not all of the articles will be of equal relevance to the specific issue being investigated here. The relative importance will be implicit in the comments concerning each article. In addition, special notation will be made of crucial articles in the bibliography.

The issue reviewed here is the manner in which nonstandard dialects differ from standard English. In other words, possible answers are explored concerning the question of *how* nonstandard dialects differ from standard dialects.

Deficiency versus Difference

Although it may seem somewhat oversimplified, the current viewpoints on how nonstandard dialects differ from standard dialects can be subsumed under two theoretical positions: either nonstandard dialects are viewed as a *deficient* form of standard English or they are viewed as a *different* but equal language system. In a *deficit* model, speech differences are viewed and described with reference to a norm and deviation from that norm. The control group for describing deviation is middle-class speech behavior. From this perspective, nonconformity to the norm is seen as an indication of retarded language acquisition or under-developed language capacity. Nonstandard pronunciation and grammatical patterns are sometimes viewed as inaccurate and unworthy approximations of standard English. Nonstandard dialects are considered as "the pathology of non-organic speech deficiencies," and the patterns of these dialects are labeled with such terms as "misarticulations," "deviations," "replacements," "faulty pronunciations," and the like.

On the other hand. the *difference* model considers each language variety to be a self-contained system which is inherently neither superior nor deficient. Nonstandard dialects are systems in their own right, with their own pronunciation and grammatical rules. Although these rules may differ from standard English, they are no less consistent or logical than the rules of the socially prestigious dialect. That one language variety is associated with a socially subordinate group and, therefore, socially stigmatized has nothing to do with the actual linguistic capacity as a communicative code.

Although the deficit perspective has enjoyed considerable popularity in a number of disciplines, it conflicts with some basic assumptions about the nature of language (Wolfram, 1969). In the first place, empirical evidence suggests that all languages are capable of conceptualization and expressing logical operations. It is therefore assumed that different surface forms for expression have nothing to do with the underlying logic of a sentence, since there is nothing inherent in a given language variety which will interfere with the development of conceptualization. This is not to say that differences between the handling of logical operations may never correlate with social class. However, social class categories cannot be explained by language differences alone, since all language varieties provide for the expression of syllogistic reasoning.

A second linguistic premise is that all languages and dialects are adequate as communicative systems. It has been established that language is a human phenomenon which characterizes every social group, and that all language systems are perfectly adequate for communication by the members of the social group. The social acceptability of a particular language or dialect, considered nonstandard because of its association with a subordinate social group, is totally unrelated to its adequacy for communication.

Another linguistic premise relating to the adequacy of all language systems is that languages are systematic and ordered. Technically speaking, there is no such thing as a "primitive" language or dialect. All languages and dialects are highly developed and complex systems in their internal organization. Furthermore, affinities between the pronunciation and grammatical patterns of related dialects are consistent and regular, not haphazard and random.

Finally, language is learned in the context of the community. All linguistic evidence points to the conclusion that children have acquired a fairly complete language system by the age of five or six, with minor adjustments in language competence sometimes occurring until eight or nine. This system is acquired from contact with individuals in the immediate environment. Whether the source for this acquisition is parental, sibling, or peer group interaction is only incidental from a linguistic viewpoint. What is more important is the fact that the rate of language development is approximately parallel across cultures and subcultures. That is, lower-class children learn nonstandard dialects at approximately the same rate as middle-class children learn standard English.

Nonstandard Dialects as Deficient

Although the linguistic premises concerning the nature of language have been basic to the discipline of linguistics for decades now, when the speech patterns of the so-called disadvantaged became an area of high priority for educators in the early sixties, it was the *deficit* model which provided a framework for this discussion. On this basis, programs were devised to describe and change the speech patterns of these children. One of the earlier programs designed to deal with the speech of these children was the Institute for Developmental Studies, founded and directed by Martin Deutsch.

Deutsch and his staff (1964) describe a "language intervention" program, an attempt to intervene with the development of speech patterns at a preschool period in order to prepare and equip the child with the linguistic capacity for success in school. In other words, the program is set up to remedy the presumed deficits of these children before entering school. Three major premises are enumerated as the theoretical basis for this program: (1) the intellectual deficit caused by early cultural deprivation cannot be made up for by putting children in a middle-class school; they need more direct emphasis on cognition; (2) to overcome deficiencies, there must be a carefully planned match between specific deficits and remedial measures; and (3) to alleviate the language handicap of disadvantaged children, they must be motivated to learn a standard and pattern.

The Deutsch model for intervention is based on the theory that environment plays a major role in the development of cognitive skills, and that language skills and cognitive skills go hand in hand. Because of a "noisy environment" and the inaccessibility of adults in the home, the language and cognitive skills of these children are deficient.

The theoretical basis of Deutsch's position suggests that behavioral characteristics different from middle-class norms are inherently lacking in culture. Such ethnocentric norms for comparison are, of course, at variance with basic understandings of the nature of culture. That ghetto culture is different is not disputed here, but a de facto interpretation that this difference is equivalent to deficiency is difficult to justify. When the implicit criteria for viewing differences as deficiencies are looked at closely, the main criterion which emerges is conformity to middle-class patterns, as if there were some inherent "correctness" in this way of doing things. Attributing speech deficiencies to the unavailability of adults for interaction, for example, takes into account only one model for language acquisition—parent-child interaction. Sibling or peer group interaction, which may be quite extensive at a relatively young age for ghetto children, is not considered.

Furthermore, the relationship of language development and cognitive development has often been misunderstood. That language is integral to the cognitive development of an individual is not at issue here, but empirical linguistic evidence demonstrates that all languages and dialects provide for syllogistic reasoning. Every bit of linguistic data points to the fact that any logical operation possible in a standard dialect is also possible in a nonstandard dialect. The linguistic expression of logical operations may be different from dialect to dialect, but the underlying logic is quite intact. For example, both standard English and nonstandard English provide for making "identity statements" such as "The box is blue," but in the dialect spoken by many lower-class Negro children, this construction is "The box blue." That the copula form *be* is not found in this instance has no effect on the ability to form an identity statement. Rather, this dialect, like languages such as Russian, Thai, and Hungarian, may not have any copula in certain types of constructions. This is not a matter of deficiency but a difference in linguistic expression.

In "The Disadvantaged Child and the Learning Process," (1963) Deutsch is somewhat more detailed in his discussion of the environmental and psychological factors which contribute to the presumed verbal deficiency. Factors such as the lack of toys and books, an unstable family life, and substandard housing may leave a child deficient in perceptual discrimination, attentional mechanisms, expectation of rewards, and the ability to use adults as sources of information. All of these tasks are skills required for learning in schools, at least those of the sixties. Due to the "nonverbal" slum home, the child may fail to acquire a language-concept system which fits the school's instructional patterns.

As we have suggested above, correlations between learning ability and the language of these children are misleading. What is considered to be a lack of syntactic organization and inadequate perceptual ability may emerge only because of the external norms of acquisition, the white middle-class behavior which serves as a measure of "normalcy." Dialect-fair and culture-fair measurements of perceptual ability and syntactic organization have only recently come under consideration. Furthermore, claims about the nonverbalness of slum homes are not based on formal research evidence. As mentioned above, the ghetto homes may well be the predominant source for verbal interaction in this cultural setting.

Cynthia Deutsch (1964) measured the auditory discrimination abilities of lower-class black children on the premise that "a particular minimum level of auditory discrimination skill is necessary for the acquisition of reading and general verbal skills." A basic assumption was that lower-class children are deficient in the development of auditory attentiveness and discrimination because of an excessively noisy, overcrowded environment.

The basis for measuring perception was the Wepman Auditory Discrimination Test, one of the standard tests for discrimination development. Several important limitations of the Wepman Test must be identified. In the first place, the Wepman Test is constructed without reference to legitimate dialect differences. Thus, the failure to discriminate between *wreath* and *reef* or *lave* and *lathe* by young black children is interpreted as indicative of underdeveloped auditory discrimination. Actually, such pairs are the result of a systematic pattern in which *th* in wreath and *f* in reef are both pronounced as *f* at the end of a word, and *th* in lathe and *v* in lave are both pronounced as *v* in the dialect spoken by many black children in the ghetto. This, however, is not the result of retarded speech development, but the result of a legitimate dialect difference which may be maintained by adults as well as children. In essence, this homophony (that is, the pronunciation of two different words alike) is no different from that of the New England middle-class child who does not discriminate between *caught,* the past tense of catch, and *cot,* the object for resting, or *taught,* the past tense of teach, and *torte,* the pastry. The learning of standard English measured by the Wepman Test is not differentiated from the language development of a different dialect. Without taking such dialect differences into account, one can only arrive at erroneous conclusions.

Even if a dialect-fair test indicated that some of these children did reveal developmental retardation, asserting that this might be attributed to the noisy home environment of the child seems to be a simplistic explanation. The social dynamics of the ghetto home, although much mentioned, are just beginning to be researched from an anthropologically valid perspective.

In "The Role of Social Class in Language Development and Cognition," Martin Deutsch (1966) attempts to identify background patterns at two developmental stages and relate them to specific cognitive and linguistic patterns. His conclusions are based on a four year "verbal survey" of 292 Negro and white children in the lower and middle socioeconomic groups. The data indicate that being lower-class and/or Negro contributes to lower language scores. On the basis of these data Deutsch suggests that there is a "cumulative language deficit." That is, language deficits become more marked as the child progresses through school, showing the increasing disparity between the school expectations and performance of these children with respect to the prescribed mold. The finding that the language deficits become more marked as the child progresses through school is significant; the assumptions and interpretations as to the cause of these differences, however, bear closer examination.

Labov and Robins (1969) for example, in their study of Harlem teenagers, have shown that there is a direct relation between peer group involvement and reading achievement. On this basis, it might more reasonably be suggested that as the child becomes older, the values of the peer group, in direct conflict with the school-imposed value system, are basically responsible for the increasing alienation of ghetto children in middle-class oriented classrooms.

John (1964) has set forth the early stages of language acquisition as they relate to social environment in "The Social Context of Language Acquisition." She suggests that a child, surrounded by a sea of words, selectively and sequentially acquires the names of objects and actions. The learning of new responses is facilitated by "the relative invariance of the environment where the social context of learning as well as the stability of the bond between word and referent is being acquired." Differences in the rate and breadth of acquisition can be influenced by the nature of verbal interaction with those caring for the child. Using the Peabody Picture Vocabulary Test as a basis for measurement, it is found that three clusters of words are difficult for low-income children: words relating to rural living, words whose referents are rare in low-income homes, and action words, particularly those dealing with gerundives (for example, lying, running); and that these children did not have difficulty in experience with the referent, but had trouble fitting the label to the varying forms of the action.

The assumptions and methods of John follow those of Deutsch; therefore, the limitations ascribed earlier to Deutsch pertain also to John: (1) the assumptions concerning the social environment of these children are not research based; and (2) the investigators fail to recognize legitimate form differences between dialects in discussing linguistic capacity. Nowhere, for example, is the possibility explored that difficulties with standard English gerundives might be attributed to form differences in the linguistic structure of the dialects investigated.

In all fairness to John and other members of the Institute for Developmental Studies, we must mention that all the above articles were written before the issue of difference versus deficiency was clearly articulated. Characteristically, these articles did not even recognize the existence of the difference alternative. However, with the more recent explication of this issue, current literature dealing with this topic must bear the full responsibility for considering and examining alternatives to the deficit view of language differences in the lower-class child in its assumptions, interpretations, and applications.

A slightly different approach to the speech of the economically impoverished is offered in Osser's "The Syntactic Structures of 5-Year-Old Culturally Deprived Children" (1966). Osser has compared the syntactic structures of middle-class children and black-ghetto children in an attempt to discover how much environmental stimulation is necessary for language development. Using the total number of sentences the children used in the experimental session, the total number of different syntactic structures, and the average "complexity score," a difference favoring the middle-class group is found. Osser also observes that the lower-class group does not show homogeneous speech behavior, a fact he interprets to support the position that environmental differences may not only account for large differences *between* divergent groups, but large differences *within* groups.

Although Osser is treated here along with other studies of nonstandard dialects from a deficit model, he shows considerably more respect for the legitimacy of nonstandard speech as a linguistic system than other approaches from this perspective. It is for this reason that he recognizes the concept of *functional equivalence* in syntactic structures. This refers to "the fact that sequences of words in one dialect may be something different in the other dialect, yet the two sequences are syntactically functionally equivalent, for example, *his sister hat* in the nonstandard dialect is functionally equivalent to *his sister's hat* in the standard dialect."

Despite the caution found in Osser's conclusions, several exceptions to his interpretations must be taken. We have already seen the need to justify statements about the influence of verbal environment on speech by correlational studies, so we need not elaborate this criticism again. The conclusions about the syntax of these children must also be viewed suspiciously, as Osser himself has cautioned. The total number of sentences used in an experimental situation may not have any direct relationship to the communicative adequacy of speech in a natural speech situation. Furthermore, the number of sentences used is significantly intercorrelated with the diversity and complexity of structures. Is, for example, the absence of relatives among the lower-class children representative of the actual linguistic capacity or a function of the failure to elicit a sufficient speech sample? Unfortunately, the legitimacy of cultural differences affecting the experimental situation has not been recognized.

Nonstandard Dialects as Different

One of the first important attempts to explicate the different approaches to the study of nonstandard speech was Cazden's "Subcultural Differences in Child Language: An Interdisciplinary Review" (1966). Although this article reflects the fact that it was written at the inception of much of the current research on nonstandard speech, it is still quite useful. Disciplines included in Cazden's review are linguistics, experimental psychology, anthropology, and sociology. Three main areas of inter-disciplinary convergence are reviewed: (1) nonstandard versus standard English; (2) stages in the developmental continuum; and (3) different modes of communication.

In her discussion of the relation of standard to nonstandard dialects, Cazden delimits several methods of describing differences, including frequency of errors, contrastive analysis, and transformational grammar. The first method, describing errors, is associated with the deficit view of language described above. Cazden is rightly skeptical of studies which assess the status of nonstandard dialects as a cognitive liability, although not as polemical as most linguists dealing with this issue might be. The other two methods, contrastive analysis and transformational grammar, assume a difference view of nonstandard languages. Cazden's distinction of contrastive analysis from transformational grammar, however, is nebulous. For one, these two approaches are not mutually exclusive. Contrastive analyses can, and often do, employ the methods of transformational analysis. Furthermore, transformational grammar is only one linguistic model which might be used in the description of a language or dialect. What is more important than the particular linguistic model is the general linguistic perspective which recognizes the structure of different languages and dialects as systems in their own right, with both similarities and differences to related varieties.

With reference to the stages of the developmental continuum, Cazden summarizes work in this area by noting that children of upper socioeconomic status are generally evaluated as more advanced than those of lower socioeconomic status. But she correctly points out that studies are only valid if evaluated in terms of the norms of a child's own speech community. In this regard, she anticipates the significance of constructing dialect-fair tests.

The final area, the different modes of communication, reviews research on both the intra- and inter- individual aspects of communication. Essentially, this concerns the importance of what, to whom, how, and in what situation we are speaking. She concludes that we know very little about differences in language function.

As a review of the literature up to 1965 on the subcultural differences in the language of children, this can be recommended as a thorough reference. It is less evaluative than might be hoped for with respect to the crucial issue of difference versus deficit, but the period in which it was written may have called for a more cautionary evaluation.

The most explicit sources on the difference/deficit issue are several papers by Joan C. Baratz. In "A Bi-Dialectal Task for Determining Language Proficiency in Economically Disadvantaged Negro Children" (1968*a*), the major dispute about this issue in the literature is outlined, and experimental evidence for her own conclusion is offered.

Baratz suggests that there are three main viewpoints concerning the linguistic system of low-income Negro children. First is the view that such children are verbally destitute, not having yet developed a functionally adequate or structurally systematic language code. This viewpoint is rejected by Baratz because of the biased testing procedures, for example, the use of middle-class testing situations such as the classroom.

The second viewpoint considers these children to have systematic but underdeveloped language behavior, their underdeveloped system leading to cognitive deficits. Again the view point is considered invalid because of the use of middle-class oriented tasks and norms which serve as a standard of normalcy.

The third viewpoint is that these children have a fully developed but different system from standard English. In support of this viewpoint,

Baratz has conducted a bidialectal test in which she assesses the proficiency of black ghetto children and middle-class white children in repeating standard English and nonstandard Negro English. The black children were significantly more proficient in repeating the nonstandard Negro dialect sentences than the white children, but when they repeated the standard English sentences there were predictable differences in their repetitions based on interference from the nonstandard dialect. When the same test was given to the white children, the standard English sentences were repeated quite adequately, but predictable differences in their repetitions of the nonstandard sentences, based on interference from the standard-English system, were observed. The results of this study show that: (1) there are two dialects involved in the educational complex of black children; (2) neither white nor black children are bidialectal; and (3) there is interference from their dialect when black children attempt to use standard English. This type of evidence, Baratz points out, indicates the bias of testing which uses standard English as a yardstick of language development.

The conclusions that Baratz reaches on the basis of her study are important support for the viewpoint which maintains that we are dealing with different but equal systems. Furthermore, the concise discussion of the deficit/difference controversy makes this one of the most essential articles for anyone interested in the issue.

A slightly different emphasis on this issue is given in Baratz's article "Language and Cognitive Assessment of Negro Children: Assumptions and Research Needs" (1968*b*). In this article Baratz examines the speech of lower-class children in relation to cognitive ability. Several of the problems confronting a primarily psychological approach to the language assessment of black children are pointed out: (1) the assumption that language development is synonymous with the acquisition of standard English; (2) the tendency to equate cognition with rationality, that is, the tacit acceptance of external norms resulting in the description of cognitive abilities of black children in terms of a developmental lag; and (3) the conclusion that some environments are inherently more adequate than others for stimulating general language and cognitive growth. The foregoing problems seem to have evolved from misconceptions of what language is and how it functions.

Like the previous article by Baratz (1968*a*), the explication of the different viewpoints in approaching the speech of low-income children makes this an invaluable contribution to the field. Without taking issue with the essential contribution of this article, it is necessary to point out one example in which the position of Englemann and Bereiter is misrepresented.

One of the prime illustrations in her refutation of the Bereiter-Englemann position of language deficits is the treatment of the *if-then* construction; they claim that children are unable to handle this construction in deductive reasoning, for example, *If this block is big, then the other is small.* Baratz understands this use of it to be the same as the "question" *if* in a sentence such as *He asked John if he could come.* Because black children may not use *if* in the second type of construction (He asked John could he come, being appropriate in the dialect of these children), she assumes that Bereiter and Englemann have interpreted a legitimate dialect difference as a cognitive liability. But one cannot argue the case of *if-then* deductions on the basis of question *if* since the two uses of *if* have quite different syntactical functions. Although Baratz's general criticism of the reasoning of Bereiter and Englemann is quite defensible, the particular example chosen to refute their position is, in this case, unfortunate.

In "Grammatical Constructions in the Language of the Negro Preschool Child" (1968*c*), Baratz and Povich compare the language development of a group of Head Start children with the results obtained for middle-class preschoolers, using Lee's *Developmental Sentence Type* model (1966). This article chronologically preceded the papers discussed above, but probably has been preempted by them in terms of relevance to the deficiency/difference issue. It is, nevertheless, important because the analytical method used by Baratz and Povich is different from that described in the articles of Baratz which were discussed in the above paragraphs.

The majority of utterances by the lower-class children are on the kernel and transformational levels of Lee's developmental model, according to the investigators. Although the language of economically impoverished Negro children indicates that their language contains a number of structures which would be considered as "restructured forms" when they are compared with standard English, they conclude that these forms are not only acceptable in lower-class dialect, but also indicate a level of syntactic development where transformations are being used appropriately. Inasmuch as the lower-class Negro child is using the same forms as the lower-class Negro adult, Baratz and Povich conclude that he has adequately acquired the forms of his linguistic environment.

Although the vast majority of the controversy over the difference/deficit model in describing speech differences concerns the speech of ghetto Negro children, Vincent P. Skinner looks at the speech of low-income families in Appalachia from this perspective in "Mountaineers Aren't Really Illiterate" (1967). Because of the paucity of material on Appalachian speech, the article is mentioned here, despite the fact that it is lacking in detail. Skinner does, however, note that this dialect is a sophisticated language which is quite effective for the communicative purposes of the community. The dialect spoken by these mountaineers tends to preserve a more archaic form of English, due to the geographical and social isolation of this group from mainstream American culture. Unfortunately, this article is much too brief and sketchy to be useful as more than an illustration of the status of white nonstandard Appalachian speech as a different but equal system.

Summary

We have seen that there is considerable difference in how nonstandard dialects are viewed as represented in ERIC documents. It should be apparent that one's view of this divergence is crucial for our educational system. For one, the view of a child's dialect will have a direct bearing on teachers' attitudes toward the dialect with which the child comes to school. The attitudinal biases toward linguistically adequate but socially stigmatized language varieties is no doubt the biggest problem we face.

There are also practical reasons for understanding how nonstandard dialects differ from standard English. With respect to testing language proficiency, it means that we must strive to design dialect-fair measures of language proficiency. Only such tests can authentically indicate where a child is in terms of language development. Our viewpoint of nonstandard dialects is also crucial if we propose teaching standard English to nonstandard dialect speakers. A thorough understanding of the systematic and regular differences between standard and nonstandard English must serve as a basis for the most effective teaching of standard English in our schools.

Bibliography

*1. Baratz, Joan C., "A Bi-Dialectal Test for Determining Language Proficiency," 1968. ED 020 519**

*2. Baratz, Joan C., "Language and Cognitive Assessment of Negro Children: Assumptions and Research Needs," 1968. Ed 020 518

3. Baratz, Joan C. and Povich, Edna, "Grammatical Constructions in the Language of the Negro Preschool Child," 1968. ED 022 157

*4. Cazen, Courtney B., "Subcultural Differences in Child Language: an Interdisciplinary Review," 1966. *Merrill-Palmer Quarterly of Behavior and Development*, 12, 185–219, ED O11 325

5. Deutsch, Martin, "The Role of Social Class in Language Development and Cognition," 1966. ED 011 329

6. Deutsch, Martin, "The Disadvantaged Child and the Learning Process," 1963. ED 021 721

7. Deutsch, Martin, et al., "The Deutsch Model—Institute for Developmental Studies," 1964. ED 020 009

8. Deutsch, Cynthia, "Auditory Discrimination and Learning: Social Factors," 1964. ED 001 116

9. John, Vera P., "The Social Context of Language Acquisition," 1964. ED 001 494

10. Labov, William and Robins, Clarence, "A Note on the Relation of Reading Failure to Peer-Group Status in Urban Ghettos" in Alfred C. Aarons, Barbara Y.

Gordon, and William A. Stewart, *Linguistic-Cultural Differences and American Education*, Special Anthology Issue, *The Florida FL Reporter*, 7, No. 1 (Spring/Summer 1969).

11. Lee, Laura L., "Developmental Sentence Types: A Method for Comparing Normal and Deviant Syntactic Development," *Journal of Speech and Hearing Disorders*, 31 (1966).
12. Osser, Harry, "The Syntactic Structures of 5-Year-Old Culturally Deprived Children," 1966. ED 020 788
13. Skinner, Vincent P., "Mountaineers Aren't Really Illiterate," 1967. *Southern Education Report*, 3, 18–19. ED 020 236

*14. Wolfram, Walter A., "Sociolinguistic Perspectives on the Speech of the Disadvantaged," 1969. ED 029 280

* Articles considered to be of crucial importance to the issue.
** Eric Document Number.

How one views the matter of dialect divergence will largely determine how one treats children who speak a nonstandard dialect in the classroom. After a review of research dealing with language acquisition in general and language acquisition among disadvantaged minority children in particular, Susan H. Houston reexamines some assumptions that educators commonly make about the language of the disadvantaged child.

The assumptions that Houston reexamines are: (1) The language of the disadvantaged child is deficient. (2) The disadvantaged child does not use words properly. (3) The language of the disadvantaged child does not provide him with an adequate basis for (abstract and other) thinking. (4) To the disadvantaged child, language is dispensable; such children tend to communicate nonverbally in preference to verbally, and (5) The language of the disadvantaged child, since it represents his culture and environment, should be left alone and not changed in any way. In dealing with the first four assumptions, Houston shakes many of the foundations on which they are based. Her approach to the fifth assumption is more pragmatic. Houston's own research and field work in this area give a particularly sound basis to her thinking.

Another excellent and highly recommended article on the same topic (the assumptions and negative attitudes that teachers have about nonstandard—specifically Negro—dialect) is Kenneth R. Johnson's "Teachers' Attitudes Toward the Nonstandard Negro Dialect—Let's Change It." *Elementary English* 48 (February 1971): 176–184.

A Reexamination of Some Assumptions about the Language of the Disadvantaged Child

Susan H. Houston

Editor's Note: After identifying the concern of educators with the matter of dialect divergence in schools, the author surveys research dealing with language acquisition in general and with language acquisition among disadvantaged or minority children.

Several conclusions may be drawn from even this brief discussion of the language-acquisition process. In particular, it will be seen that modern linguistic and psycholinguistic knowledge casts serious doubts on many standard comments about the language development of the disadvantaged child. It may be helpful to the reader for us to consider individually some of these frequently appearing notions and to make comments on them based upon what has been reviewed above and other relevant material.

1. *The language of the disadvantaged child is deficient.* Different ap-

proaches are needed to this postulate, depending on the nature of the deficiency intended. I have already discussed the invalidity of suggesting that the language of disadvantaged children is generally primitive and simple, any more than that of other children. However, a number of more specific statements along the same lines have also gained currency of late. For example, Bernstein (1961) and others have commented on the apparent great limitations of disadvantaged and minority children's language, the lack of willingness or perhaps ability of these children to use language as easily or as often as nondisadvantaged children, and the peculiar characteristics of the language they do use. Among relevant characteristics frequently cited are short utterance length, one-word replies to questions, limited expressed affect (for example, Blank and Solomon 1968, page 379), strange intonational and paralinguistics features, and similar manifestations. Such a set of characteristics is said to demonstrate either that language use somehow does not come naturally to these children, who prefer to express themselves in other ways, or that their language remains fixed at an early stage and so becomes inappropriate to their environments as they become older.

In fact, all these observations do have some basis. They are, however, apparently all due to the occurrence in disadvantaged language of a single phenomenon, that which we term "register" (Houston 1969*a*, 1969*b*). A register consists of a range of styles of language which have in common their appropriateness to a given situation or environment. Register is a broader concept than style, since there may be much stylistic variation within a single register, but it can nevertheless be viewed as one register if there are linguistic and behavioral features common to that one unified situation alone. The concept of register became relevant in a study I conducted (under the auspices of the Southeastern Education Laboratory, a regional lab of the U.S. Office of Education) of Child Black English in rural northern Florida. The children studied had at least two distinct registers, termed by us the School and the Nonschool register, because the first appeared primarily in school settings and with teachers and the second in other settings. However, the School register also was used with all persons perceived by the children as in authority over them or studying them in any way (the author excluded, for various reasons too lengthy to be detailed here) and in formal and constrained situations. A description of either register is a linguistic task of some complexity and is not relevant for our purposes. But one may note that the characteristics of the School register include most of the observations given above as indications of disadvantaged nonfluency, notably foreshortened utterances, simplified syntax, and phonological hypercorrection. It should be added that the content expressed in this register tends to be rather limited and nonrevelatory of the children's attitudes, feelings, and ideas.

It is my current opinion, then, that the majority of postulations of linguistic deficiency among speakers of Uneducated English, Black or White, are due to observation of the school register only, since the possession of two or more registers is nearly universal, among such child speakers. Clearly, most investigations and research carried out among these children involve situations in which the school register is almost certain to be used, especially when the children are black and the researcher is both white and unknown to them—and this register does give an impression of nonfluency and strange language use. But it must be borne in mind that this is neither the whole of the children's linguistic performance nor in any way representative of their linguistic competence.

In regard to performance, the Nonschool register presents an entirely different picture from the School register. It is the language which the children use naturally, with friends and family, and in which they express themselves with greatest ease and fluency. To the observer able to elicit the Nonschool register, as I did in Florida, the natural linguistic creativity and frequent giftedness of the so-called linguistically deprived child become apparent. The children worked with, perhaps because they were quite poor and had little material with which to play, engaged in constant language games, verbal contests, and narrative improvisations far removed from linguistic disability. Moreover, the Nonschool register shows a complete set of the expected syntactic patterns characteristic of children of this age, namely, about eleven years, insofar as these are known (see the works cited by Houston [1969*a*, 1969*b*] for technical details). This should come as no surprise, considering the rather minimal syntactic variation characteristic of subforms, geographic or otherwise, of any given language.

As to linguistic competence, it has been pointed out that the internalized ability to comprehend and produce an infinite variety of sentences in one's language is not mirrored isomorphically by linguistic performance. Indeed, it cannot be, since competence is open-ended and performance is finite. That the children of disadvantaged environments are able to understand outside researchers, their teachers, their parents, and each other—often four very different kinds of language—indicates that competence goes far beyond spoken performance, as is the case for all speakers.

The remark above concerning the syntax of the disadvantaged child brings up another often cited kind of language deficiency, namely, what can be described as an unusually high rate of error or deviation from "standard English" on some or all levels of language (for example, Blank and Solomon 1968; Dillard 1967; Hurst and Jones 1966). In fact, this notion contains two separate claims: Whereas it is not the case that the language of the disadvantaged child contains mistakes in the most literal sense, that is, departures from his own system of grammatical rules, it may be true that disadvantaged-child language does differ considerably from standard textbook English. It has already been pointed out that the first claim cannot be valid, since all forms of all languages are systematic. This is in the nature of a fact rather than a theory still in doubt. The second claim is somewhat more complicated to discuss, however, largely because there is almost no data save an occasional anecdote either to substantiate or disconfirm it. But there do exist some indications which cast doubt on the theory of numerous differences between disadvantaged and nondisadvantaged child language, at least on the syntactic level. One bit of evidence considered relevant by some linguists, among them myself, is that dialects or regional variants of a language tend to differ mainly in phonology. Although deeper underlying differences between dialects do exist, they are fewer in number than the phonological and lexical differences which in fact often define dialect boundaries. Whereas in a strict sense neither disadvantaged nor minority language can be called dialects, nevertheless as variants of a single language they can be expected to differ much in the same way as do dialects. Further, studies such as the one I conducted indicate that the nonstandard forms often classed as syntactic deviations might better be treated as phonological. For example, to oversimplify somewhat, one may say either that uneducated Child Black English lacks regular past-tense forms or that it lacks final /t/ and /d/. In my study I observed fewer than a half-dozen main syntactic divergences between the target language and standard English, although these divergences occur frequently in speech. Other differences between the nonstandard and standard variants of language were phonological. This implies no comment about the relative importance of phonological and syntactic differences from educated English, a problem on which almost no data have yet been collected.

2. *The disadvantaged child does not use words properly.* Several studies, for example, the widely quoted Bereiter and Englemann work (1966, for example, page 34), have stated that the disadvantaged child does not use words in the same way as the nondisadvantaged, that the former does not construct sentences from words at all but rather from differently structured units, perhaps larger conceptual groupings. Along with this proposition, it is often remarked that such children tend to omit certain words in their speech, for instance articles and prepositions. The Bereiter and Englemann discussion of this point also adds that, when one has listened to such children for awhile, one may be deceived into thinking that such items are in fact present—due, presumably, to the tendency to interpret language according to customary patterns—whereas the children invariably omit them.

Now, few observers would want to suggest that disadvantaged American children speak something other than English or, in other words, that their language differs enough from the standard to be considered a separate language. This being the case, clearly utterances in the language of the disadvantaged child must be formed the same way as utterances of standard English, whatever this method may be. No language can properly be described as a simple concatenation of words, as was held by linguists prior to the 1950s, since sentences are hierarchically constructed and manifest complicated interrelationships (Chomsky 1959 and many subsequent dates). The important point here is that the fact of hierarchical organization does not vary from language to language, so that it could scarcely be expected to vary within one single language. However disadvantaged children may use words, linearly or otherwise, all children use them in the same way.

The range of comments illustrated by statement two above seems essentially to be caused by unfamiliarity with phonological theory, and in particular with the phonology of the target children. Several phenomena acting together produce the impression described by Bereiter and Engelmann and others. First, the language of the disadvantaged black child at least differs considerably from standard White English in its phonological structure. This does not mean that the children keep making mistakes or are unable to pronounce the sounds of English. It does mean, however, that their phonological system is constructed somewhat differently, on one level, from that of the average adult White English speaker. Note that the level on which the differences occur is one of systematic performance, as we term it, rather than competence. This is manifested in the nearly universal ability among disadvantaged black children to comprehend utterances in Educated White English (if they are familiar with the lexicon used, of course). All forms of all languages are produced by regular rules, and this is true on all levels of language. Thus, the children do not eliminate sounds at random but, rather, have a regular and fully describable set of rules by which they pronounce their language. The effect of some of these rules is to eliminate certain sounds, notably final consonants and consonant clusters, /r/ and /l/, and some intervocalic nasals. Others of the rules function in determining the shape of vowels in the children's language; often the children produce vowels which do not occur in the same context in standard English, for instance, Southern Child Black English /flow/ for standard English /flɔr/ "floor."

Also, English in general shows many so-called Sandhi phenomena, or changes in the phonological shape of morphemes (minimal meaning units) when the morphemes are concatenated or strung together. The Sandhi rules of Child Black English are undoubtedly different from those of standard White English, although the latter has them also. Some of these rules are in effect what is often called elision, as when the final /d/ of the first word in "good morning" is not pronounced. They do not constitute errors, although the appearance of some of these rules seems to strike some listeners as unaesthetic. It is not known whether Child Black English, or any disadvantaged child language, has any greater preponderance of Sandhi rules than standard English. At any rate, since Child Black English does tend to eliminate many final consonants present in standard English, the former often sounds as though it has numerous elisions or omissions of phonological items. This is not equivalent to stating that speakers of this language do not use words or that they use them in an aberrant manner. Their words are simply sometimes shaped differently from the corresponding words in standard English.

Bereiter and Englemann in particular add an interesting note to their discussion when they observe that the listener may sometimes be deceived into believing that he hears some of the omitted items, whether sounds or words. The linguist would say that the reason the listener is led to believe this is that in fact he has heard something, even if it is not the same thing that he would have said in context. Rarely are items simply left out of Child Black English or other variants of language. They are almost always replaced by something, at least if the items are phonological units. Omission of final consonants, /l/ and /r/, and nasals nearly always leaves something in place of the omitted unit. This something may be a pause, a glide, a lengthening of the preceding vowel segment or syllable, or a combination of these. It is this that the listener hears.

3. *The language of the disadvantaged child does not provide him with an adequate basis for (abstract or other) thinking.* This assumption also seems to have appeared very frequently and has been stated in a form similar to this by Bernstein (1961), Blank and Solomon (1968, page 381), and others. It is most commonly presented in connection with programs designed to impart various types of abstract thinking and conceptualization to so-called disadvantaged children. The importance of this proposition is great, since it presents the underlying rationale for the majority of programs as well as a leading cause for their frequent failure (for a report on the failure of Operation Head Start, perhaps the best known of programs to aid disadvantaged children, see the reference to Westinghouse Learning Corporation 1969).

Evidence for remarks such as statement three is sometimes considered to be the children's lack of abstract terminology. This is probably the most usual basis for the notion that disadvantaged children cannot think properly, since deductions about the thought processes of the children seem to be based primarily or entirely on evidence from language. Unfortunately, this tends to render the conclusions invalid for the following reasons.

Although this fact remains largely unrecognized by persons not specializing in language science or psychology, the direction of dependence between language and cognition is still undetermined. However, it is no longer considered possible to extrapolate cognitive patterns directly from specific linguistic patterns, a notion sometimes incorrectly attributed to the 1930–1940 writing of Benjamin Lee Whorf (Whorf 1956). That a language is highly inflecting, for instance, does not necessarily indicate that its speakers are more complex or more energetic than the speakers of an isolating language such as Chinese; that a language contains many consonant clusters or velar fricatives (popularly termed gutterals) does not mean that its speakers are primitive and bestial in their thinking; and so forth. Likewise, if a language or form of language is found to lack a unitary term for a certain phenomenon, this does not indicate either that its speakers are unaware of the phenomenon or that they cannot deal with it when it occurs. It does not in fact indicate anything whatever, save that the language lacks the term. This matter has been experimentally supported on a number of occasions (for example, Lenneberg 1961). Thus, a lack of specific lexical items on the part of disadvantaged children does not imply a lack of sophisticated cognition, nor does their putative failure to use abstract terms necessarily imply inability to conceptualize in this manner.

An additional difficulty with assertions such as statement three above is that it is not at all clear precisely what constitutes abstract thinking or how one is to determine whether a subject is engaging in it at a given moment. Abstract thinking is sometimes said to consist of the ability to generalize and categorize. Such abilities are usually considered innate, however, and are implied in the use of language itself; it is not certain that portions of language can be considered more abstract than other portions, or more involved with categorization and generalization. Presumably, grammatical utterances could not be constructed at all without internalized notions of grammatical category, and novel utterances could not be formed without generalization from previously experienced patterns. Furthermore, it is not the case exactly that language provides a conceptual base for thinking, abstract or otherwise; more accurately, the innate ability to abstract, generalize, conceptualize, and so forth is necessary in order for language, generically speaking, to be present. In all members of the human species, save the genetically damaged, these abilities do exist, although of course they show a developmental progression with age, since their ontogenesis is maturationally determined. But the universal existence of these abilities implies, among other things, that much of language is impregnable to environmental forces and that those environmental forces which do in some way act upon language nevertheless fail to alter the innate component of intellection.

In regard to child language and the ability, or lack of it, to generalize, it has been proposed (for example, Blank and Solomon 1968, page 382) that the disadvantaged child is unable to use his language efficiently enough to extract information from what is said to him. This is presumably either because such children are unable to think in this way since their language does not provide them with the necessary tools or simply because they have not been taught to do so. The following small example of this assertion comes from Blank and Solomon (1968). It purports to demonstrate the disadvantaged child's lack of a linguistic framework for extracting information from the environment and consists of a dialogue between such a child and his teacher: "For example, the teacher put on her coat at the end of a session. The child said, 'Why are you going home?' The teacher replied, 'How do you know I am going home?' to which the child said, 'You're not going home?' This response meant that the child had dropped any attempt at reasoning; he had interpreted the teacher's query to mean that he must negate his earlier inference."

The problem demonstrated by the above instance is not technically one of linguistics but rather of psychology; it is, however, rather typical of the incidents cited by teachers and others to substantiate statement three above. However, there is actually nothing anomalous in the child's use of language in this situation. Of the large number of ways the teacher's query could have been answered, it seems to me that the child chose the most sensible. At the point where the teacher asked how the child knew she was going home, there is little else that he could have inferred except that his original answer had been wrong, since this is one of the standard ways in which a teacher indicates this. In other words, the child was making a rather subtle and complex generalization from past experience with teachers, a process quite distant from "dropping any attempt at reasoning." It is not especially the case that the disadvantaged child communicates in peculiar ways, except insofar as these are necessitated by his environment. It should be recognized that a school setting is utterly alien to any other setting in regard to the child's linguistic interaction with the teacher and to his permitted interaction with his age mates. To be sure, the child's remark would have been inappropriate, or at the very least, facetious, in most other social contexts, but for that matter the teacher's question would have been considered quite rude under ordinary social circumstances. The concept of rudeness applied to adult-child conversations is an unusual one. It is clear that this is a unique communication situation in which different rules apply for both parties. One should also bear in mind that children in a school setting are tacitly or otherwise threatened with far more sanctions for incorrect behavior than are participants in most other types of social interaction. Had the child in the above example not been fearful of being "wrong," it is doubtful that he would have needed his original deduction verified. And once again, the entire incident was described in such detail here because it strikes me as representative of teachers' comments about the behavior of the disadvantaged child, behavior cited as atypical and demonstrative of conceptualization deficiencies. It is our purpose to indicate that such incidents can often be interpreted in a number of ways, some of which often show extremely adaptive and reasoned behavior.

4. *To the disadvantaged child, language is dispensable; such children tend to communicate nonverbally in preference to verbally.* It is, of course, scarcely necessary to point out that language is dispensable to nobody and is not used because of choice or necessity. This is because language acquisition is not a skill—neither is it acquisition of a skill—and so does not depend on environmental exigencies, except in that children must hear a language in order to learn it. But it is natural for children to learn and employ language, which they do without regard to their needs. Probably all children's use of language is similar in some respects (McNeill 1966*a*). On the other hand, it is also clear that verbal proficiency and skill at handling words are differently valued in many communities here and elsewhere (Kochman 1969; Labov and Cohen 1967) and that the rules of communication must differ in different social groups. Many children's games are nonverbal and are based primarily on physical contact. It is not known whether this is more typical of the disadvantaged child than of the nondisadvantaged. However, the nondisadvantaged child is almost by definition far better supplied with actual things with which to play and so is less constrained to develop any sort of game on his own. Contact between individuals is either verbal or nonverbal; the disadvantaged children I observed engaged in much ritualized fighting and roughhousing, and they also engaged in constant verbal play. There are few other alternatives open to the child without playthings, after all.

It should not be thought, on the other hand, that we wish to deny the possibility that the use of language differs among disadvantaged children. There is simply no solid evidence on this point to date. One might wish to ascertain, for instance, whether parent-child use of language is qualitatively or quantitatively different in this setting, as has been proposed by Bernstein (1961) and many others. The researcher must remember the existence of register, however; perhaps one of the reasons why these children have been said to use language strangely or in limited ways is that only the limited register has been perceived by outside researchers.

5. *The language of the disadvantaged child, since it represents his culture and environment, should be left alone and not changed in any way.* This proposal, at the opposite end of the spectrum from the proposals considered previously, is sometimes expressed by linguists and others in the spirit that the sociolinguist Charles Ferguson has characterized as "sentimental egalitarianism." Now, it is perfectly correct to state that the language of the disadvantaged child is useful to him, systematic and regular in its rules of construction, not syntactically or semantically deficient, and as good a basis for thinking and conceptualization as any

other form of language. However, statement five above does not follow from these facts, because there are other considerations which must be taken into account by educators.

In the first place, it is quite conceivable that the disadvantaged child, especially if rural, may lack some of the lexicon he needs in order to succeed at school, read newspapers, get professional or managerial jobs, and so forth. If this is found to be the case, then disadvantaged children must be taught those items they do not know. However, this is a weighty "*if*." It is possible that the target child may be able to comprehend such lexicon even though he never uses it. This means in effect that he already "knows" it in some sense and must be given contexts in which to use it along with encouragement to do so. Or, possibly, he both understands and uses it already, only not in a school setting but rather in other registers. It is very difficult to ascertain this, but it is a possibility which must not be overlooked, especially with the prevalence of television and the expanded linguistic environment which it provides.

A far more important consideration, although one more difficult to deal with, is the status of the target child's language in relation to others and standard-English speakers' perception of it. Although *Webster's Dictionary* (third edition) has removed the label of substandard from such items as *ain't,* nevertheless it is a sociolinguistic fact that some forms of language are an irrevocable block to social, academic, economic, and even geographic upward mobility. If some social prejudice is based on language, as seems to be the case, then this is all the justification necessary for altering those features which elicit such reactions. Note that one can speak of Educated and Uneducated English, a distinction obtaining throughout the English-speaking world regardless of other factors, and that no particular dialect or regional set of characteristics is in itself substandard or uneducated, although some may be considered as unesthetic by speakers from other regions. It should also be pointed out here that there is Uneducated White English and Uneducated Black English, as well as Educated varieties of each (Houston 1969*a*). In order to proceed rationally with programs of language change in the schools, it is of course necessary to discover precisely which features of the language of the disadvantaged child are likely to be deleterious (not, I might note, "debilitating"). This is not known at present.

Finally, it has been suggested (for example, Blank and Solomon 1968) that a useful task might be to lead the disadvantaged child to an awareness that he possesses language and to impart to him sensitivity to differences in the ways people talk. This is obviously a most worthwhile goal. There is no reason to confine it to the disadvantaged child, either, since an awareness of the diversity and functioning of language can be of inestimable value to any child. The way in which this should be done, I believe, is as directly as possible. If the disadvantaged or other child is to be taught about how he talks, he should be told that he is being taught this and should be encouraged to perceive and discuss language itself.

The usual proposed alternative to this suggestion seems to be to engage in a series of word games in which the child is asked to first draw something and then draw something else belonging to a different class from the first object drawn, told to select "two red blocks and one green block" (Blank and Solomon 1968, page 383) from a pile in order to become habituated to the selective use of adjectives, directed to repeat commands aloud before obeying them, and so on. None of these activities is the least bit atypical of programs designed to augment the linguistic capacity of the disadvantaged child, and none of them is, furthermore, at all likely to achieve this goal, because they are merely exercises to the child and not learning activities. As Joos (1964, page 207) has pointed out, to most children school requires a whole new way of thinking and is unrelated to any real situation encountered elsewhere. Thus, a child will accept the necessity for stacking blocks and following other commands which seem silly to him because school activities are designed for this purpose. It "never occurs to him that there is such a thing as a geography of his home town, or a rhetoric of persuasion within his circle of friends" (Joos 1964). If it is found that the language of the disadvantaged child actually needs certain types of augmentation, which I presume would be in lexicon, this can be done through conversation; if such children are to be made aware of language, this should be done through direct reference to language. Most likely, the linguistic aid they need most is encouragement to use their nonschool or natural language in the presence of adults, teachers, and otherwise, since this register of language often turns out to possess all the features said to be lacking in the language of the disadvantaged child.

References

Bereiter, C., and Englemann, S. *Teaching Disadvantaged Children in the Preschool.* Englewood Cliffs, N. J.: Prentice-Hall, 1966.

Bernstein, B. "Social Structure, Language, and Learning." *Educational Research* 3 (1961): 163–176.

Blank, M., and Solomon, F. "A Tutorial Language Program to Develop Abstract Thinking in Socially Disadvantaged Preschool Children." *Child Development* 39 (1968): 379–389.

Chomsky, N. *Syntactic Structures.* The Hague: Mouton, 1959.

Dillard, J. L. "Negro Children's Dialect in the Inner City." *Florida FL Reporter* (Fall 1967): 1–3.

Houston, S. H. "A Sociolinguistic Consideration of the Black-English of Children in Northern Florida." *Language* 45 (1969): 599–607. (*a*)

Houston, S. H. *Child Black English: the School Register.* Paper presented to the 44th Annual Meeting of the Linguistic Society of America, San Francisco, 1969. (*b*)

Hurst, C. C., and Jones, W. L. "Psychosocial Concomitants of Sub-standard Speech." *Journal of Negro Education* (Fall 1966): 409–421.
Joos, M. "Language and the School Child." *Harvard Educational Review*, 34 (1964): 203–210.
Kochman, T. " 'Rapping' in the Black Ghetto." *Trans-action* 6(4) (1969): 26–34.
Labov, W., and Cohen, P. "Systematic Relations of Standard and Non-standard Rules in the Grammars of Negro Speakers." *Project Literacy Reports* 8 (July 1967): 66–84.
Lenneberg, E. H. "Color Naming, Color Recognition, Color Discrimination: A Reappraisal." *Perceptual and Motor Skills* **2** (1961): 375–382.
McNeill, D. "Developmental Psycholinguistics." In F. Smith and G. A. Miller (Eds.), *The Genesis of Language*. Cambridge, Mass.: M.I.T. Press (1966): 15–84.
Westinghouse Learning Corporation. *The Impact of Headstart*. Washington, D. C.: Westinghouse, 1969.
Whorf, B. L. *Language, Thought and Reality*. Cambridge, Mass.: M.I.T. Press, 1956.

Kenneth S. Goodman has probably written more on the topic of linguistics for teachers than any other current author. In the following article he sees the function of linguistics as providing input for a language curriculum suited to children's needs. He puts linguistics in perspective with other disciplines and identifies specific contributions that linguistics can make in building a relevant curriculum. Although the article was written to relate to language programs in the elementary school, much of what he has to say applies to secondary school language programs as well.

Goodman's several articles on dialect divergence and what it means to classroom teachers—"Let's Dump the Uptight Model in English" *(Elementary School Journal* October 1969), "The Language Children Bring to School" *(Grade Teacher* March 1969), "On Valuing Diversity in Language" *(Childhood Education* December 1969), among others—are down-to-earth presentations on the topic and have a great deal of relevance for teachers.

Linguistics in a Relevant Curriculum

Kenneth S. Goodman

When you start out on a trip, the first decision you need to make is where you're going. Everything else, all the other decisions involved in planning the trip, flow from the decision about the destination. Furthermore, the means of conveyance, the route, the time required to get there, cannot be determined unless the destination is continuously kept in mind.

So it is with the elementary language curriculum. First you must decide on objectives, the purposes for the curriculum, before any other decisions are possible or meaningful. The wise choice of objectives will require many kinds of input, not the least of which is values. What does the school, and the community which has chartered the school, want for its children? What should it want for them? There are other sources of input; the children themselves and basic disciplines like psychology, sociology, and linguistics.

If there is a single test which all objectives and the curricula built to achieve them should meet, it is the test of relevancy. A curriculum must be relevant to the society, to the times, but most of all, it must be relevant to the learners. This is true in every area of education, but it is most vital in the area of language, because language is central to all communication, learning, and thought.

But language programs have often been the least relevant aspects of the curriculum. Frequently children are asked to learn things which are neither useful to them in any sense nor true in relation to their own language.

To be relevant, a language program must be consistent with the prior language of the learners. It must offer them insights into language as it really is or it must make it possible for them to use language more effectively. It must expand and facilitate language use and not put artificial restrictions on its use.

The Need for Linguistics

Linguistics makes no promises in this endeavor and thus need keep no promises. Linguistics is input for curriculum making, but like all such input, it may be used in varying ways and it may be misused. As a discipline, it is concerned with the scientific study of language and not with language instruction. A language curriculum cannot be built without dealing with linguistic matters, just as a bridge cannot be built by engineers without dealing with the laws of physics. But knowing the laws of physics does not determine how the bridge may be built, or where, or when, or in fact whether it should be built at all. Similarly, linguistics does not directly answer the key curricular questions.

Three kinds of input are provided by linguistics for use in building elementary curricula in language:

1. Concepts to be used and dealt with in making decisions about method, scope, sequence, procedures.

2. Knowledge: to enlighten teachers and to form the base of language content for the learners.

3. New vantage points for looking at language and language users. One such useful vantage point comes from descriptive linguistics: language is viewed as the product of human activity. Another different and useful vantage point comes from generative-transformational linguistics which views language as a human process.

Such input neither can nor should be ignored in building elementary language curriculum. It cannot be ignored, either, in evaluating existing curricula and methodology. But new decisions do not come from substituting new input for old. The new and the old must be accommodated so that what emerges is consistent with that which is valid from both. Language programs can be linguistically valid; they cannot simply be linguistic, for that would imply that linguistics as such is capable of generating language programs with no assistance from philosophy, learning theory, child development, sociology, or pedagogy. What makes a program linguistically valid is that it utilizes linguistic input when dealing with linguistic matters. But that does not guarantee that it is consistent within itself or relevant.

The Goals of School Language Programs

It is in the context of relevancy that I would like to examine the objectives of the elementary language program and the linguistic input which will prove useful in building a relevant program. This is an era in which educators had better be able to answer when parents, community groups, and the learners themselves ask us why.

School language programs have three basic purposes:

1. *They seek to help learners become more effective users of language.* Since this is a direction in which the learners have constantly been moving since they began as infants to acquire language, it is a key objective and one easily made relevant to the learners. It is most important, however, that we do not presume that certain kinds of instruction or learning activities lead to more effective language use when in fact they do not. To take a simple example, handwriting becomes more effective as it becomes more legible. Beauty or conformity to a model of perfection may either not contribute to effectiveness or may in fact reduce it.

2. *They seek to provide the learners with knowledge about language.* A distinction always needs to be made in building school curricula between *knowing that* and *knowing how*. Language is an exciting and important aspect of human activity. It is worth studying, in order to understand *that* it works in certain ways. But, such knowledge has little to do with the knowledge of *how to use language*. Studying grammar, whether conventional school grammar or one of the new linguistic grammars, has little effect on actual language used by the learner. Fortunately, he has already learned the grammatical system of his language. He is his own resource on language when he examines it. Inquiry and discovery techniques can help him to examine his own language in relevant ways. It does not matter what social status his language enjoys, it still has the characteristics of language that the school wants him to understand. Language study, to be relevant, must deal with language "like it is."

3. *School language programs seek to expand the language of learners.* Often, misunderstanding the nature of language difference, we have sought to change children's language: to eliminate bad language and substitute good language. Now we are coming to understand that language difference is legitimate and expected. We are coming to understand that it is neither necessary nor desirable to demand that a child give up his native dialect in order to learn a dialect with higher social status. We are coming to understand that the goal is to help the learner achieve the linguistic flexibility that will serve his communicative needs at all stages of his life. We are coming also to understand that the learner must be a willing partner in this enterprise (not cajoled, threatened, or conditioned into cooperation) and that it must at all stages be relevant to his *current* needs.

Language moves at all stages toward more effective use. Less effective forms tend to give way to more effective ones. This is the essential motivational force behind language learning. When it comes to expanding language there is a direct relationship between motivation to learn and the communicative needs of the learner. Relevancy is critical.

In planning activities and curricula to achieve these three ends, we have often confused them and confused ourselves about the reason why we engage in certain activities. Here we are very much entangled in old misconceptions. Perhaps the deepest rooted of these and one of the most destructive is that we teach children language in school. We have tended to ignore the tremendous language resources that children have already acquired and flattered ourselves that when we are teaching grammar lessons, we are teaching children how to use their language. At best, if our grammar lessons are well conceived, we are providing children with insights into the whys that language works—and that has little or nothing to do with their effectiveness as users of language.

Time and time again research has confirmed the intuitive discovery of many teachers: the way to improve language effectiveness both in oral and written forms is to stimulate children to use language frequently, freely, and confidently.

A related error comes from the elitist view that dialects can be arranged hierarchically, which leads teachers and material writers to assume that children who don't speak standard English are speaking a corrupt or sloppy form of it, or at least a lesser form. They confuse difference with deficiency and thereby create a wholly irrelevant curriculum. They insist to the learner that what sounds right to him is wrong and what sounds wrong is right. Instead of expanding his language, the curriculum they create has the effect of putting it into a linguistic straight jacket.

Linguistics as Input

If we remember that linguistics is a source of input in the curricular and teaching decisions, we must make it a method or a set of materials; if we remember that this input must be synthesized with input from many other disciplines to aid in solving our problems, then we are ready to consider the specific ways that this input can help to build a more relevant curriculum.

1. Linguistics can help us—the educators—to understand how language works and to appreciate its functions in communication, thought, learning.
2. Linguistics can help us to understand the language of the children we teach and to appreciate its form, system, and legitimacy.
3. Linguistics can help us to see the child as an expert language user and eliminate our illusions about where language is learned.

4. Linguistics can be a source of content when we build curriculum about language.

5. Linguistics can be a source of insight to the teacher in dealing with all language areas: reading, spelling, composition, literature, oral expression.

We must always strive in our schools for more effective, more relevant methods and materials. But no New English program, no new language-arts series, no programmed learning materials can fully expoit the applications of linguistics to building a relevant curriculum. This can only be accomplished by enlightened teachers who work in direct contact with the learners for whom the curriculum must be relevant.

Postscript

How Can Linguistics Be Put to Work in the Classroom?

Each field within the linguistic domain suggests language learning activities for the classroom.

The first step in scientific inquiry is observation of phenomena and the collection of data. So it is with the scientific study of language, both inside and outside of the classroom. The linguist begins with a *corpus,* a body of language collected from informants who are native speakers. The teacher's starting point can be the corpus of language used by children in the minisociety of the classroom. Letting children explore the language that they use in daily life, rather than forcing something out of a textbook upon them is likely to heighten their excitement and awareness in language matters.

What's language good for, anyway? We tend to take language for granted. To focus pupils' attention on the importance and function of language, let them try to convey a message without using any language (in a sort of classroom charade or pantomime). They will be able to convey some meaning without words, of course, and this can lead to an interesting discussion of *kinesics*; that is, the facial expressions, body movements, and gestures that are such an integral part of oral communication. Other means of communicating messages (for example, Morse code, semaphore signals, signs commonly found in airports, and the like) can also be discussed. This type of activity will likely lead to an awareness of the usefulness and advantages of language over nonlanguage signals as a way of conveying great amounts of information to others.

Phonology

In the linguist's eyes, speech is the first form of language. In the teacher's eyes, speech can be the first focus of language instruction. Directing children's attention to their own speech can make them more aware of certain speech features that can be useful in later language and reading instruction (long and short vowels, digraphs, blends, each syllable has a vowel sound, and so on). Although exact phonetic transcription takes a great deal of technical knowledge and skill, your class might have fun representing their more obvious speech characteristics in writing; for example, "We've bin talkin' to Missus Smith 'bout dat." This type of writing is what linguists call *eye dialect* and what many fourth grade composition teachers call everyday writing for some of their pupils.

While children do not need a technical knowledge of the sound system of American English, such a knowledge is helpful for the kind of speech therapy that teachers are sometimes called upon to do in the classroom. For foreign language teachers, an adequate knowledge of the sound system is essential. The same can be said for teachers of standard English as a second language.

Standards of usage in speech can be another focus. You can suggest that your class try to discover the prevailing standards of speech in their own communities. (How often do they hear the expression *ain't* used? By whom? Under what conditions?) Further suggestions for this type of activity will be presented in the postscript for part II.

Intonation—the pitch, stress, and juncture that Burns defined earlier—has a lot to do in determining meaning in speech. Remember, you're not *teaching* the pupil the intonation system. He is already in command of this by virtue of the fact that he can speak English. What you're aiming at is leading your pupils to realize the part that intonation plays in their language.

"It's not what he said but how he said it." How would you say *m-m-m-m-m* if you:

> were tasting a piece of delicious apple pie
> were trying to figure out the answer to a tough math problem
> had just figured out the answer

How would *That's fresh*! sound when said by:

> a fruit salesman talking about a watermelon
> an angry teacher
> a girl who had just been whistled at (and who liked it—or didn't)

Have the pupils think of examples like *that's beautiful* when said sarcastically or genuinely. Have them put the stress on different words in sentences such as, *Is that how you make your money*? or *I like that*! to convey different meanings.

Both phonological and syntactic elements combine to convey meaning in certain expressions. Some old hackneyed plays on words are—Did you ever see a match box? A board walk? A house fly?—Do your pupils know any newer ones or can they make up some original ones?

Juncture contrasts such expressions as ice cream and I scream, a name and an aim, illegal and ill eagle. And try this one: Diddle, diddle dumpling, Mice on John. How many similar minimal pairs can your pupils list?

Phonology relates directly to reading as well, and will be taken up again later in this book.

Dialect

Observing sound features in language can lead directly into an examination of the rich variety of American-English dialects. Children are already aware of dialect differences, if from no other source than the hours of television that they watch.

An interesting activity might be to trade original tapes with a class in another part of the country, having a sort of "tape pal" exchange. (Surely, someone you graduated with is now teaching in Maine or Missouri or New Mexico!) In what respects do the children in your tape-pal class sound different? ("No, Charlie, they don't talk funny; just differently than we do.") Do the consonants sound the same? The vowels? Exactly what differences can we identify? The more tapes you collect from different dialect areas, the greater sets of contrasts you will find.

Do the children in our tape-pal class use different words than we do? This might result in making a glossary of terms used in different dialect areas. It might be expanded to words and expressions in what some linguists call "temporal dialects"; that is, differences in the speech of different age groups—teenagers and their parents, for example.

Morphology

The branch of linguistics that suggests exercises and activities for understanding old words and for building new ones is morphology.

For example, adding the suffix *-or* or *-er* to verb base words can produce nouns: *sail* becomes *sailor*, *teach* becomes *teacher*, *play* becomes *player*, and so on. (On a popular television talk show a couple of years ago, one guest angrily said, "Someone has made allegations against me and I'm going to find out who is the alligator!") Similarly, morphemes such as *-ee* (payee), *-tion* (examination), *-ent* (dependent), and so forth, can be added to bases to form nouns. The first time I tried this type of exercise, I asked for a word ending in the noun-marking suffix *-ee*, and the first word a fifth grader came up with was *tree*. Afterward, they got the idea.

Other suffixes can be added to form (or mark) verbs. Marcia Brown, in *Once a Mouse*, tells about the proud animal who "peacocked around the forest." And the three-year old working diligently on a piece of paper, when asked if she was coloring, replied, "No, I'm chalking." *Peacocked* and *chalking* are new words that were formed merely by adding common morphemes, but they carry a clear meaning.

Suffixes such as *-ify* (glorify), *ize* (sympathize), *-en* (darken), and so on, form verbs. The suffixes *-able* (comfortable), *-ary* (honorary),

-ful (careful), and others mark adjectives; and *-time* (anytime), *-ward* (homeward), and of course *-ly* (quickly) mark adverbs. Prefixes also mark certain conventional parts of speech in much the same way. It is important to remember that some morphemes are used in more than one part of speech, as, for example, the *-en* in *darken* (verb) and *wooden* (adjective). With a glossary of affixes (prefixes and suffixes), the pupils can start building their own words.

The kind of exercise described above can lead to a study of how words were adopted from other languages into English. A *sailor* is one who sails, but is a *tailor* one who tails? The base word in tailor is tail, all right, but it is a word derived from an old French word meaning "to cut." This base can also be found in words such as *detail* and *retail.* How many other words like this can you and your class find?

Historical Linguistics

Tracing the source of words (as in the activity suggested above) is part of historical linguistics. Another concern of the historical linguist is the origin of language.

Although no one is absolutely certain exactly how language began, there are a number of theories. One is the bow-wow theory, which holds that language originated with the imitation of natural sounds. Another is the go-go theory, which suggests that language started with commands. Still another is the pooh-pooh theory, which says that language got started with expressions of human feelings and emotions. Perhaps your class could discuss and/or write their own version of how language began. While the result will probably be more like science fiction than science, the activity will serve to focus their attention on the origins of language.

In the upper elementary, junior high, or high school grades, some pupils might be interested in looking up the Lord's Prayer or some other sample of language written in Old English or Middle English and comparing it with a modern version of the same passage. Records of Chaucer's work read in Middle English dialect are available. The history of language might be a good research project or term paper for students who are interested.

Our English vocabulary is a hybrid of words from many languages. Finding out how words came into the language is a fascinating activity for all of us, old and young alike. Since English is a direct descendent of West Germanic, the Germanic element is a fundamental element in our vocabulary. Basic words such as come, go, eat, drink, meat, fish, hand, arm, and other words can be traced to our Teutonic heritage. The French-speaking Normans brought words such as crown, prince, sermon, defense, fashion, leisure, (and other words important to the Norman nobility) in the eleventh, twelfth, and thirteenth centuries. The majority of our words are derived from Latin, either directly or via French, a Romance language. Lunatic, aqueduct, prevent, and transport reflect the Latin influence. Greek influence is apparent in words such as psychology and telephone. Words were borrowed wholesale and unchanged from other languages: colleen (Irish), kindergarten (German), cargo (Spanish), not counting all those words that were borrowed and Anglicized. There is hardly a language that has not made its contribution to the English lexicon.

Place names and family names are fun to trace because these are words that are personally important to children. Many of our state names come from the American Indians (Dakota, Michigan, Illinois). Other state names came from French and Spanish, from locations in the Old World, from famous historical personages. Our land is studded with picturesque place names of interesting origins. What's the origin of the name of the state and the town where you teach? Surnames come from occupations (Baker, Smith, Miller), personal characteristics (Strong, Stout, Hardy), father's names (Robertson, O'Brien, Fitzgerald), place names (English, Welsh, Hollander), and other sources. Kids usually have a few laughs tracing my name: Savage. The origin of brand names (of automobiles, for example), days of the week, months of the year, and other proper names can be traced too.

Often, somebody's family name becomes part of our language because of an invention he made or because some peculiar characteristic or event is associated with that person. Antoine Sax, for example, invented the saxaphone. Louis Pasteur discovered pasteurization. General Burnside popularized a whisker style known as sideburns. Anthony Van Dyke popularized a whisker style too. The meaning of words sometimes changes in the process of development. Dunce came from a brilliant thirteenth century Scottish teacher who was born in Duns. Guppy, diesel, boycott, sandwich, and teddy bear are just a few of the words that can be traced to famous people. Can your class make up their own eponyms (words derived from proper names)? "Murphyism" might come from the name of your pupil, Joe Murphy, who is the class politician. "Mitchelling" might be a verb derived from Charley Mitchell's name, the kid who never sits still. Who knows, maybe one of your pupils will some day lend his name to the language. McCarthyism became a recent eponym, didn't it?

Slang is defined as an informal and supposedly temporary form of language. But after a period of widespread use, many slang expressions become part of the standard lexicon of the language. Hubbub and bump were slang expressions in Shakespeare's day. Jalopy, cop (for policeman, not as in "cop out", although this too is slang), and grapevine(source of information) all originated as slang expressions. Some expressions, of course, never make it. (How many of your pupils have ever heard of "the cat's pajamas"?) Not too long ago, a teacher friend told me that her superintendent only recently sanctioned the use of the word *goofed* in the classroom because prior to this he had considered it as slang and thus unworthy of classroom use. Kids and teachers alike had been using it for years, because it became a legitimate part of our language some time ago.

All of this kind of word-tracing activity focuses children's attention on language matters, and this is actually the *practice* of linguistics in the classroom. Among many excellent sources of this kind of information for teachers are Mario Pei's two books, *The Story of Language* (Lippincott, 1965) and *The Story of English* (Lippincott, 1952). Many clues to etymological derivations can be found in dictionaries such as Webster's *Third International* and the Random House *Dictionary of the English Language.*

Syntax

Most of the work done in syntax is under the banner of grammar. The arrangement of words to convey and change meanings, however, can be looked at in any part of the language program. The order in which words are arranged in a sentence determines the meaning. Use this example with your class (a sliding mask on an overhead transparency is an effective device for presentation):

> *Only* John went to school yesterday.
> John *only* went to school yesterday.
> John went *only* to school yesterday.
> John went to school *only* yesterday.
> John went to school yesterday *only.*

In each sentence, the words are the same, but the movement of *only* alters the meaning. No other word in the sentence, however, has the mobility that *only* does without completely destroying the meaning of the sentence.

Using examples from their own speech, children will discover a lot about word placement. For example, articles always occur before nouns. we say *the* teacher, *a* pupil, never teacher *the*, pupil *a.* In normal speech, the place of adjectives in the word order of sentences is fairly well set; they appear before nouns (although they also appear after verbs, as in *Joe is strong*). Adverbs, however, are more mobile. Consider these sentences:

I. With Adjectives	II. With Adverbs
A. He saw the *big* dog.	A. Joe ran *quickly* home.
B. *Big* he saw the dog.	B. *Quickly*, Joe ran home.
C. He saw the dog *big.*	C. Joe ran home *quickly.*

The locations of the modifiers in both sets of sentences are parallel.

Sentence I–A is the conventional English form; I–B and I–C don't make sense. All three sentences in II make perfect sense. In I, if we replace *he* with *George*, then II–B would make sense (*Big George saw the dog*), but then *big* modifies *George*, not *dog*.

Letting pupils rearrange words in this way will convey the importance that word order has in English sentences.

Semantics

The meaning of words is important to both oral and written expression, and this a branch of linguistics that is applicable at any grade level. There are different shades of meaning in words such as fat, stout, chubby, robust, rotund. What's the difference between a person who is *strong willed* and one who is *pig headed*? Can your pupils think of other ways to say: This tastes terrible, Your ball team stinks, or He's lazy? (How many times have you tried to express this latter sentiment in different terms at report card time?)

The meaning any word has for a person will often depend on his experiences and the attitudes he has toward the word. What associations do your pupils bring to such words as candy, homework, kitten? The class might make a list of words with commonly pleasant connotations (television, baseball game, summer) or negative ones (skunk, bedtime, punishment).

Critical listening demands semantic decoding, and television commercials provide excellent vehicles for this activity. Which words with pleasant connotations do advertisers use to make their products seem more appealing? Which propaganda devices do they use?

Comparative Linguistics

Beyond third grade (even before that in some newer curricula) children study people in other lands as part of social studies. The language of these people can be studied too. How does it differ from ours? What words have we borrowed from that language? What words have they borrowed from us? What would each child's name be in the language of the country they are studying? This comparative study can certainly focus on vocabulary, and, depending on your own knowledge of language structure, can be extended to include a comparison of sound and syntax as well. Since language is such an integral part of the social system of any people, it seems that language study ought to be built into social studies at every grade level.

Besides obvious sound differences, words differ from one part of the

English-speaking world to another. We have different words for the same thing (in England, a truck is called a lorry, an elevator is called a lift, and so on) and the same word for different things (in England the word corn refers to what we call wheat, and in Scotland to what we call oats). This is in part why one Paris shopkeeper posted a sign in his window: "English spoken here. American also understood." How many examples of such linguistic variants can your pupils find from one part of the English-speaking world to another?

Conclusion

It is safe to say that ideas generated by the linguist can be used with varying degrees of sophistication at every grade level. Even the youngest child brings to school a vast store of language. Each field of linguistics has something to offer the classroom teacher. The suggestions contained in this postscript are only a few of the many that any creative teacher who is reasonably cognizant of linguistics can think of and use. Paul Burns has given some classroom suggestions in his article. More and more materials intended for children's use are beginning to contain suggestions from linguistics, and so are methods texts designed for language-arts teachers. See Carl A. Lefevre's *Linguistics, English, and the Language Arts* (Allyn and Bacon, 1970) as a good example.

Although the kinds of activities discussed here don't promise miracles in language learning, they do make pupils more aware of their language and they also give them something more to do than underline items in inane exercises that too often pass under the guise of language instruction. The kinds of activities suggested give children the opportunity to investigate and draw conclusions about the language they speak. Besides, such activities are great fun, both for teachers and pupils. Try them. You'll like them!

One More Step

Questions and activities for further learning.

1. Examine one or two books from an English or Language Arts series currently being used in the elementary or secondary grades. (Be sure to check the copyright date!) What evidence or reflection of "New English" do you find in the content or in the approach used?
2. At a curriculum meeting, Charlie Grammar shouts, "Linguistics is eroding our English curriculum. All that these linguists do is condone falling standards and place their seal of approval on sloppy language."

"That's right," says Miss Information. "We've been getting along very well all these years without the linguist's fancy terminology and faulty theory. The linguists are doing nothing more than dehumanizing our beautiful tongue."

Defend the poor, maligned linguist.

3. Having read the article by Brown and Bellugi, choose your own Adam and Eve (or Cain and Abel) and conduct your own research on language acquisition. Keep a record of such items as vocabulary growth, use of word endings, auxiliary verbs, modifiers, the arrangement of words in sentences, and the like.

On a short term basis, listen to a five-year old speaking (a tape recorder will be a great help) and note the phonological, morphological, and syntactic features of his speech. How does his speech differ from your own adult speech? From the speech of another child the same age?

4. In view of the language that children have already learned by the time they come to school, what modifications would you suggest in existing conventional nursery school, kindergarten, and first grade language-arts programs?

5. Kenneth Goodman argues for linguistics on the grounds of *relevancy*. What specific ways can you think of in which your curriculum could be made more relevant with the inclusion of linguistic content or approach?

(lĭng gwĭs′

Part II

Linguistics and Grammar

Introduction

The scene: A cocktail party.

The time: Any time.

Act I

Host: Well, John, what do you do for a living?

John: I'm an English teacher.

Host: Oh, oh! When I'm talking to you, I'd better be careful about using prepositions to end sentences with. Hey Charlie! John here is an English teacher.

Charlie: Oh God! I've always hated English. . . .

And so it goes. Scenes similar to the above have long been familiar to any English teacher honest, brave, foolish, and/or naive enough to admit his true profession in out-of-school company. When people hear that we are English teachers, they shun us as they would if we used too much "Brand X". They fear we'll correct them for splitting an infinitive or dangling a participle. Or they heap abuse on us in some sort of cathartic effort to purge themselves of pent-up hostility brought about by years of diagramming sentences; identifying parts of speech; memorizing rules, rules, and more rules; writing weekly themes in good handwriting, in ink, on paper carefully lined with one-inch margins all around (only to have them corrected in red pencil for grammatical errors). Or more legitimately they may still be resenting the feeling of being put down by teachers who admitted to only one acceptable way of speaking—theirs.

Grammar has long held the place of honor in English instruction. As H. A. Gleason points out, "the study of language has been segregated as 'grammar'," so much so that "grammar teaching" and "English teaching" have come to be synonymous in the minds of most. And with what consequences? Because of the heavy emphasis that has been placed on grammar in schools, many people (like Charlie at the cocktail party) have come to profess that they hate English: the language that they use from the time they get up in the morning until they go to bed at night—their mother tongue. Rather than hate the language, what many people have done is build up a resistance to the way language is taught—in an atmosphere of fear and criticism, with emphasis all the time on grammar and learning in-school rules that plainly have little application or relevance to language outside of school.

Like happiness, grammar is different things to different people. The term has been subject to various interpretations and has been used in many ways. W. Nelson Francis makes a very useful distinction of what people mean by grammar on pages 135–151.

Grammar has been conventionally (and is still widely) seen as the device we use for achieving correctness in language. Most people conceive of grammar as a set of rather dogmatic rules governing which words can and cannot go together, which expressions are proper and which are not, and how language is to be used "correctly."

The newer concept of grammar is that of the internal structure of language. Grammar is seen as the system by which a language operates; something linguists refer to as *inner form* in language.

The way in which a teacher defines grammar will largely determine the kind of grammar he adheres to and how he handles it in the classroom. As we shall see later, Robert Lowth, an eighteenth-century grammarian, defined grammar as the act of rightly expressing our thoughts by words, and grammarians who followed perpetuated this concept. Charles Fries defines grammar as those devices that signal structural meaning, and he articulates a model known as *structural grammar.* Noam Chomsky defines grammar as that device by which all the grammatical sentences in a language and none of the ungrammatical ones are generated, and he formulated a model known as *transformational-generative grammar.*

Grammar Past and Present

Grammar past. Grammar has had at least a two-thousand year tenure in schools. Aristotle concerned himself extensively with defining the parts of speech. Later, the Greek grammarian Dionysius Thrax listed eight parts of speech and defined a sentence as "a combination of words expressing a thought complete in itself,"[1] in a grammar that has notable similarities to more recent grammars now being taught in some schools. Roman grammarians built upon the work done by their earlier Greek counterparts and adapted the Greek grammar to fit their Latin language. It was this Latin grammar that was the staple of the curriculum in English schools through the seventeenth century, and beyond. In Shakespeare's *Henry VI, part II,* Jack Cade says "... thou has men about thee that usually talk of a noun and a verb, and such abominable words as no Christian ear can endure to hear." Grammar would seem to have been no more popular in pre-Elizabethan and Elizabethan days than it is today.

Eighteenth century England witnessed what has been called a "Midsummer madness of grammar." As was pointed out in the introduction to part I of this book, a large number of English grammars were produced during this era. Grammarians at the time were concerned with codifying the principles of English and reducing it to rules in an attempt to settle disputed points about language usage, to apply logical thinking to language

---

[1] Charles V. Hartung, "The Persistence of Traditional Grammar." *Quarterly Journal of Speech* 48 (October 1954): 178.

matters, and to bring order to a language that was thought to be "copious without order, energetic without rules." A new middle class sought standards of correctness in language matters, and rules aplenty were provided to fill this passion for preciseness.

Where did eighteenth-century grammarians get their rules for English? Largely from Latin. The education of the eighteenth-century grammarian was steeped in a classical tradition that included Latin grammar. As Francis points out, the early English grammarians "were conditioned from their earliest school days to conceive of the classical languages as superior to the vernaculars. . . . Hence it was natural for these men to take Latin grammar as the norm, and to analyze English in terms of Latin." English grammar was based on a Latinate model. Rules and terminology were borrowed wholesale from Latin. In cases where English didn't conform to Latin, new rules were concocted to make English fit in a procrustean way. Some English authors went so far as to translate what they had written into Latin to check the grammatical propriety of what they wrote.

This, then, is the legacy that we have inherited, the model upon which traditional grammar is based.

Grammar present. The term "new grammar" can be misleading. It implies that there is one single model to which all modern grammarians adhere, one unitary theory of grammar that is universally accepted. This is not the case. Several models of new grammar have been set forth. Out of this grammatical pluralism, the relatively recent theory known as transformational-generative grammar has emerged as the one currently most widely accepted and taught, and thus it has come to be equated with "new grammar." It is important to remember, however, that other newer theories have had their place in the sun at various times, although their place was neither prominent nor enduring enough to make their presence felt to any great extent in elementary and secondary school classrooms.

While there are some differences among these various theories of new grammar, all theories differ from traditional grammar in several ways. Besides the basic difference in the definition and conception of grammar (a device for achieving correctness in language versus the internal structure of language), new grammar is, by and large:

• *descriptive rather than prescriptive.* Traditional grammar is prescriptive; that is it contains "the notion that a rule of grammar is competent, in and of itself, to determine whether a usage is correct or incorrect." (H. A. Gleason) Grammar was seen as the device which set up rules that told us how language *ought* to be used. It was primarily concerned with dos and don'ts regarding language matters.

By contrast, new grammar is descriptive; that is, it attempts to describe how language works rather than prescribing how it should work.

Grammar in this sense expresses no preference and creates no standards. It describes language as it is actually used by native speakers.

• *based on English rather than a Latinate model.* As was pointed out earlier, traditional grammar borrowed heavily from Latin grammar in establishing its rules and definitions. (How many times have you heard the expression: I never really learned English grammar until I began to study Latin?) Newer theories of grammar have been formulated based on the observation of the English language as it is used by native speakers. New grammars provide theories about our language based on the observation of that language.

There is, to be sure, a relation between English and Latin. For one thing, both are believed to have sprung from the same ancient language (Indo-European) but they came from different branches of the tree. Latin came from the Italic descendents of Indo-European; English, from the Germanic branch of the tree. There has also been a heavy Latin influence on our vocabulary, though not on our grammar. The grammar—the "frame" of our language—remained Germanic, while the words—the "shingles" that we put on the frame—were influenced by Latin.

New grammar, then, can be said to be more accurate in that it is based on observation of the language that it purports to describe, not on the basis of the observation of another language.

• *based on the concepts and aspects of language that have emerged and have been highlighted as the result of modern linguistic science.* Some of these concepts are: (1) language is speech; (2) language changes; (3) users of a language determine standards of that language.

1. Traditionally, grammar was most often thought of and taught in connection with writing. But whenever we use language in its spoken or written form, we follow the structure (or grammar) of the language. New grammar theories are based on language as it is used in its spoken form, because speech is the first form of language.

2. Language is dynamic. Standards of language change. An expression that may have been considered inappropriate at one point in time (*where it's at,* for example) might be appropriate at another point in time. It has been said that whenever enough people make the same mistake, it becomes a rule. A grammar must be flexible enough to permit these changes.

3. The commonly agreed on standards that any group of native speakers adhere to, not any authoritative rules sent down from above, determine the appropriateness of a language. There is no absolute, infallible, ultimately authoritative book of grammar. There is no Bureau of Nouns and Verbs modeled after the Bureau of Weights and Measures. The ultimate authority for language is the people who use it. Grammar does not exist outside of language.

The differences between traditional and modern grammar may be illustrated by the expression It is I (or me). Traditionally, the rule governing this expression was "use the nominative case after the verb *to be*," a rule borrowed directly from Latin. Now, in English, the subject-predicate-object arrangement in a sentence is common and the objective form of the first person personal pronoun is *me*, not *I*. According to the structure of English, then, *me* rather than *I* fits the pattern (or grammar) of the language. This is the form that most people normally used in their day-to-day speech. By now, *It is I* has become a rather archaic form of expression and has already departed from most school grammar books. Although the expression is still used, the "rule" is no longer considered to be incontrovertible.

An example such as It is I is not terribly difficult for most teachers to accept, since it has all but taken its leave from the grammatical scene. But when we apply the same logic to expressions like *ain't* and use of the double negative, eyebrows are raised and heads are bowed. And yet it is not inconceiveable that the same type of thing may happen to these perpetual sources of annoyance for the composition teacher.

Is this to say that anything goes? Are there no standards left in language matters? Yes, there are standards, but these are social standards applied to linguistic matters. They are not standards of grammar but standards of usage.

Grammar and usage. Although they are often confused in the minds of many people (including teachers), the distinction between grammar and usage is an important one to the linguist.

Grammar is the structure or system of a language, something that is inherent within the language itself. Usage, on the other hand, refers to the prevailing standards of acceptable language in a community, something that is outside the language. The difference between grammar and usage has been compared with the difference between behavior and etiquette. Behavior identifies what people do; etiquette sets up standards by which the stamp of approval or disapproval is put on people's actions. Usage is the Grammar 3 that Francis refers to. In fact, he uses the term "linguistic etiquette" to identify this concept of grammar.

The linguist does not talk about "good grammar" or "bad grammar" in the traditional sense. To illustrate, take an example used by Paul Burns in part I of this book: I done it. This expression is "grammatical" in that it conforms to the order and structure underlying English. The expressions Done it I or It done I would be considered "ungrammatical" in that they do not conform to English syntax or structure. While the linguist would say that I done it is grammatical, no linguist would recommend that the expression ought to be used by anyone trying to make a good impression on educated speakers. The expression is not considered good usage. The "goodness" or "badness" of an expression, then, is not inherent in the language itself but in the opinion of those who speak the language. Grammar and usage are different. Grammar is a matter of language structure; usage, one of preference or ethical judgment.

Two Models of New Grammar

As was said earlier, several models of new grammar have been postulated and published. Two that have had the most effect on schools are presented here. *Structural grammar* was fairly widely studied in post-secondary education during the middle to late 1950s and is still adhered to by some language scholars. Although it did not achieve widespread popularity in the grades, some of the content of structural grammar is extremely useful to the language arts teacher. *Transformational grammar* is a slightly newer model that has achieved enormous popularity among language scholars. It has come to be the "new grammar" presented in most modern English or grammar texts.

Naturally, it is impossible to do little more than scratch the surface of the rationale and content of these grammars in a book of this size and nature. References are, however, provided for further reading on each of these models of new grammar.

Structural grammar. As the name indicates, structural grammar is based on structural linguistics, the scientific study of language. Structural grammarians aim at producing a description of English based on the analysis of the language as it is used by native speakers. Charles Fries, who presented a comprehensive and formal account of structural grammar in *The Structure of English*[1], recorded many hours of telephone conversations and built his description on the analysis of the transcription of these conversations. (Fries, of course, had been studying people's language long before he formalized his theory.)

Like any linguist, the structural grammarian begins with speech. He defines a sentence as the segment of speech found between final terminal junctures, points in the stream of speech where the rising or falling of the voice indicates a sense of completeness. Thus, intonation and other parts of phonology are important aspects of his grammar. Also, structural grammar contains a different classification of sentences than traditional grammar does. The expression *A quarter* standing alone does not make much sense, but in response to *How much do I owe you?* it is a sentence. (In this example, *A quarter* would be called a "response sentence.")

Sentence patterns are an important part of structural grammar. These patterns are identified from the analysis of the order in which speakers

---

[1] New York: Harcourt, Brace and World, 1952.

place words in their everyday use of language. Some of the most common sentence patterns in English are: (D) N V* (*People talk.*); (D) N V (D) N (*John hit the ball.*); (D) NV (D) N (D) N (*The boy gave the girl a gift.*); (D) N V Adv-p (*His family lives here.*); (D) N V Adj (*The pupil seems young.*); (D) N be (D) N (*My brother is a sailor.*); (D) N be Adj (*My sister is pretty*); and so on. After the structural grammarian identifies these patterns, he classifies and describes the words used in them in very precise ways.

In dealing with parts of speech, structural grammar departs significantly from the traditional definitions that we are used to. The structural grammarian describes parts of speech according to structural features—that is, word order in the sentence, affixes, and the relationship of one word to the others in the sentence. For example, if we were to hear the sentence *The glings glongled glorgily in the goag,* we would probably identify *glings* and *goag* as nouns, *glongled* as the verb, and *glorgily* as an adverb. Why? Because of their respective positions in the sentence. Because we know that *the* procedes nouns in normal conversation. Because we are familiar with the morphemes [-s], [-ed], and [-ly] which usually mark nouns, verbs, and adverbs respectively. In other words, we identify these parts of speech on the basis of their structural characteristics, not because they are "names of persons, places, or things" or "action words" or "words that modify verbs, adjectives, and other adverbs." The example of *Jabberwocky* and some ideas on using the structuralists' techniques with pupils will be presented later in the postscript.

In *The Structure of English,* Fries avoids the traditional parts-of-speech labels (noun, verb, adjective, adverb, preposition, conjunction, interjection) altogether. Instead, he classifies words as *form words* and *function words.* He identifies four classes of form words and he labels and describes them as follows: *Class 1 words:* words that pattern like *boy, concert, building,* and so on; *Class 2 words:* words that pattern like *run, see, seem,* and so on; *Class 3 words:* words that fit the pattern The ——— ——— (noun) is ———————. (The *beautiful* girl is *beautiful,* for example); and *Class 4 words,* words that fit the frame The ——————— (noun) ——————— (verb) the ——————— (noun) ———————. (The boy ate the apple *quickly,* or The boy hit the ball *hard,* for example.) Function words are classified and labeled as *Group A:* words that pattern like *a* and *the* in English sentences (including such words as my, every, three, and so on); *Group B:* words that pattern like *is* (as an auxiliary), will, must, and so on; *Group C,* and so on. The distinction between form and function words in structural grammar is analagous to

---

* The Symbols used are: D = Determiner; ( ) = may or may not be used; N = Noun; V = Verb; Adv-p = Adverb of Place; Adj = Adjective; be = the appropriate form of the verb *to be.*

bricks and mortar in building a wall: the bricks make up the bulk and substance of a wall, while the mortar holds the bricks solidly in place. Similarly, in building sentences, the form words carry the bulk of the meaning, while function words are used to "cement" these form words together to produce the total meaning of the sentence. The implication of Fries' form-function word distinction will be explained more fully in the postscripts following this part and part three of this book.

There's a lot more to structural grammar than has just been presented. The articles by W. Nelson Francis and by Carl A. Lefevre present more of the rationale and content of this model of grammar. *The Structure of English* has already been mentioned as a valuable source of information. Paul Roberts' *Patterns of English* (New York: Harcourt Brace and World, 1955) and Norman Stageberg's *An Introductory English Grammar* (second edition, New York: Holt, Rinehart, & Winston 1971) are two other texts of structural grammar that teachers will find valuable.

Transformational grammar. "Transformational-generative grammar" (to be more exact) introduced a new orientation, a new dimension, and new content in language study. Like structural grammar, it was formulated on the basis of the analysis and description of the English language. But the transformationalist observes that structural grammar is based on a finite corpus; that is, sentences that have already been used. Yet we can both produce and recognize an unlimited number of grammatical sentences that we have never experienced before. Consider, for example, this sentence: Green and white striped aardvarks who are addicted to chocolate will some day land on the dark side of a planet in outer space. Although you've probably never heard or seen this sentence before, it can be recognized as being grammatical. It doesn't make much sense, of course, but it is a grammatical sentence in that it conforms to the standard form and order of English.

Thus, the transformalist's aim is to produce a system of explicit rules that will explain the system of language, a set of logical principles about the way a language operates. Language has system. Transformational grammar sets out to discover and describe this system.

A distinction needs to be made here between the way "rule" is used in traditional and in transformational grammar. Traditionally, a rule implies something that should be followed in order to produce a sentence that is considered good grammar. "Rules" in transformational grammar are designed not to dictate but rather to explain how language operates. In producing sentences, the native speaker follows these rules intuitively. The function of transformational grammar is to identify the rules that explain his intuition.

The pioneer of transformational grammar is Noam Chomsky, who has also been the most dominant figure in English linguistics for the past ten years or so. Chomsky introduced his formal theory of transformational grammar in *Syntactic Structures.*[2] His latter-day theory is in part presented in Ved Mehta's article, based on extensive interviews with Chomsky.

Transformational grammar begins with phrase-structure rules, rules that describe the parts and relations of elements in simple declarative sentences. The first phrase-structure rule is S → NP + VP, which is to say "A sentence can be rewritten as a noun phrase and a verb phrase." Each element is then further broken down and spelled out according to its components and sequences:

$$NP \rightarrow \begin{Bmatrix} \text{Prop N} \\ D + N \\ \text{Pro} \end{Bmatrix}$$

(Noun phrase can be rewritten as either a proper noun, determiner plus noun, or pronoun); VP → Aux + V (Verb phrase can be rewritten as an auxiliary plus verb); and so on. (More phrase-structure rules are given in articles that follow.

We know, of course, that we don't just speak in simple declarative sentences, so transformational grammar provides rules for *single base transformations* and *double base transformations* that explain the structures of our more complex utterances.

Single-base transformations provide for the rearrangement, addition, deletion, or combination of linguistic elements in sentences. For example, the Yes/No Question Transformation Rule is:

$$NP + t + M + X \rightarrow t + M + NP + X$$

(that is, noun phrase plus tense plus modal plus other optional parts of the expression can be rewritten as tense plus model plus noun phrase plus optional parts of the expression). Let's apply the rule. From the simple *kernel* sentence: John is going (to the party), we produce: Is John going (to the party)? This is the rule that we intuitively follow whenever we form a question requiring a simple *yes* or *no* answer. Other single base transformation rules explain the negative, the passive, the use of *there* in There is a man at the door (generated from the kernel A man is at the door), and other language operations.

Double-base transformations explain our more complex utterances. These are the ones that we follow in producing longer and intricate sentences that characterize most of our speech and writing. For example, in the sentence The children at the library were reading books, the basic *(matrix)* sentence is The children were reading books. Into this matrix sentence is *embedded* a sentence called a *constituent,* The children were at the library. Any number of these constituents can be embedded to produce longer utterances. Examples of how these transformational rules may be used in the classroom are presented in the postscript.

---

[2] The Hague: Mouton, 1957.

On first brush, all of these transformational rules seem rather complicated, perhaps needlessly so. But it must be remembered that language itself is a complicated phenomenon that precludes a simplistic description. What the transformalist does is provide ordered rules describing what the native speaker does automatically and unconsciously as he uses language.

Transformational grammar also introduced another concept that Chomsky refers to in Mehta's article, that Jacobs alludes to, and that Simons uses in part 3 as his basis for reading comprehension; that is, *surface structure* and *deep structure*. Surface structure is the way a sentence is spoken; deep structure is the underlying relationships that are expressed. While the deep structure is not always apparent, it is something that the native speaker knows by intuition. The examples that have been used by Chomsky and thereafter have been repeated ad nauseam are:

John is easy to please. John is eager to please. The surface structure—the arrangement of words—is parallel but the deep structure is very different. In the first, John is (to use an old familiar expression) the potential receiver of the action. In the second, John is the one who is doing (or wants to do) the pleasing. This concept will be explained more fully in the articles referred to at the beginning of this paragraph.

Besides Ved Mehta's article, some of the rationale and content of transformational grammar is presented in three selections that follow: Roderick A. Jacobs' "A Short Introduction to Transformational Grammar," Charles and Mary Ross' "Linguistics in the Elementary School Classroom," and Frank J. Zidonis' "Incorporating Transformational Grammar into the English Curriculum." For further reading, Owen Thomas' *Transformational Grammar and the Teacher of English* (New York: Holt, Rinehart, & Winston, 1965) is a tailor-made reference. *English Syntax* by Paul Roberts (New York: Harcourt, Brace and World, 1964) has a programmed edition that presents the essentials of the transformational theory. Also, Norman Stageberg's *An Introductory English Grammar* (cited earlier) contains an excellent section on transformational grammar written by Ralph M. Goodman.

But What's New Grammar Good For?

Once again, we come to the practical questions for teachers: What's new grammar good for? and Will it produce results that are any better than the ones produced by traditional grammar? While there is a growing body of research literature aimed at answering these questions, early evidence suggests that new grammar will not improve children's ability in speaking and writing any more than traditional grammar has done. And then there are those who point out that language improvement is not the purpose of new grammar, that the information it produces about the structure of language is worth knowing in and of itself.

Practical claims for teaching any brand of grammar have always been questionable. Since the work of Franklin Hoyt in the early part of this century, one research study after another has proven that the intensive study of grammar has little if any positive effect on helping pupils speak or write better English. Nor has it ever been proven conclusively that the study of traditional grammar helps pupils appreciate or interpret literature any better, improve reading ability, or improve pupils' language behavior in functional situations. Moreover, research has shown that students forget at an amazing rate the grammar they have been taught.[3]

What can be said of new grammar on these grounds? During the past few years, the research literature has contained a growing number of reports on the effectiveness of linguistic grammars. Irma Gale, for example, found that fifth graders can understand the concepts of structural and transformational grammars and this knowledge can enable them to construct longer structures of greater complexity.[4] Ruthellen Crews also worked with fifth graders and found that pupils in the experimental (that is, linguistic) groups made certain gains in measures of sentence structure, but the gains were not so significant as to suggest a wholesale shift to the linguistic grammar.[5]

Zidonis tested the effectiveness of transformational grammar at the ninth and tenth grade levels. In a two-year experimental study, he found that a knowledge of transformational grammar helped students to increase the proportion of well formed sentences they wrote and to reduce the occurrence of errors in their writing. His results suggest that transformational grammar might be a useful first step in improving composition skills.[6] Ronald Wardhaugh worked with high school students as well, but concluded that students' knowledge of transformational grammar is but poorly related to the ability to write, just as a knowledge of traditional grammar is.[7] Similar studies report results similar to those reported above.

---

[3] Many books cite research along these lines, but two references that highlight the futility of teaching traditional grammar for practical purposes are the 1950 edition of *The Encyclopedia of Educational Research* (an article by John R. Searles and G. Robert Carlsen) and *Four Problems in Teaching English: A Critique of Research* by J. Stanley Sherwin (Scranton, Pa.: International Textbook Co., 1969).

[4] Irma F. Gale. "An Experimental Study of Two Fifth Grade Language Arts Programs: An Analysis of the Writing of Children Taught Linguistic Grammars Compared to Those Taught Traditional Grammars." Unpublished EdD. Dissertation. Muncie, Ind.: Ball State University, 1967, ERIC Document ED 015 197.

[5] Ruthellen Crews. "A Linguistic versus a Traditional Grammar Program—The Effects on Written Sentence Structure and Composition." *Educational Leadership* 5 (November 1971): 145–149.

[6] Frank J. Zidonis, "Generative Grammar: A Report on Research." *English Journal* 54 (May 1965): 405–409.

[7] Ronald Wardhaugh, "Ability in Written Composition and Transformational Grammar," *The Journal of Educational Research* 60 (May–June 1967): 427–429.

Despite the inconclusiveness of research on the matter, most authors who write about new grammar do make practical claims. For example, Lefevre on structural grammar: "Effective use of clause markers is a specialty of the successful writer . . . Mastery of the system can contribute a great deal to the development of writing style." Francis on structural grammar: " . . . it seems probable that a realistic, scientific grammar should vastly facilitate the teaching of English, especially as a foreign language." Jacobs on transformational grammar: "Teachers have been studying transformational grammar . . . as a possible aid in the teaching of composition." Ross and Ross on transformational grammar: "The evidence indicates that raising the use of transformation to a conscious level helps pupils write more maturely at an earlier age." The claims are mostly guarded, laced with such terms as "probable" and "possible", but they are present nevertheless. To be sure, the more one knows about his language, the more tools he will have at his disposal in teaching and using that language. But great writers have written and great orators spoken without any formal knowledge of grammar at all.

So from a practical point of view, it might be said that research has shown that pupils are capable of learning new grammar and that this learning many result in some improvements in their writing. The evidence that has been gathered up to this point, however, does not seem to justify any grammatical model—traditional or modern—on practical grounds alone. But with the proven futility of achieving practical ends with traditional grammar, it seems that new grammar deserves at least an equal chance.

Knowledge for its own sake is another justification given for the study of new grammar. Francis speaks to this point: " . . . the superseding of vague and sloppy thinking (traditional grammar) by clear and precise thinking (structural grammar) is an exciting experience in and of itself." So do Ross and Ross: "For the teacher, the new English promises great rewards because it provides a true subject matter (which) . . . will mean for many a new satisfaction." According to this point of view, practical claims alone are irrelevant. New grammar meets the "learning *about* language" objective of the language-arts curriculum. New grammar provides an accurate and up-to-date picture of language, a model that is based on observation of and discoveries about one's native tongue. This knowledge may be justification enough for studying new grammar.

H. A. Gleason, Jr. is one of the best known, most widely read, and highly respected linguists of our time. In the article that follows, Gleason suggests some lines along which we ought to be building a grammar for schools.

He begins with a critical look at school grammar, or rather a critical look at the way grammar has been handled in schools. He sees the need for a shift in grammar from a narrow utilitarianism to a more broadly conceived approach, humanistic in its orientation.

Gleason conceives of grammar as an all-encompassing part of the language curriculum. He finds grammar to be "a part of the fundamental equipment essential to the whole process of stylistic study." After making some important distinctions and observations about the difference between traditional and linguistic grammarians, Gleason identifies some deterrents to teaching new grammar in the classroom, mainly centering on the lack of materials available and a review of those materials that were available when the article was originally published (1964).

Gleason identifies five needs for strengthening a grammar program: to treat grammar in a less superficial way, which requires a deeper knowledge on the part of teachers; to extend the concern of grammar beyond the level of the sentence; to widen the concern of grammar beyond standard English; to broaden the language curriculum beyond English and into foreign language to illustrate linguistic principles; to change the method of presenting grammar.

What Grammar?

H. A. Gleason, Jr.

An educated man should be able to think rationally and incisively about his environment and about his human situation. Yet the ideal of the educated man is seldom approached in one of the most significant facets of his life: language. Adult Americans are badly informed about language and endemically prone to naive reasoning on any linguistic question. Moreover, they have no better insight into their own English tongue than into language in general, and this is, perhaps, the most serious failure of liberal humanistic objectives in American education.

This lack of insight is the more disturbing when it is remembered that our schools devote a larger part of the educational effort to "language arts" and to "English" than to any other subject matter. It might appear that the shortcomings cannot have arisen simply from lack of attention. But on closer examination, we find that language itself actually receives little direct consideration in most segments of this sadly riven curriculum and is totally neglected in others. The result of this prevailing neglect is an anomaly: Within what is often called the language curriculum the study of language is segregated as grammar.

To note this strange situation is neither to excuse it nor to explain it. There is grave presumption of some basic underlying fault which must be deeply embedded in the fundamental structure of our language curriculum and in the views on which it is based, since no superficial reform seems to have been able to correct it. The symptoms themselves suggest that part, at least, of the trouble must be in an antihumanistic orientation of some crucial component. This would certainly produce serious strains within a curriculum often considered as the bulwark of the humanities in our educational system.

In the study of grammar we would expect some solid effort to wrestle with language as, in itself, a subject worthy of study, and give to the students some of the perspectives they will need for clear linguistic thinking. Such expectations are not met. Of the subjects in the curriculum, grammar is one of the least liberally conceived. It is seldom mentioned when the values of the teaching of English are discussed. Rather than being simply indifferent to the values of the humanities, the current teaching of grammar is actively hostile. Not only does it contribute nothing to the announced objectives of English teaching, but it goes a long way toward rendering the whole ineffective. Grammar is that crucial component with the antihumanistic orientation.

Several courses of action suggest themselves. They range from simply elimination of grammar, to a radical restructuring of the place and function of grammar in the curriculum. Today the discussion in the English teaching profession centers largely on an intermediate proposal, the replacement of the present system of grammar with some other. Several candidates are currently being advocated, often with the enthusiasm of a political campaign. Hence, the question that stands as a title over this paper is a real question and it must be faced, but it must be considered in a broader context.

Seldom is the basic difficulty recognized. "School grammar" is more than a system of description of a language; it is also a view of grammar, of its nature and function. The American curriculum has had a long and tortuous development. It has given grammar a conspicuous but marginal and ineffectual place. The grammatical system used has developed slowly during the same period, largely innocent of any contact with scholarly research on language. Hence it has been amenable to moulding by the same complex interaction of forces that produced the American curriculum. This parallel development under the same influences has resulted in a peculiarly close adaptation of one to the other. We have endowed school grammar with the very narrow and shallow view appropriate to its assigned place. We have shaped it to the parochial instrumentalism which has dominated the curriculum. We have shrunk from any involvement, other than the most superficial, of school grammar in any other segment of the whole structure. In so doing, we have accepted and confirmed grammar's assignment to marginality.

It is a popular pastime to look at school grammar out of its context and to condemn it soundly. Yet we must recognize that school grammar is very nearly the ideal type for the existing curriculum in English. Conversely something very much like that curriculum is the only environment likely to be congenial to school grammar as we know it. Both the type of grammar and the place assigned to it must be accepted or rejected together. To change either alone would be futile. If we do desire a curriculum which is liberally humanistic in its orientation, rather than simply instrumental or even heavily tainted with antiintellectualism, we must find both a new, more broadly conceived grammar, and a new, less constricted frame for it. That this is so, is perhaps best seen by starting from an observation not quite so basic: School grammar is closed. By various devices it excludes from view all unsettled and unsettling questions. It gives artificially unambiguous answers to the questions it can accept as appropriately grammatical, and no help at all with others.

There are many possible ways to delimit the scope of grammar. School grammar and the conceptions underlying our present curriculum concur in a position that approaches one extreme. The assumption is made that questions are either wholly grammatical, or not grammatical at all. That is, in some instances grammar alone is adequate to answer them; in others, grammar has nothing to contribute. Borderline cases, where grammar can provide only part of a solution, are seldom recognized. In order to give grammar absolute dominion within its assigned limits, the scope must be very narrowly conceived. This black-or-white dichotomy is a chief source of our difficulties with grammar. The consequences are serious, both when responsibility is denied and when it is arrogated.

One consequence is *prescriptivism,* the notion that a rule of grammar is competent, in and of itself, to determine whether a usage is correct or incorrect. No other consideration—kind of writing, public, social context, or anything else—is thought to be relevant. This is a dangerous oversimplification. Moreover, the imputing of such authority to grammar inevitably deprives it of any humanistic values. The result is the dry-rot that has spread through the entire English curriculum from this focus of infection.

The antidote is to recognize, first, that the real standard is elsewhere, perhaps in some corpus of literature generally considered excellent, and, second, that grammar is one of several tools that must be used to compare any given sample of English with that standard. This comparison must be made by the joint use of a number of devices (for example, rhetorical analysis), since the standard of good English must involve much more than mere mechanical correctness, and since the various components of quality cannot be separated absolutely either from one another or from various social dimensions.

The inflexibility of school formulations of grammar are a concomitant of prescriptivism. If the rules are the standard, they must be protected as jealously as the standard meter in Paris, and like it, they must be made of the most immutable materials available. Any basic restructuring is certain of rejection, and the most minor adjustments arouse intense suspicion. But if the rules cease to be the standard, new formulations may make possible more incisive comparisons. Openness in the grammar is then no longer a peril to good English, but a promise of more effective teaching, and hence of higher standards.

An example of the other sort of consequences is the estrangement of grammar from literature and composition, with the resulting fragmentation of the English curriculum. The separation is not absolute—there is one familiar application: Certain difficulties in student writing (for example, the incorrect agreement of verbs) are looked upon as purely grammatical problems. When found in a paper, they are marked as errors, and the student is referred to the appropriate rule. If this procedure has the hoped-for result, the paper is brought to a minimum mechanical correctness—minimum because some matters of mechanical correctness are not provided for in the rules, for example, many aspects of the use of the article. In some instances the student ultimately acquires the ability to produce work that consistently meets these simple standards. Important as such an attainment may be, there is certainly much more that a composition teacher must aim at. Traditional composition teaching relates grammar only to the first step toward writing competence. From the point of view of ultimate goals, therefore, its contribution is only marginal or superficial.

Grammar has had even less place in the literature class. The application of canons of correctness to well-regarded writings has seemed either unnecessary or slightly embarrassing. Moreover, the attention has seldom been focused on details of structure within sentences, the only place where most formulations of grammar might apply. Teachers have seldom even raised the issue of the relevance of grammar instruction to literary learning.

The shortcomings have left the English curriculum disjointed. Grammar relates only superficially to composition and hardly at all to literature. It is generally felt that there is more connection between composition and literature, but this has always been very difficult to formulate clearly and precisely. This last fact may be as much a result of the restricted view of the scope of grammar as of any basic difficulty in either composition or literature. The lack of cohesion within the English curriculum seems to reflect a single basic disjunction.

This last suggestion certainly requires some discussion, even if it is necessarily something of an excursus. The central problems in composition and literature are very similar or even basically identical. They are commonly viewed, of course, from opposite directions, so that they can easily be stated in contrasting forms, thus disguising their unity. Nevertheless those of one field are mirrored in the other. If in either they were precisely formulated, the relationships should become clearly visible. As it stands, few can be stated with the requisite exactitude, and this community of fundamentals can be recognized only in rather general propositions (such as that wide reading is reflected in better writing).

Advancement in any field of learning comes most often from sharper definition of problems or from more incisive techniques for studying them. Certainly these, rather than the accretion of more data, seem to hold the real promise in either literature or composition. Within English studies, sharpening of definition should be especially fruitful, since it may well bring hitherto separate questions into relationship. If the insights painfully reached in the study of literature can be opened up to composition, and vice versa, the interchange will be most profitable.

Grammar and Stylistics

The complex of problems commonly designated "style" may be taken as representative. There is far more agreement in the identification of stylistic problems than in their definition. They seem to merge imperceptibly into one another and to deal largely with subjective evaluations in which no two investigators can find common ground. Some results have been obtained, but all together they seem a small yield for the tremendous labor that has been expended, and even so, most of them are less firmly established than we might expect. It would seem that the vagueness of formulation of the problems is the ground of much of the difficulty with either research or teaching in stylistics. One prerequisite for further progress is simply to extricate, from this mass, manageable topics of study, and to state them precisely.

Nebulous as style is, we may expect that it comprehends more than one type of problem. Among them it would seem certain that many involve the patterning of choices among alternatives presented by the structure of the language. At every point the writer makes a choice—some deliberately and some unconsciously. These cannot be made at random if the result is to be good writing. Nor can there be dead uniformity. What is required is an artful patterning. This latter is, therefore, one essential component of style. Composition teaching involves developing the ability to make these choices effectively. Literature teaching might[1] include developing understanding and appreciation of style as choice. Here is an

---

[1] There is a recurrent debate as to how much technical literary criticism (of any sort) should be included in the school curriculum. If students were adequately equipped with some basic understanding of language structure, the question would be shifted to very different ground.

opportunity of correlation—perhaps even integration—of composition and literature around a specific problem.

To study this aspect of stylistics requires knowledge of the choices that are presented (for example, of the denotatively equivalent and grammatically related alternative forms of sentences), of their connotative implications, and of the valences for combination with other sentences into larger units. Two of these are grammatical problems, if grammar is conceived broadly enough, and the remaining one must be rooted in the grammatical structure of the passage. This means that stylistics is not simply a point of contact between composition and literature, but equally between these two and grammar.

If this matter is looked at strictly from outside grammar, it might be concluded that stylistics is merely a place where grammar can make a useful contribution to the other two major subdivisions of English study. One of their needs seems to be for precise formulation of problems. This grammar can provide, in some cases. It can sort out the alternatives, put them into some sort of systematic ordering, and so provide a framework within which the literary student can approach some stylistic problems. For composition, the contribution seems to be even more directly practical: grammar can provide a sharper diagnosis of written infelicities, a terminology by which the teacher can discuss them with the student, and in some cases even procedures for improvement.

However, it would be a mistake to take so strictly instrumental a view. The help that can be provided by grammar is much more basic, not simply assistance with problems already familiar, but the finding of new and more revealing questions to examine. Nor is grammar a tool to be called in when needed, but rather a part of the fundamental equipment essential to the whole process of stylistic study. Moreover, it should not be thus narrowly viewed as an outsider to any part of the English curriculum. The proper subject of the English curriculum is English, a language. Every language has certain basic characteristics which influence its uses and functions. Conspicuous among these is structure, the proper subject of grammatical study. The act of writing, like the act of reading, is rooted in this structure, and skill in either can only be based in a comprehension (perhaps informal) of structure. Grammar has a relevance in the study of literature and composition simply because it deals in a systematic way with the same basic stuff which these use as their medium. It is a central component in a comprehensive English curriculum.

Such centrality is beyond the capacity of grammar as we have known it in the American schools. No small alteration, either in the system of grammar itself or in our view of its place, will allow effective focusing on the basic problems. We cannot build an English curriculum worthy of its professed subject without a grammar more capable of broad application and more compatible with the liberal tradition of the humanities. What is at stake here is not simply the grammar segment of the curriculum, but the whole—literature and composition as well.

While the peculiar kind of grammar familiar in American schools was growing in close adjustment to the curriculum limitations that grew with it, English grammar was also developing quite independently, in the very different climate of university scholarship. The result has been the gradual amassing of a very large body of facts and theory and the building of several alternative frameworks for organizing the whole into a more or less coherent system. Every aspect of the language has been examined from various directions, though not in all cases with equal productiveness. The university grammarians have tended to set the boundaries of their work as wide as possible, and nothing like the deceptively neat delimitation of school grammar has appeared. Indeed, traditional grammars (as they are best called[2]) have tended to ramble slightly. Nor have there been the same forces for uniformity that have been so strong in the schools. On the contrary, the work has gone on in the most diverse environments under men of varied backgrounds. There is no one, but several traditional grammars[3], though all have been in the continual interaction with each other.

Another group of grammars has arisen as descriptive linguists have turned their attention to English in the last two decades.[4] This recency should not obscure the much older roots. Linguistics as a tradition is as old as grammar. Its theory and methods have grown gradually through many decades of work with a wide range of problems in a still wider assortment of languages. The continuity of efforts and the dependence on the past is much greater than either outsiders or most linguists realize. What is new is largely the application of these methods, worked out in

---

[2] Unfortunately, there has been a tendency to apply the label "traditional grammar" both to this and to what is here called "school grammar." The resulting confusion has led to a common nonsequitur, justifying school grammar on the basis of the evident advantages of scholarly traditional grammar. If schools had been committed to traditional grammar (in this sense) most of the present vacuity would never have arisen.

[3] The two most familiar are the work of Jespersen, a Dane, most conveniently seen in Jens Otto Harry Jespersen, *Essentials of English Grammar* (London: George Allen and Unwin, Ltd., 1933); and that developed by a group of Dutch scholars including Poutsma and Kruisinga and most conveniently seen in Reinard William Zandvoort, *A Handbook of English Grammar* (London: Longsmans, Green, 1957).

[4] The following represent basic works in a variety of approaches, the first much closer to traditional gramar than the others: Charles Carpenter Fries, *The Structure of English.* (New York: Harcourt, Brace and World, 1952.) George L. Trager, and Henry L. Smith, Jr. *An Outline of English Structure.* (Washington, D. C.: American Council of Learned Societies, 1951.) Eugene Albert Nida, *A Synopsis of English Syntax..* (Norman, Okla.: Summer Institute of Linguistics, 1960.) Noam Chomsky, *Syntactic Structures* ('s-Gravenhage Mouton, 1957). Harold E. Palmer and F. G. Blandford. *A Grammar of Spoken English.* (Cambridge: W. Heffer and Sons, 1939).

other contexts, to English. Though they have been designated as "new grammar," there is really none of the radical rootlessness that this term often suggests.

The Traditional Grammarians and the "Linguist"

There is a significant difference between the traditional grammarians and the "linguists."[5] The two groups have tended to concentrate on different aspects of the problem. Traditional grammarians have inherited a framework for the structure of English. They have modified this whenever they have found it necessary to do so, but their chief attention has been focused on details of structure and usage. The linguists, on the other hand, have come to English with an interest more in the general theory of language and, in any specific language, more in the overall framework than in the minor details. They have, therefore, tended to concentrate on the broader issues rather than on the small points central to the interests of the traditional grammarians. The results attained by the two groups are, therefore, largely complementary.

This fact is widely realized by those active in English grammar research. As linguists work downward from the general structure toward the details, they are making increasing use of the work of the traditional grammarians. The recent work of the latter, of course, takes critical cognizance of that of the linguists. The distinction between "traditional grammars" and "linguistic grammars" is beginning to blur, and may be expected soon to become irrelevant.

This does not mean, however, that all the various grammars are merging into one, but only that the two groups are losing their group identities. Indeed, the variety of grammars is proliferating, and will probably continue to do so in the immediate future, as linguists continue to experiment with new descriptive techniques and fresh theoretical insights.

The most recent major development has been transformational-generative grammar. This first came to wide attention with the publication in 1957 of Noam Chomsky's *Syntactic Structures*,[6] but has had tremendous growth in the few years since, and now is the framework for more research on English grammar than any other position. It has come to be regarded by many teachers of English as a third great movement alongside

---

[5] The contrast between the labels "linguist" and "grammarian" is an artificial one. One kind of "linguist" is merely a research grammarian, and the traditional grammarians are, in fact, fully entitled to be called "linguists."

[6] Noam Chomsky, *Syntactic Structures*. ('s-Gravenhage: Mouton, 1957). This book is not so much a grammar of English as a tract on linguistic theory. Its examples, however are drawn from English and it gives an abridged outline grammar which suggests possible lines of development.

traditional grammars and linguistic grammars. Currently, much of the theoretical debate in the linguistic profession centers around issues raised by transformational-generative grammar. It is unquestionable that this approach has called attention to certain very significant questions previously neglected, and that it has made some valuable contributions to linguistic theory, as well as to our understanding of English grammar. But these facts should not lead anyone to believe that transformational-generative grammar has supplanted structural grammar any more than that the latter has supplanted traditional grammar. Each still has some significant contribution to make.

Sharp as the contrast between the transformational-generative position and that of the "old-line" linguists may seem to be, it is already clear that the differences are beginning to be dulled. Ways are being found to incorporate certain of the newer findings into other general schemes. At the same time, the transformational-generative model is beginning to divide into competing varieties—a most healthy condition, of course. Totally new systems built on still other premises are in the process of formation, some of which may turn out to have distinct advantages. Just as the dichotomy between traditional and structural is beginning to be meaningless, that between transformational-generative and structural may be expected first to weaken and then to disappear.

The present situation, therefore, is that there are a considerable number of grammatical systems held by various workers in the field. They are all in interaction, and the lines of demarcation are constantly shifting. Debate is sharp, and naturally tends to highlight the points of disagreement, pushing the much larger areas of agreement into the background. The discussion involves both general points of theory and the treatment of individual points of structure. It is to this complex of systems and theories that the curriculum reformer must look for material if he desires to replace the conventional school grammar.

Deterrents to Change

It might seem that the choice would be difficult only because of the large number of alternative grammars available. The situation, however, is quite otherwise. None of the systems produced by traditional grammarians or modern linguists is, in its present form, suitable for classroom use. Academic specialists write, for the most part, for scholars of their own kind. A different organization and a different style of presentation are required in the schools. At the minimum, the textbook writer or curriculum planner must completely restate any grammar that he might select. This, in itself, can be a complicated and tedious task; actually, much more is required. Most of the grammars are fragmentary. If they do not actually omit treatment of certain topics, they almost always slight some. Many of the grammars are designed for very restricted functions. The choice is presented then, not so much in the form of an assortment of fully worked out comprehensive grammars, as a copious mass of materials from which the elements can be selected. It is up to the people primarily concerned with the curriculum to build an integrated system out of the materials available.

The favored solution in recent years can be exemplified by Paul Roberts' two high-school textbooks, both landmarks in the movement for grammatical reform in the schools. The approach is eclectic. In his *Patterns of English,*[7] the greater part of the grammatical material is based on C. C. Fries' work, *The Structure of English,*[8] with only relatively minor and quite straightforward modification. However, Fries gives no attention to phonology. For this, Roberts followed the work of George L. Trager and Henry Lee Smith, Jr., *An Outline of English Structure.*[9] If these two sources are compared as wholes, they will be seen to take very different positions on many basic points. The incompatibility is not directly evident in Roberts' book, however, since the phonology is from one and the syntax from the other and the two areas of study are not very tightly interrelated.

This particular pattern, in numerous minor variations, has been so widely used that, for many English teachers, new grammar or linguistic grammar, or, even linguistics[10] is identified with a system of this kind—basically Fries' syntax with Trager and Smith's phonology.

Roberts' later book, *English Sentences,*[11] follows much the same approach, but adds to it a number of ideas which he found in Noam Chomsky's *Syntactic Structures.*[12] The book is often said to have abandoned the "structural grammar" of its predecessor for the new "transformational grammar," but this is clearly not the case. Most of the old remains, obscured by a quite fortunate return to a more conservative

---

[7] Paul Roberts, *Patterns of English.* New York: Harcourt, Brace and World, 1956.

[8] Charles Carpenter Fries, *The Structure of English.* New York: Harcourt, Brace and World, 1952.

[9] George L. Trager and Henry L. Smith, Jr. *An Outline of English Structure.* Washington: American Council of Learned Societies, 1951.

[10] It is perhaps futile to protest, but this use of "linguistics" has led to serious confusion. Linguistics is the systematic study of language, particularly language structure. It is a large, rapidly growing, and highly technical body of knowledge, within which English grammar constitutes only a small part. In particular, it involves a body of fundamental theory about language in general which underlies and gives method and meaning to research on any individual language. Something of the breadth of the subject (even before some significant recent developments) can be seen in John Bissel Carroll, *The Study of Language.* Cambridge: Harvard University Press, 1953.

[11] Paul Roberts, *English Sentences.* New York: Harcourt, Brace and World, 1962.

[12] Noam Chomsky, *Syntactic Structures* ('s-Gravenhage: Mouton, 1957).

terminology.[13] To this has been added the conception of a transformation as a process converting one sentence to another. The treatment at this point shows a significant departure from that in *Syntactic Structures.* Chomsky—quite appropriately for his purpose—applies transformations not to sentences but to "strings" underlying sentences. For school use the less abstract treatment is certainly preferable. In a sense, *English Sentences* follows the same eclectic approach as does *Patterns of English,* only weaving in one more source. However, the material is much better integrated, the book seems more of a unity, and—probably as a consequence of this—it is a much more successful attempt.

Roberts' two books and a few others[14] like them are significant steps forward. They go a long way toward establishing the usefulness of "modern grammar" in the schools and demonstrating one possible way in which the work can be presented. However, in a broader context, they must be considered primarily as pilot projects. As such they suggest the feasibility of further large scale undertakings along the same general lines. Expansion will be needed in several directions if modern grammar is to find its proper place in the total curriculum.

So far we have only isolated one-year textbooks. There is as yet no series that can carry a consistent grammar program from the initial stages to some suitable culmination.* There is, therefore, a serious problem of articulation, both with the work of previous years and, most particularly, with that of following years. A true evaluation of the new approach cannot be made until an on-going program can be tested. Moreover, we cannot expect to reap the full benefit of the change until it is built, with a revitalized sequence in literature and composition, into an articulated program from kindergarten to grade twelve.

Another limitation is in breadth. None of these modern books makes much effort to extend the outreach of grammar toward composition and literature. This is perhaps inevitable at this point in history. The reaction

---

[13] *Patterns of English* follows Fries in designating classes of words by arbitrary numbers or letters. This has been very widely misunderstood. For many people, the mere substitution of "Word of Form Class 1" for "Noun" has seemed like progress, and "modern grammar" has been trivialized to a mere juggling with terminology. Fries had very much deeper reasons for the change than are generally credited to him, but these reasons have been lost sight of by most advocates of "linguistic grammar."

[14] The only other yet widely circulated is: Neil Postman, Harold Morine, and Greta Morine, *Discovering your Language.* New York: Holt, Rinehart & Winston, 1963. Several others have appeared on limited circulation, and additional ones are currently in various stages of preparation.

**Editor's Note:* This article was written in the early 1960s. Since that time, several multigrade textbook series incorporating at least parts of new grammar have been published for use in schools.

against prescriptivism has attenuated the one thread of application of grammar to composition. We have not yet had time to build new and significant connections. The reintegration of the English curriculum and the reestablishment of basic humanistic values throughout its whole structure is the most urgent task before the profession today, but it is equally clearly a long-term undertaking in which only the next steps may be seen at this time. These next steps demand certain specific strengthenings in the grammar program. We can mention only five.

Needs for a Strengthened Grammar Program

Our accustomed treatment of grammar has been notably superficial. The first need, then, is for greater depth at many places. Recent efforts at reform have done something to bring about new content in addition to reconstructing the old. Roberts' *English Sentences,* for example, presents much more material than the books it supplants. Teachers who have made the effort to understand it thoroughly before attempting to use it in the classroom have found that the additions can be taught successfully. With a sound foundation in previous years a great deal more could be covered effectively than is now possible with the meager background students have when they are introduced to a book using a "modern approach." There is certainly room for increase in content, if it can be accompanied by improved efficiency in the use of the available time.[15] Moreover, such an increase is demanded either by the purely liberal objective of building an understanding of language, or by the determination to integrate the English curriculum about its proper language center.

In some topics the needed information is readily at hand, requiring only organization to conform it to the rest of the scheme into which it must be embedded. An example is the distinction between mass and count nouns, seldom mentioned in older textbooks. While there remain some unclear details, the basic facts are now well established. Many details of the behavior of determiners are heavily dependent on this distinction so that it has a significant place in an integrated grammar course. In other cases, the required information is just coming to light, and will be necessary for the curriculum designer to follow new research results closely and critically. An example here is the classification of the adverbs and the

---

[15] The endless review and excessive drill traditional in English grammar teaching result in an extremely low amount of learning-per-hour expended. Simply bringing the efficiency up to the average level prevailing in other subjects would allow a very substantial increase in content. Grammar has been assigned enough time in most school systems to accomplish everything here suggested without imposing any undue pressure on the students. We have simply wasted that time in meaningless activity.

treatment of their places in sentence structure. This has long been a source of confusion in teaching. Recent books clarify the matter somewhat by segregating intensifiers (words like "very"), but there remain numerous difficulties, and some creative new work here is urgently needed.

Grammar has often been thought of as the description of sentence formation. Even when not so defined, the sentence has in practice been the upper limit of concern for most grammarians. In a sense, however, this is just barely across the threshold of real interest in composition and literature study. A second need, then, is for an upward extension of the scope of grammar. Scattered work in very recent years has shown that it is both feasible and useful to study larger patterns by methods that are upward extensions of the grammatical methods used in describing sentence structure.[16] Most of this work has been done on languages other than English, and most of it is fragmentary. Yet its importance must not be underestimated. Details of the techniques are being worked out through experimentation. Our ability to handle phenomena extending beyond sentence boundaries is steadily, if still slowly, increasing. We seem to be on the brink of very significant new developments which may bring rapid acceleration of progress. With it will certainly come penetrating new insights of great importance in composition teaching and the study of literature.

It is a particularly difficult task to build very recent results into a school curriculum, but it can also be a very rewarding one. Experience in some of the recent science curriculum projects indicates the usefulness of this sort of material if broadly liberal educational goals are sought. The random bits already known must be given more prominent places in future school materials, and textbook writers and curriculum planners must follow new developments appreciatively, always watching for new results that will be useful in the classroom. Such are certainly on the way.

Grammar teaching has always been narrowly focused on one form of standard English, the infinite variety of speech and writing habits receiving only silent neglect. Such a partial picture is so unreal as to have cast doubt in the minds of many on the whole structure of grammar. The third need, then, is to broaden the concern of grammar teaching to comprehend more than a single form of the language. Something of this sort is already underway and, increasingly, this segment of the whole is being referred to as *language* rather than as *grammar*. What is being done is generally good, but often far too limited. Both geographical and social

---

[16] The following are more or less random exemplifications of the approaches used:
Zellig S. Harris, "Discourse Analysis." *Language* XXVIII (1952): 18–23.
Eugene E. Loos, *Capanahua Narration Structure*. Texas Studies in Literature and Language IV. Austin, Texas: University of Texas (1963): 699–742.
Leslie H. Stennes, *An Introduction to Fulani Syntax*. Hartford Studies in Linguistics, No. 2. Hartford, Conn.: Hartford Seminary Press, 1961.

dialects are worthy of attention, as is the situational variation in speech that is so important in maintaining social adjustments.[17] The historical dimension also requires attention, and this on a much broader basis than the familiar discussion of meaning changes and word histories. The study of language variation is an important point of contact with the study of literature. Dialect is a favorite device of many writers, and they often use it with a subtlety that is totally lost on many readers. Not only is this so, but in some instances the use of regional and social varieties of language passes completely unnoticed. This is eminently the case with Shakespeare, who was a master of dialect writing. In his works, this dimension lies buried for most readers under the general strangeness even of his normal language. If this can be missed, how much more must remain hidden in his plays? Full understanding of Shakespeare certainly requires a historical dimension in language study that has been almost entirely lacking at the level where his works are first studied.

Grammar must, then, be expanded to become a full study of the English language comprehending both its structure and the variation in its patterns. But the issue is still wider. English is a special case of that most intriguing phenomenon, language. It is best understood in this framework. The fourth need, then, is to broaden the language curriculum beyond English. The syntax, phonology, dialectology, and historical development of the students' own language are clarified—and hence most easily taught—from a perspective of general linguistics. Contrasts with other languages can frequently illuminate points as no amounts of discussion restricted to English can possibly do.

With increasing teaching of foreign languages in American schools, material is becoming more readily at hand. The English class should make full use of these new opportunities. But in addition, examples from more exotic languages can and should be introduced simply to provide contrast and to illustrate significant general principles. That is, the language section of the English curriculum must be expanded to include a considerable amount of general linguistics. This, of course, has values beyond what it contributes to English. In a world of increasingly frequent and increasingly significant multilingual contacts, the general principles of language are profoundly important.

Grammar has tended in the past to be a body of incomprehensible rules handed down with authority to be learned without question—usually with a minimum of explanation. The fifth need, then, is for a total change in the method of presentation of grammar. Two things must be done here. First, we must introduce students to the techniques by which grammatical formulations are arrived at, and show them how these

---

[17] Martin Joos, *The Five Clocks*. Publication of the Research Center in Anthropology, Folklore, and Linguistics, No. 22. Bloomington, Ind.: Indiana University, 1962.

statements are rooted in observations of language. This is most easily done by what is now often called inductive teaching, the leading of students to discover principles for themselves. Grammar happens to be a specially suitable subject for this kind of work, since the data are readily available and generally familiar. Second, our students must not only be made to be critical about language, but equally critical about our understanding of language. At suitable places they must see that there is more than one way to describe a significant point of structure. They should have at least a basic understanding of the major approaches to syntax. They should know something of school grammar, in part because it is assumed in so many places, but equally because its basic assumptions are worth examining. Names like Lowth, Jespersen, Bloomfield, de Saussure should mean as much to them as do Faraday, Mendeleyev, or Pasteur, and they should know Priestly from both Chemistry and English—and understand the significance of his wide-ranging activities. The history of linguistics, like the history of other systems of notable ideas, should be within the purview of an educated man.

Some readers undoubtedly looked at the title at the head of this discussion, "What Grammar?" and mentally translated it "Traditional Grammar, Structural Grammar, or Transformational Grammar?" Such a question ought to receive a fairly straightforward answer in only a few thousand words. But of course it is not the real question, and no such easy answer can be given. All that we can do is to suggest some lines along which to work in building a grammar for the schools. The actual result will have to be hammered out slowly, laboriously, and as a work of craftmanship in the schools themselves. That will take time, knowledge, imagination, and deep understanding of the educational process. To attempt to foresee the result in full outline would be presumptuous.

But what I have suggested, I would like to claim, is realistic. It is based on some, albeit limited, experience in the classroom, mostly in the observation of teachers who are already moving ahead along the five directions proposed. Those who have gone farthest are the most eager to go on. They have seen that every step has taken them farther toward restoring the relevance and the intellectual challenge of the English curriculum, toward its integration and the reaffirmation of a broadly liberal outlook.

W. Nelson Francis' article reprinted here is a classic. It has been reprinted in over twenty anthologies and is probably the most widely quoted article on new grammar ever written. The grammatical revolution referred to in the title is one of structural grammar. The article was originally published in 1954 (the year before Chomsky's *Syntactic Structures)* and in Francis' own words in a telephone conversation I had with him, "A lot of water has gone under the bridge since that time." Nevertheless, a great deal of what Francis has to say is as important and relevant in the 70s as it was in the 50s.

He begins with a useful distinction between various interpretations of the word grammar. He identifies the fundamental tenets and premises on which structural grammar is built, briefly sketches the history of traditional grammar, and points to some of the inadequacies of the traditional model. He then presents some of the rationale and content of structural grammar, with illustrations of how we use the structural devices contained in our language. The final section addresses itself to the two questions: What is the value of this new system? and How can the change from one grammar to the other be effected?

Revolution in Grammar

W. Nelson Francis

I

A long overdue revolution is at present taking place in the study of English grammar—a revolution as sweeping in its consequences as the Darwinian revolution in biology. It is the result of the application to English of methods of descriptive analysis originally developed for use with languages of primitive people. To anyone at all interested in language, it is challenging; to those concerned with the teaching of English (including parents), it presents the necessity of radically revising both the substance and the methods of their teaching.

A curious paradox exists in regard to grammar. On the one hand it is felt to be the dullest and driest of academic subjects, fit only for those in whose veins the red blood of life has long since turned to ink. On the other, it is a subject on which people who would scorn to be professional grammarians hold very dogmatic opinions, which they will defend with

* This paper was written nearly twenty years ago. During the intervening time, theories of grammar and the views of grammarians, including the author, have changed drastically. But the article reflects faithfully the views of a structural grammarian of his time.

considerable emotion. Much of this prejudice stems from the usual sources of prejudice—ignorance and confusion. Even highly educated people seldom have a clear idea of what grammarians do, and there is an unfortunate confusion about the meaning of the term "grammar" itself.

Hence it would be well to begin with definitions. What do people mean when they use the word grammar? Actually the word is used to refer to three different things, and much of the emotional thinking about matters grammatical arises from confusion among these different meanings.

The first thing we mean by grammar is "the set of formal patterns in which the words of a language are arranged in order to convey larger meanings." It is not necessary that we be able to discuss these patterns self-consciously in order to be able to use them. In fact, all speakers of a language above the age of five or six know how to use its complex forms of organization with considerable skill; in this sense of the word—call it Grammar 1—they are thoroughly familiar with its grammar.

The second meaning of grammar—call it Grammar 2—is "the branch of linguistic science which is concerned with the description, analysis, and formulization of formal language patterns." Just as gravity was in full operation before Newton's apple fell, so grammar in the first sense was in full operation before anyone formulated the first rule that began the history of grammar as a study.

The third sense in which people use the word grammar is "linguistic etiquette." This we may call Grammar 3. The word in this sense is often coupled with a derogatory adjective: we say that the expression "he ain't here" is bad grammar. What we mean is that such an expression is bad linguistic manners in certain circles. From the point of view of Grammar 1 it is faultless; it conforms just as completely to the structural patterns of English as does "he isn't here." The trouble with it is like the trouble with Prince Hal in Shakespeare's play—it is bad, not in itself, but in the company it keeps.

As has already been suggested, much confusion arises from mixing these meanings. One hears a good deal of criticism of teachers of English couched in such terms as "they don't teach grammar any more." Criticism of this sort is based on the wholly unproved assumption that teaching Grammar 2 will increase the student's proficiency in Grammar 1 or improve his manners in Grammar 3. Actually, the form of Grammar 2 which is usually taught is a very inaccurate and misleading analysis of the facts of Grammar 1; and it therefore is of highly questionable value in improving a person's ability to handle the structural patterns of his language. It is hardly reasonable to expect that teaching a person some inaccurate grammatical analysis will either improve the effectiveness of his assertions or teach him what expressions are acceptable to use in a given social context.

These, then, are the three meanings of grammar: Grammar 1, a form of behavior; Grammar 2, a field of study, a science; and Grammar 3, a branch of etiquette.

II

Grammarians have arrived at some basic principles of their science, three of which are fundamental to this discussion. The first is that a language constitutes a set of behavior patterns common to the members of a given community. It is a part of what the anthropologists call the culture of the community. Actually it has complex and intimate relationships with other phases of culture such as myth and ritual. But for purposes of study it may be dealt with as a separate set of phenomena that can be objectively described and analyzed like any other universe of facts. Specifically, its phenomena can be observed, recorded, classified, and compared; and general laws of their behavior can be made by the same inductive process that is used to produce the "laws" of physics, chemistry, and the other sciences.

A second important principle of linguistic science is that each language or dialect has its own unique system of behavior patterns. Parts of this system may show similarities to parts of the systems of other languages, particularly if those languages are genetically related. But different languages solve the problems of expression and communication in different ways, just as the problems of movement through water are solved in different ways by lobsters, fish, seals, and penguins. A couple of corollaries of this principle are important. The first is that there is no such thing as "universal grammar," or at least if there is, it is so general and abstract as to be of little use. The second corollary is that the grammar of each language must be made up on the basis of a study of that particular language—a study that is free from preconceived notions of what a language should contain and how it should operate. The marine biologist does not criticize the octopus for using jet-propulsion to get him through the water instead of the methods of a self-respecting fish. Neither does the linguistic scientist express alarm or distress when he finds a language that seems to get along quite well without any words that correspond to what in English we call verbs.

A third principle on which linguistic science is based is that the analysis and description of a given language must conform to the requirements laid down for any satisfactory scientific theory. These are (1) simplicity, (2) consistency, (3) completeness, and (4) usefulness for predicting the behavior of phenomena not brought under immediate observation when the theory was formed. Linguistic scientists who have recently turned their attention to English have found that, judged by these criteria, the traditional grammar of English is unsatisfactory. It falls down badly on the first two requirements, being unduly complex and glaringly inconsistent within itself. It can be made to work, just as the Ptolemaic earth-centered astronomy can be, but at the cost of great elaboration and complication. The new grammar, like the Copernican sun-centered astronomy, solves the same problems with greater elegance, which is the scientist's word for the simplicity, compactness, and tidiness that characterize a satisfactory theory.

III

A brief look at the history of the traditional grammar of English will make apparent the reasons for its inadequacy. The study of English grammar is actually an outgrowth of the linguistic interest of the Renaissance. It was during the later Middle Ages and early Renaissance that the various vernacular languages of Europe came into their own. They began to be used for many kinds of writing which had previously always been done in Latin. As the vernaculars, in the hands of great writers like Dante and Chaucer, came of age as members of the linguistic family, a concomitant interest in their grammars arose. The earliest important English grammar was written by Shakespeare's contemporary, Ben Jonson.

It is important to observe that not only Ben Jonson himself but also those who followed him in the study of English grammar were men deeply learned in Latin and sometimes in Greek. For all their interest in English, they were conditioned from earliest school days to conceive of the classical languages as superior to the vernaculars. We still sometimes call the elementary school the grammar school; historically the term means the school where Latin grammar was taught. By the time the Renaissance or eighteenth-century scholar took his university degree, he was accustomed to use Latin as the normal means of communication with his fellow scholars. Dr. Samuel Johnson, for instance, who had only three years at the university and did not take a degree, wrote poetry in both Latin and Greek. Hence it was natural for these men to take Latin grammar as the norm, and to analyze English in terms of Latin. The grammarians of the seventeenth and eighteenth centuries who formulated the traditional grammar of English looked for the devices and distinctions of Latin grammar in English, and where they did not actually find them they imagined or created them. Of course, since English is a member of the Indo-European family of languages, to which Latin and Greek also belong, it did have many grammatical elements in common with them. But many of these had been obscured or wholly lost as a result of the extensive changes that had taken place in English—changes that the early grammarians inevitably conceived of as degeneration. They felt that it was their function to resist further change, if not to repair the damage already done. So preoccupied were they with the grammar of Latin as the ideal that they overlooked in large part the exceedingly complex and delicate system that English had substituted for the Indo-European grammar it had abandoned. Instead they stretched unhappy English on the Procrustean bed of Latin. It is no wonder that we commonly hear people say, "I didn't really understand grammar until I began to study Latin." This is eloquent testimony to the fact that the grammar "rules" of our present-day textbooks are largely an inheritance from the Latin-based grammar of the eighteenth century.

Meanwhile the extension of linguistic study beyond the Indo-European and Semitic families began to reveal that there are many different ways in which linguistic phenomena are organized—in other words, many different kinds of grammar. The tone-languages of the Orient and of North America, and the complex agglutinative languages of Africa, among others, forced grammarians to abandon the idea of a universal or ideal grammar and to direct their attention more closely to the individual systems employed by the multifarious languages of mankind. With the growth and refinement of the scientific method and its application to the field of anthropology, language came under more rigorous scientific scrutiny. As with anthropology in general, linguistic science at first concerned itself with the primitive. Finally, again following the lead of anthropology, linguistics began to apply its techniques to the old familiar tongues, among them English. Accelerated by the practical need during World War II of teaching languages, including English, to large numbers in a short time, research into the nature of English grammar has moved rapidly in the last fifteen years. The definitive grammar of English is yet to be written, but the results so far achieved are spectacular. It is now as unrealistic to teach "traditional" grammar of English as it is to teach "traditional" (that is, pre-Darwinian) biology or "traditional" (that is, four-element) chemistry. Yet nearly all certified teachers of English on all levels are doing so. Here is a cultural lag of major proportions.

IV

Before we can proceed to a sketch of what the new grammar of English looks like, we must take account of a few more of the premises of linguistic science. They must be understood and accepted by anyone who wishes to understand the new grammar.

First, the spoken language is primary, at least for the original study of a language. In many of the primitive languages,[1] of course, where writing is unknown, the spoken language is the *only* form. This is in many ways an advantage to the linguist, because the written language may use conventions that obscure its basic structure. The reason for the primary importance of the spoken language is that language originates as speech, and most of the changes and innovations that occur in the history of a given language begin in the spoken tongue.

Secondly, we must take account of the concept of dialect. I suppose most laymen would define a dialect as "a corrupt form of language spoken in a given region by people who don't know any better." This introduces moral judgments which are repulsive to the linguistic scholar. Let us approach the definition of a dialect from the more objective end, through the notion of a speech community. A speech community is merely a group of people who are in pretty constant intercommunication. There are various types of speech communities: local ones, like "the people who live in Tidewater Virginia"; class ones, like "the white-collar class"; occupational ones, like "doctors, nurses, and other people who work in hospitals"; social ones, like "clubwomen." In a sense, each of these has its own dialect. Each family may be said to have its own dialect; in fact, in so far as each of us has his own vocabulary and particular quirks of speech, each individual has his own dialect. Also, of course, in so far as he is a member of many speech communities, each individual is more or less master of many dialects and shifts easily and almost unconsciously from one to another as he shifts from one social environment to another.

In the light of this concept of dialects, a language can be defined as a group of dialects which have enough of their sound-system, vocabulary, and grammar (Grammar 1, that is) in common to permit their speakers to be mutually intelligible in the ordinary affairs of life. It usually happens that one of the many dialects that make up a language comes to have more prestige than the others; in modern times it has usually been the dialect of the middle-class residents of the capital, like Parisian French and London English, which is so distinguished. This comes to be thought of as the standard dialect; in fact, its speakers become snobbish and succeed in establishing the belief that it is not a dialect at all, but the only proper form of the language. This causes the speakers of other dialects to become self-conscious and ashamed of their speech, or else aggressive and jingoistic about it—either of which is an acknowledgment of their feelings of inferiority. Thus one of the duties of the educational system comes to be that of teaching the standard dialect to all so as to

---

[1] "Primitive languages" here is really an abbreviated statement for "languages used by peoples of relatively primitive culture"; it is not to be taken as implying anything simple or rudimentary about the languages themselves. Many languages included under the term, such as native languages of Africa and Mexico, exhibit grammatical complexities unknown to more "civilized" languages.

relieve them of feelings of inferiority, and thus relieve society of linguistic neurotics. This is where Grammar 3, linguistic etiquette, comes into the picture.

A third premise arising from the two just discussed is that the difference between the way educated people talk and the way they write is a dialectical difference. The spread between these two dialects may be very narrow, as in present-day America, or very wide, as in Norway, where people often speak local Norwegian dialects but write in the Dano-Norwegian *Riksmaal.* The extreme is the use by writers of an entirely different language, or at least an ancient and no longer spoken form of the language—like Sanskrit in northern India or Latin in Western Europe during the Middle Ages. A corollary of this premise is that anyone setting out to write a grammar must know and make clear whether he is dealing with the spoken or the written dialect. Virtually all current English grammars deal with the written language only; evidence for this is that their rules for the plurals of nouns, for instance, are really spelling rules, which say nothing about pronunciation.

This is not the place to go into any sort of detail about the methods of analysis the linguistic scientist uses. Suffice it to say that he begins by breaking up the flow of speech into minimum sound-units, or phones, which he then groups into families called phonemes, the minimum significant sound-units. Most languages have from twenty to sixty of these. American English has forty-one: nine vowels, twenty-four consonants, four degrees of stress, and four levels of pitch. These phonemes group themselves into minimum meaningful units, called morphemes. These fall into two groups: free morphemes, those that can enter freely into many combinations with other free morphemes to make phrases and sentences; and bound morphemes, which are always found tied in a close and often indissoluble relationship with other bound or free morphemes. An example of a free morpheme is "dog"; an example of a bound morpheme is *un-* or *ex-*. The linguist usually avoids talking about "words" because the term is very inexact. Is "instead of," for instance, to be considered one, two, or three words? This is purely a matter of opinion; but it is a matter of fact that it is made up of three morphemes.

In any case, our analysis has now brought the linguist to the point where he has some notion of the word-stock (he would call it the *lexicon*) of his language. He must then go into the question of how the morphemes are grouped into meaningful utterances, which is the field of grammar proper. At this point in the analysis of English, as of many other languages, it becomes apparent that there are three bases upon which classification and analysis may be built: form, function, and meaning. For illustration let us take the word *boys* in the utterance "the boys are here." From the point of view of form, *boys* is a noun with the plural ending *s* (pronounced like *z*), preceded by the noun-determiner *the*, and tied by concord to the verb *are*, which it precedes. From the point of view of function, *boys* is the subject of the verb *are* and of the sentence. From the point of view of meaning, *boys* points out or names more than one of the male young of the human species, about whom an assertion is being made.

Of these three bases of classification, the one most amenable to objective description and analysis of a rigorously scientific sort is form. In fact, many conclusions about form can be drawn by a person unable to understand or speak the language. Next comes function. But except as it is revealed by form, function is dependent on knowing the meaning. In a telegraphic sentence such as "ship sails today"[2] no one can say whether *ship* is the subject of *sails* or an imperative verb with *sails* as its object until he knows what the sentence means. Most shaky of all bases for grammatical analysis is meaning. Attempts have been made to reduce the phenomena of meaning to objective description, but so far they have not succeeded very well. Meaning is such a subjective quality that it is usually omitted entirely from scientific description. The botanist can describe the forms of plants and the functions of their various parts, but he refuses to concern himself with their meaning. It is left to the poet to find symbolic meaning in roses, violets, and lilies.

At this point it is interesting to note that the traditional grammar of English bases some of its key concepts and definitions on this very subjective and shaky foundation of meaning. A recent English grammar defines a sentence as "a group of words which expresses a complete thought through the use of a verb, called its predicate, and a subject, consisting of a noun or pronoun about which the verb has something to say."[3] But what is a complete thought? Actually we do not identify sentences this way at all. If someone says, "I don't know what to do," dropping his voice at the end, and pauses, the hearer will know that it is quite safe for him to make a comment without running the risk of interrupting an unfinished sentence. But if the speaker says the same words and maintains a level pitch at the end, the polite listener will wait for him to finish his sentence. The words are the same, the meaning is the same; the only difference is a slight one in the pitch of the final syllable—a purely formal distinction, which signals that the first utterance is complete, a sentence, while the second is incomplete. In writing we would translate these signals into punctuation: a period or exclamation point at the end of the first, a comma or dash at the end of the second. It is the form of the utterance, not the completeness of the thought, that tells us whether it is a whole sentence or only part of one.

---

[2] This example is taken from C. C. Fries, *The Structure of English*. New York: Harcourt, Brace, 1952, p. 62. This important book will be discussed later.

[3] Ralph B. Allen, *English Grammar*. New York: American Book Company, 1950, p. 187.

Another favorite definition of the traditional grammar, also based on meaning, is that of *noun* as "the name of a person, place, or thing"; or, as the grammar just quoted has it, "the name of anybody or anything, with or without life, and with or without substance or form."[4] Yet we identify nouns, not by asking if they name something, but by their positions in expressions and by the formal marks they carry. In the sentence, "The slithy toves did gyre and gimble in the wabe," any speaker of English knows that *toves* and *wabe* are nouns, though he cannot tell what they name, if indeed they name anything. How does he know? Actually because they have certain formal marks, like their position in relation to *the* as well as the whole arrangement of the sentence. We know from our practical knowledge of English grammar (Grammar 1), which we have had since before we went to school, that if we were to put meaningful words into this sentence, we would have to put nouns in place of *toves* and *wabe*, giving something like "The slithy snakes did gyre and gamble in the wood." The pattern of the sentence simply will not allow us to say "The slithy arounds did gyre and gimble in the wooden."

One trouble with the traditional grammar, then, is that it relies heavily on the most subjective element in language, meaning. Another is that it shifts the ground of its classification and produces the elementary logical error of cross-division. A zoologist who divided animals into invertebrates, mammals, and beasts of burden would not get very far before running into trouble. Yet the traditional grammar is guilty of the same error when it defines three parts of speech on the basis of meaning (noun, verb, and interjection), four more on the basis of function (adjective, adverb, pronoun, conjunction), and one partly on function and partly on form (preposition). The result is that in such an expression as "a dog's life" there can be endless futile argument about whether *dog's* is a noun or an adjective. It is, of course, a noun from the point of view of form and an adjective from the point of view of function, and hence falls into both classes, just as a horse is both a mammal and a beast of burden. No wonder students are bewildered in their attempts to master the traditional grammar. Their natural clearness of mind tells them that it is a crazy patchwork violating the elementary principles of logical thought.

V

If the traditional grammar is so bad, what does the new grammar offer in its place?

It offers a description, analysis, and set of definitions and formulas—rules, if you will—based firmly and consistently on the easiest, or at

---

[4] Ibid., p. 1.

least the most objective, aspect of language, form. Experts can quibble over whether *dog's* in "a dog's life" is a noun or an adjective, but anyone can see that it is spelled with *'s* and hear that it ends with a *z* sound; likewise anyone can tell that it comes in the middle between *a* and *life.* Furthermore he can tell that something important has happened if the expression is changed to "the dog's alive," "the live dogs," or "the dogs lived," even if he doesn't know what the words mean and has never heard of such functions as modifier, subject, or attributive genitive. He cannot, of course, get very far into his analysis without either a knowledge of the language or access to someone with such knowledge. He will also need a minimum technical vocabulary describing grammatical functions. Just so the anatomist is better off for knowing physiology. But the grammarian, like the anatomist, must beware of allowing his preconceived notions to lead him into the error of interpreting before he describes—an error which often results in his finding only what he is looking for.

When the grammarian looks at English objectively, he finds that it conveys its meanings by two broad devices: the denotations and connotations of words separately considered, which the linguist calls *lexical meaning*, and the significance of word-form, word-groups, and arrangements apart from the lexical meanings of the words, which the linguist calls *structural meaning.* The first of these is the domain of the lexicographer and the semanticist, and hence is not our present concern. The second, the structural meaning, is the business of the structural linguist, or grammarian. The importance of this second kind of meaning must be emphasized because it is often overlooked. The man in the street tends to think of the meaning of a sentence as being the aggregate of the dictionary meanings of the words that make it up; hence the widespread fallacy of literal translation—the feeling that if you take a French sentence and a French-English dictionary and write down the English equivalent of each French word you will come out with an intelligible English sentence. How ludicrous the results can be, anyone knows who is familiar with Mark Twain's retranslation from the French of his jumping frog story. One sentence read, "Eh bien! I no saw not that that frog has nothing of better than each frog." Upon which Mark's comment is, "if that isn't grammar gone to seed, then I count myself no judge."[5]

The second point brought out by a formal analysis of English is that it uses four principal devices of form to signal structural meanings:

1. Word order—the sequence in which words and word-groups are arranged.

---

[5] Mark Twain, "The Jumping Frog; the Original Story in English; the Retranslation Clawed Back from the French, into a Civilized Language Once More, by Patient and Unremunerated Toil," *1601 . . . and Sketches Old and New* (n.p. 1933), p. 50.

2. Function-words—words devoid of lexical meaning that indicate relationships among the meaningful words with which they appear.
3. Inflections—alternations in the forms of words themselves to signal changes in meaning and relationship.
4. Formal contrasts—contrasts in the forms of words signaling greater differences in function and meaning. These could also be considered inflections, but it is more convenient for both the lexicographer and the grammarian to consider them separately.

Usually several of these are present in any utterance, but they can be separately illustrated by means of contrasting expressions involving minimum variations—the kind of controlled experiment used in the scientific laboratory.

To illustrate the structural meaning of word order, let us compare the two sentences "man bites dog" and "dog bites man."—The words are identical in lexical meaning and in form; the only difference is in sequence. It is interesting to note that Latin expresses the difference between these two by changes in the form of the words, without necessarily altering the order: "homo canem mordet" or "hominem canis mordet." Latin grammar is worse than useless in understanding this point of English grammar.

Next, compare the sentences "the dog is the friend of man" and "any dog is a friend of that man." Here the words having lexical meaning are *dog*, *is*, *friend*, and *man*, which appear in the same form and the same order in both sentences. The formal differences between them are in the substitution of *any* and *a* for *the*, and in the insertion of *that*. These little words are function-words; they make quite a difference in the meanings of the two sentences, though it is virtually impossible to say what they mean in isolation

Third, compare the sentences "the dog loves the man" and "the dogs loved the men." Here the words are the same, in the same order, with the same function-words in the same positions. But the forms of the three words having lexical meanings have been changed: *dog* to *dogs, loves* to *loved*, and *man* to *men*. These changes are inflections. English has very few of them as compared with Greek, Latin, Russian, or even German. But it still uses them; about one word in four in an ordinary English sentence is inflected.

Fourth, consider the difference between "the dog's friend arrived" and "the dog's friendly arrival." Here the difference lies in the change of *friend* to *friendly*, a formal alteration signaling a change of function from subject to modifier, and the change of *arrived* to *arrival*, signaling a change of function from predicate to head-word in a noun-modifier group. These changes are of the same formal nature as inflections, but because they produce words of different lexical meaning, classifiable as different parts of speech, it is better to call them formal contrasts than inflections. In other words, it is logically quite defensible to consider *love*, *loving*, and *loved* as the same word in differing aspects and to consider *friend*, *friendly*, *friendliness*, *friendship*, and *befriend* as different words related by formal and semantic similarities. But this is only a matter of convenience of analysis, which permits a more accurate description of English structure. In another language we might find that this kind of distinction is unnecessary but that some other distinction, unnecessary in English, is required. The categories of grammatical description are not sacrosanct; they are as much a part of man's organization of his observations as they are of the nature of things.

If we are considering the spoken variety of English, we must add a fifth device for indicating structural meaning—the various musical and rhythmic patterns which the linguist classifies under juncture, stress, and intonation. Consider the following pair of sentences:

Alfred, the alligator is sick.
Alfred the alligator is sick.

These are identical in the four respects discussed above—word order, function-words, inflections, and word-form. Yet they have markedly different meanings, as would be revealed by the intonation if they were spoken aloud. These differences in intonation are to a certain extent indicated in the written language by punctuation—that is, in fact, the primary function of punctuation.

VI

The examples so far given were chosen to illustrate in isolation the various kinds of structural devices in English grammar. Much more commonly the structural meaning of a given sentence is indicated by a combination of two or more of these devices: a sort of margin of safety which permits some of the devices to be missed or done away with without obscuring the structural meaning of the sentence, as indeed anyone knows who has ever written a telegram or a newspaper headline. On the other hand, sentences which do not have enough of these formal devices are inevitably ambiguous. Take the example already given, Fries's "ship sails today." This is ambiguous because there is nothing to indicate which of the first two words is performing a noun function and which a verb function. If we mark the noun by putting the noun-determining function-word *the* in front of it, the ambiguity disappears; we have either "the ship sails today" or "ship the sails today." The ambiguity could just as well be resolved by using other devices: consider "ship sailed today," "ship to sail today," "shipping sails today," "shipment of sails today," and so on. It is simply a question of having enough formal devices in the sentence to indicate its structural meaning clearly.

How powerful the structural meanings of English are is illustrated by so-called "nonsense." In English, nonsense as a literary form often consists of utterances that have a clear structural meaning but use words that either have no lexical meanings, or whose lexical meanings are inconsistent one with another. This will become apparent if we suggest a rather famous bit of English nonsense to formal grammatical analysis:

All mimsy were the borogoves
And the mome raths outgrabe.

This passage consists of ten words, five of them words that should have lexical meaning but don't, one standard verb, and four function-words. In so far as it is possible to indicate its abstract structure, it would be this:

All. . . .y were the . . . . .s
And the . . . . . .s. . . . . . .

Although this is a relatively simple formal organization, it signals some rather complicated meanings. The first thing we observe is that the first line presents a conflict: word order seems to signal one thing, and inflections and function-words something else. Specifically, *mimsy* is in the position normally occupied by the subject, but we know that it is not the subject and that *borogroves* is. We know this because there is an inflectional tie between the form *were* and the *s* ending of *borogroves*, because there is the noun-determiner *the* before it, and because the alternative candidate for subject, *mimsy*, lacks both of these. It is true that *mimsy* does have the function-word *all* before it, which may indicate a noun, but when it does, the noun is either plural (in which case *mimsy* would most likely end in *s*), or else the noun is what grammarians call a mass-word (like *sugar*, *coal*, *snow*), in which case the verb would have to be *was*, not *were*. All these formal considerations are sufficient to counteract the effect of word order and show that the sentence is of the type that may be represented thus:

All gloomy were the Democrats.

Actually there is one other possibility. If *mimsy* belongs to the small group of nouns which don't use *s* to make the plural, and if *borogroves* has been so implied (but not specifically mentioned) in the context as to justify its appearing with the determiner *the*, the sentence would then belong to the following type:

(In the campaign for funds) all alumni were the canvassers.
(In the drought last summer) all cattle were the sufferers.

But the odds are so much against this that most of us would be prepared to fight for our belief that *borogroves* are things that can be named, and that at the time referred to they were in a complete state of *mimsyness.*

Moving on to the second line, "And the mome raths outgrabe," the first thing we note is that the *And* signals another parallel assertion to follow. We are thus prepared to recognize from the noun-determiner *the*, the plural inflection *s*, and the particular positions of *mome* and *outgrabe*, as well as the continuing influence of the "were" of the preceding line, that we are dealing with a sentence of this pattern:

And the lone rats agreed.

The influence of the *were* is particularly important here; it guides us in selecting among several interpretations of the sentence. Specifically, it requires us to identify *outgrabe* as a verb, since it lacks the characteristic past-tense ending *d* or *ed*. We do this in spite of the fact that there is another strong candidate for the position of verb: that is, *raths*, which bears a regular verb inflection and could be tied with *mome* as its subject in the normal noun-verb relationship. In such a case we should have to recognize *outgrabe* as either an adverb of the kind not marked by the form-contrast *ly*, an adjective, or the past participle of a strong verb. The sentence would then belong to one of the following types:

And the moon shines above.
And the man stays aloof.
And the fool seems outdone.

But we reject all of these—probably they don't even occur to us—because they all have verbs in the present tense, whereas the *were* of the first line combines with the *And* at the beginning of the second to set the whole in the past.

We might recognize one further possibility for the structural meaning of this second line, particularly in the verse context, since we are used to certain patterns in verse that do not often appear in speech or prose.

The *were* of the first line could be understood as doing double duty, its ghost or echo appearing between *raths* and *outgrabe*. Then we would have something like this:

All gloomy were the Democrats
And the home folks outraged.

But again the odds are pretty heavy against this. I for one am so sure that *outgrabe* is the past tense of a strong verb that I can give its present. In my dialect, at least, it is *outgribe*.

The reader may not realize it, but in the last four paragraphs I have been discussing grammar from a purely formal point of view. I have not once called a word a noun because it names something (that is, I have not once resorted to meaning), nor have I called any word an adjective because it modifies a noun (that is, resorted to function). Instead I have been working in the opposite direction, from form toward function and meaning. I have used only criteria which are objectively observable, and I have assumed only a working knowledge of certain structural patterns and devices known to all speakers of English over the age of six. I did use some technical terms like *noun*, *verb*, and *tense*, but only to save time; I could have got along without them.

If one clears his mind of the inconsistencies of the traditional grammar (not so easy a process as it might be), he can proceed with a similarly rigorous formal analysis of a sufficient number of representative utterances in English and come out with a descriptive grammar. This is just what Fries did in gathering and studying the material for the analysis he presents in the remarkable book to which I have already referred, *The Structure of English.* What he actually did was to put a tape recorder into action and record about fifty hours of telephone conversation among the good citizens of Ann Arbor, Michigan. When this material was transcribed, it constituted about a quarter of a million words of perfectly natural speech by educated middle-class Americans. The details of his conclusions cannot be presented here, but they are sufficiently different from the usual grammar to be revolutionary. For instance, he recognizes only four parts of speech among the words with lexical meaning, roughly corresponding to what the traditional grammar calls substantives, verbs, adjectives and adverbs, though to avoid preconceived notions from the traditional grammar Fries calls them Class 1, Class 2, Class 3, and Class 4 words. To these he adds a relatively small group of function-words, 154 in his materials, which he divides into fifteen groups. These must be memorized by anyone learning the language; they are not subject to the same kind of general rules that govern the four parts of speech. Undoubtedly his conclusion will be developed and modified by him and by other linguistic scholars, but for the present his book remains the most complete treatment extant of English grammar from the point of view of linguistic science.

VII

Two vital questions are raised by this revolution in grammar. The first is, "What is the value of this new system?" In the minds of many who ask it, the implication of this question is, "We have been getting along all these years with traditional grammar, so it can't be so very bad. Why should we go through the painful process of unlearning and relearning grammar just because linguistic scientists have concocted some new theories?"

The first answer to this question is the bravest and most honest. It is that the superseding of vague and sloppy thinking by clear and precise thinking is an exciting experience in and for itself. To acquire insight into the working of a language, and to recognize the infinitely delicate system of relationship, balance and interplay that constitutes its grammar, is to become closely acquainted with one of man's most miraculous creations, not unworthy to be set beside the equally beautiful organization of the physical universe. And to find that its most complex effects are produced by the multilayered organization of relatively simple materials is to bring our thinking about language into accord with modern thought in other fields, which is more and more coming to emphasize the importance of organization—the fact that an organized whole is truly greater than the sum of all its parts.

There are other answers, more practical if less philosophically valid. It is too early to tell, but it seems probable that a realistic, scientific grammar should vastly facilitate the teaching of English, especially as a foreign language. Already results are showing here; it has been found that if intonation contours and other structural patterns are taught quite early, the student has a confidence that allows him to attempt to speak the language much sooner than he otherwise would.

The new grammar can also be of use in improving the native speaker's proficiency in handling the structural devices of his own language. In other words, Grammar 2, if it is accurate and consistent, *can* be of use in improving skill in Grammar 1. An illustration is that famous bugaboo, the dangling participle. Consider a specific instance of it, which once appeared on a college freshman's theme, to the mingled delight and despair of the instructor:

Having eaten our lunch, the steamboat departed.

What is the trouble with this sentence? Clearly there must be something wrong with it, because it makes people laugh, although it was not the intent of the writer to make them laugh. In other words, it produces a completely wrong response, resulting in total breakdown of communication. It is, in fact, "bad grammar" in a much more serious way than are mere dialectal divergences like "he ain't here" or "he never seen none," which produce social reactions but communicate effectively. In the light of the new grammar, the trouble with our dangling participle is that the form, instead of leading to the meaning, is in conflict with it. Into the position which, in this pattern, is reserved for the word naming the eater of the lunch, the writer has inserted the word *steamboat.* The resulting tug-of-war between form and meaning is only momentary; meaning quickly wins out, simply because our common sense tells us that steamboats don't eat lunches. But if the pull of the lexical meaning is not given a good deal of help from common sense, the form will conquer the meaning, or the two will remain in ambiguous equilibrium—as, for instance, in "Having eaten our lunch, the passengers boarded the steamboat." Writers will find it easier to avoid such troubles if they know about the forms of English and are taught to use the form to convey the meaning, instead of setting up tensions between form and meaning. This, of course, is what English teachers are already trying to do. The new grammar should be a better weapon in their arsenal than the traditional grammar since it is based on a clear understanding of the realities.

The second and more difficult question is, "How can the change from one grammar to the other be effected?" Here we face obstacles of a formidable nature. When we remember the controversies attending on revolutionary changes in biology and astronomy, we realize what a tenacious hold the race can maintain on anything it has once learned, and the resistance it can offer to new ideas. And remember that neither astronomy nor biology was taught in elementary schools. They were, in fact, rather specialized subjects in advanced education. How then change grammar, which is taught to everybody, from the fifth grade up through college? The vested interest represented by thousands upon thousands of English and speech teachers who have learned the traditional grammar and taught it for many years is a conservative force comparable to those which keep us still using the chaotic system of English spelling and the unwieldy measuring system of inches and feet, pounds and ounces, quarts, bushels, and acres. Moreover, this army is constantly receiving new recruits. It is possible in my state to become certified to teach English in high school if one has had eighteen credit hours of college English—let us say two semesters of freshman composition (almost all of which is taught by people unfamiliar with the new grammar), two semesters of a survey course in English literature, one semester of Shakespeare, and one semester of the contemporary novel. And since hard-pressed school administrators feel that anyone who can speak English can in a pinch teach it, the result is that many people are called upon to teach grammar whose knowledge of the subject is totally inadequate.

There is, in other words, a battle ahead of the new grammar. It will have to fight not only the apathy of the general public but the ignorance and inertia of those who count themselves competent in the field of grammar. The battle is already on, in fact. Those who try to get the concepts of the new grammar introduced into the curriculum are tagged as "liberal" grammarians— the implication being, I suppose, that one has a free choice between "liberal" and "conservative" grammar, and that the liberals are a bit dangerous, perhaps even a touch subversive. They are accused of undermining standards, of holding that "any way of saying something is just as good as any other," of not teaching the fundamentals of good English. I trust that the readers of this article will see how unfounded these charges are. But the smear campaign is on. So far as I know, neither religion nor patriotism has yet been brought into it. When they are, Fries will have to say to Socrates, Galileo, Darwin, Freud, and the other members of the honorable fraternity of the misunderstood, "Move over, gentlemen, and make room for me."

Carl A. Lefevre's article is a more recent and less comprehensive account of structural grammar than the preceding article. He sees the value of structural grammar as providing "a heightened consciousness of English language structure."

In his presentation of structural grammar, Lefevre highlights four subsystems of structural features in language—intonation, sentence patterns, structure words, and word-form changes—briefly describes each, and makes passing reference to the usefulness of some of these structural features in improving language performance.

A Concise Structural Grammar

Carl A. Lefevre

"Every teacher an English teacher" is not so much a slogan as a fact of life. Unfortunately, native ability to speak and write a language, any language, does not qualify anyone to teach that language. This is as true of English speakers teaching English to English-speaking children as it is, say, of French speakers teaching French to the same children. Language teaching, whether of a first language or a second language, is a professional specialty; modern language teaching is based on linguistics, the descriptive study of language.

But all teachers, if they want to, can learn enough about applied English linguistics to do greater good than harm to the emergent English skills of their students. This article points the way by presenting a concise modern grammar drawn from structural linguistics. This description relies upon the native linguistic ability and intuitions of born English speakers. It makes no pretense of probing all the subtleties and intricacies of the language; for our purposes such probing is not only unnecessary, it might well prove destructive. Enough is enough.

What Is "Correct" English?

There is no one single correct English, but a variety of English styles, patterns, and usages for various speakers and writers in their varied writing and speaking situations.

Wherever you go in the English-speaking world, you will find a standard national or regional version of English speech. Standard English has been defined as the language in which the main business of any community is carried on. So much for spoken English.

There is a much broader area of agreement throughout the world on standard written English. The written form of our language tends to iron out regional and even national differences. Written English in its standard forms is known all over the world today. A heightened consciousness of English language structure will prove helpful to both teachers and pupils in their search for keys to literacy.

English: Its Four Subsystems

The English language is a commonly understood system of vocal symbols by means of which we communicate with one another; for convenience, we may divide it into four subdivisions, as follows:

1. *Intonation.* Intonation means the speech rhythms and melodies of native speech; a "foreign" intonation marks the foreigner: we recognize him as nonnative by his smaller speech sounds. Intonation gives the overall configuration to the spoken sentence; it is very important in the "silent" language-related processes of writing and reading.

The elements of intonation are levels of pitch, degrees of stress (loudness, or accent), and junctures (or pauses). These three elements pattern together in overall intonation patterns.

2. *Sentence Patterns.* The typical English sentence pattern has a subject (Noun part), a verb (Verb part), and a complement (Completer). Four important sentence patterns exist for making statements, the "declarative sentences" of school grammar. These patterns may be infinitely expanded and varied by inversion, by substitutions within patterns, and by pattern transformation, such as passive constructions. Other common patterns are questions, requests, and commands.

3. *Structure Words.* Structure words (or function words) primarily show grammatical and syntactical relationships within sentence patterns; structure words have minimal reference to the real (nonsymbolic) world of meaning outside the language system itself. The most important structure words are noun markers, verb markers, clause markers, phrase markers, and question markers.

4. *Word-Form Changes.* Word-form changes include the *inflectional endings* of the four word classes, or parts of speech (noun, including the forms of pronouns; verb, adjective, and adverb); they also include the *derivational prefixes* and *suffixes* that modify the meanings of words or convert words from one form class to another. (For example, the *-y* suffix converts the noun *steel* to the adjective *steely*.)

Intonation

For clarifying the language-related processes of reading and writing, probably the most important intonation feature is the normal dropping of the voice at the end of each sentence. This is a *structural feature* that signals termination, or completion of the utterance; it is normally heard *only once* in each sentence pattern, *at the end.* Ordinarily it does not occur within a sentence pattern except in a written sentence with a semi-colon between clauses, where the dropping of the voice would be normal. The effect of dropping the voice more than once is to fragment the statement, destroying both structure and meaning.

The dropping of the voice is also normal for a great many questions, such as "How far away is the sun?" While some questions end with a rising tone, this commonly signifies some special emphasis or intent. (Try asking the above question with both a rising voice and a dropping voice; the two questions will signify different meanings.) There is no flat rule of English as to whether the voice drops or rises at the end of a question. On the other hand, we can convert a statement in English to a question by using a rising tone instead of a falling tone at the end; for example, "This is tender steak?"

A good rule of writing is to read a composition aloud, listening for normal intonation patterns, sentence patterns, word order, grouping, phrasing, general movement and rhythm. Sometimes it is better to have someone else read a composition aloud to the writer. "It just doesn't sound right" is often an excellent criticism, and an adequate basis for revision. Reading aloud also highlights or makes more apparent the general organization and development of the whole composition.

Sentence Patterns

Sentence Parts. Along with the common categories of subject, predicate, and various kinds of complements, sentence formulas can be presented to pupils, such as *N V N (Man bites dog.),* the most common pattern in English. Here *N* means *Noun part, V* means *Verb part,* and the second *N* means *Noun Completer.* Such sentence parts, *Noun parts* in particular, may be expanded almost indefinitely.

There is a correspondence between the four word classes and the four sentence parts with corresponding names—*noun, verb, adective, adverb*—but the two categories are quite different. While single members of word classes may occasionally fill sentence parts, as in Man bites dog, a sentence part may be composed of a group or cluster of considerable complexity and length. Note this expansion of Man bites dog.

Expanded N V N Sentence:

Noun part
A Madison Avenue man in a gray flannel suit
(noun headword)
Verb part
only very, very exceptionally bites
(verb headword)
Noun completer
the clipped, curled, dyed, and manicured French poodle dog designed as
(noun headword)
an accessory for an ensemble worn on certain occasions by a female member of his social set.

NV, NVNN, NLvN Patterns:

N V N V
Other common patterns are N V (Dogs bark); N V N N (Sarah sold
N N N V N
Ebenezer a pig in a poke); N V N N (The class elected Genevieve
N
Queen of the May); and N Lv N—Lv is a symbol for Linking verb—
N Lv N
(Joe is the bartender). There are variants of all four patterns that use *Adjective completers* and *Adverb completers* in the complement position.

Structure Words

Structure words number around three hundred, yet they are used with greater frequency than all others words in the language. They serve as joints and fasteners within sentence patterns—standard, interchangeable parts—connecting one pattern part with another. Structure words not only *may* be used over and over again without dullness and monotony, they *must* be used over and over again. This does not mean that a writer will achieve variety by a monotonous use of a few sentence patterns, ad nauseum; it does mean that to write effectively a writer must use the structure words effectively.

Noun Markers. Noun markers include the articles *(a, an, the),* and all other words that may be used to mark nouns, or to signal that a noun is approaching; noun markers include the cardinal numbers (*one*, *seventeen*, and so on); the "possessive pronouns" of school grammar (*my*, *your*, *his*, and so on), and such words as *another* and *most.* Any word that marks a noun or signals that a noun is coming, no matter how far down the line, is a noun marker.

Verb Markers. Verb markers include the auxiliary, or "helping" verb, the forms of *be,* and *do,* and *have,* mainly, as well as the modals such as *can, could, may, might, must, shall, should, will, would, could,* and *ought to.* Other verbs also serve as verb markers occasionally, such as *get, go, keep,* and *start.* Verb groups often are quite complex, using many verb forms to fill the pattern; for example, *were to have been completed,* or *had been having to remain.* An attentive writer can achieve considerable variety through a sensitive use of the various verb-group patternings.

Clause Markers. Clause markers are words and word groups that *identify clauses* usually by their distribution in the starting position; they also signify *specific relationships* between two or more clauses; clause markers shift from one structure-word classification to another; they are designated clause markers only when they fill the clause marking position and/or function. Effective use of clause markers is a specialty of the successful writer.

Three Groups. We may think of clause markers as comprising three groups: so-called coordinating conjunctions, with *and* as the prototype (this group includes correlative conjunctions); sentence pattern connectors, with *therefore* as the prototype; and so-called subordinating conjunctions, with *because* as the prototype. The terms *coordinating* and *subordinating* do not describe the relationships of the clauses marked and connected by these two sets of clause markers; in particular, they do not describe the content or meaning relationships.

Coordinating conjunctions are used in compound sentences with two or more sentence patterns separated by commas, or no punctuation if the patterns are very short. The seven of common school grammar are *and, but, for, nor, or, so, yet.* This is not an especially logical grouping. Notice these characteristics:

> *and* is a simple connector of equal elements, a plus sign
> *but* and *yet* signify contrast
> (*but* also serves as a preposition: *Everyone came but George.*)
> (*yet* also doubles as an adverb: *He is not here yet.*)
> *nor* and *or* may signify either contrast or alternation.
> *for* and *so* signify causal relationships (*for* may also be a preposition: *for the nonce*)
> (*so* may also be an intensifier: *not so hot*)
> Five of the seven in this group—*and, but, nor, or, yet*—may connect single words and word groups as well as clauses.

Correlative conjunctions are important for attaining balance and parallel constructions in well-written exposition. A few examples are *both . . . and; either . . . or; if . . . then; not only . . . but also; while . . . still; while . . . yet.* Like the so-called coordinating conjunctions, correlative conjunctions may connect a variety of sentence elements: single words, phrases, clauses. Effective control of conjunctions can make all the difference between plain, dull mediocrity and effective writing that makes clear and explicit the relationships among pattern parts.

Sentence-pattern connectors may be used in compound sentences with two or more sentence patterns connected by semicolons; sometimes between two sentences separated by a period (in speech, both would be terminated by a dropping of the voice). They have the special trait of signaling quite specific relationships between sentence patterns; often they mark the beginning of a second or a third clause, but they are also movable within the clause. In meaning, they commonly signify cause, contrast, or addition. We may take *therefore* as the prototype; others are *consequently, furthermore, hence, however, indeed, moreover, nevertheless, otherwise.* These words may also be used within single sentence patterns, but usually with reference back to an earlier sentence pattern in the paragraph.

Subordinating conjunctions. In the "complex" sentences of school grammar, clause markers start clauses that are connected in specific ways—by the choice of marker—to other pattern elements: single words, word groups and clusters, entire sentence patterns. Some of these clause markers may also serve as question markers. *Because* is the prototype; others are *if, that, how, when, which, since, why.* (Note that *for* and *so* might logically be included in this group.) *However* is a sentence-pattern connector that may also serve as a clause marker of this set: *However hard I try, I cannot do it right.*

Phrase Markers. Phrase markers are the prepositions of traditional grammar. They include single words and combinations of words that pattern, or distribute, in phrase-marking positions within sentence patterns. Because prepositions have such variety of structure and specificity in expressing relationships, mastery of the system can contibute a great deal to the development of writing style.

A number of prepositions may also pattern as clause markers, or as adverbs; they are designated "phrase markers" only when they fill phrase-marking positions. Discriminating among these structural positions and functions is a part of mastering not only the system of prepositions, but the other structure-word systems as well.

Phrase markers introduce a great variety of phrases that may expand all sentence parts. Prepositions may also take adverb positions; most of the prepositions that school grammar forbids us "to end a sentence with" are in fact adverbs, or at least prepositions in adverbial positions. Interesting parallel constructions can be devised using contrasting pairs of prepositions in contrasting parallel phrases: above, below; after, before; for, against; in, out; inside, outside; into, out of; over, under.

Question Markers. Question markers include those words that begin questions and thus mark questions, or signal that a question pattern should be anticipated. They include such words as *how, however, what, whatever, when, whence, where, wherever, which, whichever, whither, who, whoever, whom, whose* (the *-ever* forms are colloquial).

Question markers may introduce inverted sentence patterns, such as "How did he do it?" Inverted patterns in themselves are often used as questions, as in "Did he do it?" Note, however, that the question without the marker *how* does not have the same meaning as the question with *how.*

Word-Form Changes

Word-form changes have two main divisions: (1) grammatical inflections of the four word classes; and (2) derivational prefixes and suffixes.

Grammatical Inflections

Noun Inflections. For writing standard English sentence patterns, the most important inflections are those for nouns, including the pronoun forms, and verbs. One structural test for nouns is the ability of a word to take the regular *-s* plural, as in *dog, dogs;* singular and plural nouns require corresponding verb inflections, as in *A dog barks* and *Dogs bark.*

Adjective and Adverb Inflections. Another important set of inflections for standard written English are the adjective endings, *-er* and *-est,* as in *warm, warmer, warmest;* some adjectives use *more* and *most* for the same purpose, as in *beautiful, more beautiful, most beautiful.* Adverbs, also, may have comparative and superlative forms that are identical with the adjective forms.

Verb Inflections. Verbs have a number of inflections in addition to those signaling (and requiring) singular and/or plural agreement with nouns. The most important of these verb inflections are the *-ed* ending for the past, as in *Dogs barked;* the *-ed/en* ending for the past participle, as in *Dogs have barked* or *Men have taken*; and the *-ing* ending for the present participle, as in *Dogs are barking.* Some verbs have five different forms, or parts, as in *ride, rides, rode, riding, ridden;* others have as few as three parts, some of which must double for the "missing" parts, as in *set, sets, setting.*

The form changes of certain verbs include a vowel change, as in *sink, sank, sunk;* or a vowel change plus a change of ending, as in *think, thought,* or *creep, crept.* Even such "irregular" verbs, however, have forms for grammatical agreement with singular and plural nouns. In addition to the above word-form changes, the forms of pronouns for various functions are important in standard written English (*I, me, my, mine,* and so on). Often the difference between standard literacy and illiteracy lies in these distinctions.

Derivational Prefixes and Suffixes

The remarkable subsystem of derivational prefixes and suffixes, whereby word bases (or roots) may shift from one word class to another, is very important for the development of precise diction in writing, and for precision of meaning in reading. A noun base plus certain endings will form an adjective; for example, *peace* plus *-able* forms *peaceable.* Similarly, a verb base plus certain endings will also form an adjective; *adapt* plus *-able* forms *adaptable.*

Other common derivational suffixes that convert nouns to adjectives are *-ar, -ic, -ish, -ly, -al, -ary, -ical, -ous, -ine;* any teacher or pupil can make up his own list from reading. A few common derivational suffixes that convert verbs to adjectives are *-al, -ate, -ory, -ent, -some, -ful, -ive;* just as with suffixes that convert nouns to adjectives, anyone can make suffixes that convert verbs to adjectives.

The English Sentence

These four subsystems—intonation, sentence patterns, structure words, and word-form changes—comprise the main features of the basic communication pattern of the English language: the sentence. The more conscious we are of the way this language system works, the better equipped we are to use it well in all the language arts. English is not an impenetrable mystery. Schools, including esoteric schools of linguists, should not treat it so.

Roderick A. Jacobs' article is similar to the preceding selection, in that it presents a general overview of a new grammatical model along with some basic content from its grammar.

Jacobs summarizes the idea behind transformational grammar; that is, it "makes explicit those relationships that the native speaker of a language perceives intuitively." He presents and briefly explains some of the rewrite rules of transformational grammar, and shows how these rules work in generating sentences. He bases part of his appeal for transformational grammar on the projection that it "may lead us eventually to a deeper understanding of the great and amazing powers of the human mind, through which language functions."

A Short Introduction to Transformational Grammar

Roderick A. Jacobs

Transformational grammar—or generative grammar as it is often called—is undoubtedly the most significant development in linguistics in the past thirty years. Psychologists such as George Miller, Roger Brown, and John B. Carroll have found the grammar a useful cognitive model.[9,10] Philosophers, particularly the natural language philosophers, have become interested in the insights offered for the philosophy of language. And teachers have been studying transformational grammar as an intellectually coherent theory of language offering itself not only as challenging subject matter in itself but also as a possible aid in the teaching of composition and logical reasoning.[6,7]

Many of the ideas underlying transformational grammar—indeed many of the actual rules—are not new. Traditional grammarians such as Jespersen[8] saw these transformational relationships. Although attacked by Leonard Bloomfield for its prescriptivism,[2] the *Grammaire générale et raisonée*[1] of the Convent of Port-Royal which appeared in 1660 presents, in fact, as clear and useful a description of language as any that have since appeared. Its closeness to transformational grammar is astonishing.[4]

However, it was Noam Chomsky of M.I.T. who first formalized the notion of this kind of grammar, notably in his *Syntactic Structures.*[3] His more recent work has so modified and advanced the theory of grammar that it is now able to account for linguistic phenomena never before explained.[5]

Explaining Underlying Relations

Basically, transformational grammar makes explicit those relationships that the native speaker of a language perceives intuitively. For example, in the sentences

(1) John was eager to please.
(2) John was easy to please.

we should sense that, logically, *John* is the subject of *please* in (1) and the object of *please* in (2). A sound grammar should be able to account for these intuitive relationships. Traditional grammarians have noted them in their compendiums of language, but the structural linguist seems to have ignored them, focusing his attention on procedures for dividing and labeling sentences.

A Sentence Grammar

Chomsky found that a more powerful device than the listing of sentence frames, form-class, and function words was necessary in order to account for human language. The key unit of language is the sentence. We are able to create or generate an infinite number of understandable sentences.

The underlying structure of any sentence (S) consists of a position for a noun phrase (NP) acting as the subject, an auxiliary phrase containing at least the unit *TENSE,* and one for a verb phrase (VP), sometimes containing a noun object. We can write this as a sentence formation "rule":

[1] S = NP—Aux.—VP

These positions underlie *any* sentence of English, though the positions may be filled by transforming sentences into clauses and inserting them into the subject and postverb positions, for example:

What worried me	was John's being sick.
(Something worried me)	(John was sick)

On the other hand, words can be deleted, for example, from the imperative *You will go home*! to form *Go home*! The native speaker knows intuitively that the words missing are "understood" as the traditionalists so accurately claimed. When necessary he can fill them in: *Go home, will you!* but never *Go home, has he!*

But let us start with a very simple sentence. The noun phrase consists of a noun place and a place for a determiner (words such as *the, this, two, some*). The verb phrase must contain a verb, and possibly another noun phrase. Our sentence is *The boy saw the dog*. We can represent the formation of this structure in an ordered way called a Phrase Structure Grammar:

[1] S → NP—Aux—VP
[2] NP → Det—N
[3] Aux → Tense
[4] VP → V—NP
[5] Det → the
[6] N → boy, dog
[7] Tense → Past
[8] V → see

This structure can also be represented by a family tree diagram with Sentence (S) at the top, dividing to the three branches—NP, Aux, and VP. Each of these branches in turn is subdivided, as the formation rules show. But this is not a very powerful grammar. Using it we can produce or *generate* only four sentences:

The boy saw the dog.
The dog saw the boy.
The boy saw the boy.
The dog saw the dog.

—not very useful, it seems. But we can make the grammar generate eight sentences by changing rule seven to read

$$[7]\ \text{Tense} \rightarrow \begin{cases} \text{Past} \\ \text{Present} \end{cases}$$

so that the present tense can also be used for each of the sentences. Allowing another verb, *like,* makes our grammar generate sixteen sentences. Other nouns can be added, the verb category subdivided into transitive, intransitive verbs, and so forth, and the noun phrase in rule four made optional for some verbs:

[4] VP → V (NP)

Simple Transformations

Soon our grammar is generating thousands of sentences. But it cannot generate all and only the grammatical structures of English. The complex ones, with their complex interrelations, require a more powerful kind of rule. Our grammar should show that *The boy saw the dog* has the same underlying structure as *The dog was seen by the boy* and, hence, the same basic meaning.

In the passive the auxiliary word *be* does not change the meaning. It acts as one of the pointers which indicated to us that it was the boy who did the "seeing" (that is, was the "logical subject") and the dog that was seen (that is, "logical object"). What the relation is between these two sentences is seen by a comparison of their arrangement. The first is structured

$$NP_1—Past—V—NP_2.$$

The second is structured

$$\underset{\text{was}}{NP_2—Past—BE}—\underset{\text{seen}}{En—V}—\text{by } NP_1$$

In the second, NP_1, though the grammatical object of the preposition, actually bears the same intuitive relation to its verb as does NP_1 to the verb in the first sentence. Logically both are the *subject* of the verb, just as "dog" is logically the *object* of the verb in both sentences.

Since the grammatical and logical relations are identical in the first sentence, it is reasonable to assume that this structure is the primary one. We can describe the second as a rearrangement or *transformation* of the first. To transform the first structure into the second, we may simply interchange the two noun phrases, insert *be* and the past participle ending (denoted *En*) before the verb, and *by* before NP_1, as shown. This type of transformation, operating on single sentence-structures, is called a *singularly* transformation.

Complex Transformations

Phrase Structure rules (often called Formation Rules) may also produce two structures like those underlying *John is eager* and *John pleases someone,* but transformational rules combine these kernel structures into one: *John is eager to please.*

The logical relation between *John* and *please* in the transformed sentence is the same as the grammatical one in one of the underlying ones—subject and verb. On the other hand, the two kernel structures underlying *It is easy* and *Someone pleases John* can be combined into *It is easy to please John* and then to *John is easy to please.*

In these two transformed sentences *John* is the logical object of the verb, *please.* And, sure enough, in one of the kernel structures we find the same verb-object relationship shown grammatically. Such transformational rules, combining two or more sentence-structures are called *generalized* transformations.

Grammar and Mind

The rules described so far are only a small, slightly simplified part of the incredibly systematic set of rules capable of generating all the sentences of English, rules that reflect man's own incredible capacity to generate a rich system of language. Research is still going on. It is believed that the same kinds of rules can generate any human language. Turkish, Hebrew, Japanese, Mohawk, Spanish and Russian are among the languages already being described in this way.

More important perhaps is the probability that whatever structure is common to all language is an innate property of the human mind. Knowledge of this kind may lead us eventually to a deeper understanding of the great and amazing powers of the human mind, through which language functions.

References

1. Arnault. *Grammaire générale et raisonnée.* Paris, 1660, pp. 66–83.
2. Bloomfield, Leonard. *Language.* New York: Holt, Rinehart & Winston, 1963, p. 6.
3. Chomsky, Noam. *Syntactic Structures.* The Hague: Mouton, 1957.
4. Chomsky, Noam. *Current Issues in Linguistic Theory.* The Hague: Mouton, 1964, pp. 15–16.
5. Chomsky, Noam. *Aspects of the Theory of Syntax.* Cambridge, Mass.: M.I.T. Press, 1965.
6. Jacobs, R. A. Review Article on H. A. Gleason's "Linguistics and English Grammar," in *Harvard Educational Review.* Summer, 1965.
7. Jacobs, R. A. "Language Study and Grammar in the High School" (to be included in forthcoming text series, Harper and Row, Evanston, Ill.)
8. Jesperson, Otto. *A Modern English Grammar.* London: Allen and Unwin, 1963, 2.283, 12.12.
9. Miller, G. and Chomsky, N. "Finitary Models of Language Users." Luce, Bush and Galanter, ed. *Handbook of Mathematical Psychology.* New York: John Wiley, 1963, pp. 476–488.
10. Miller, G. and Isard, S. "Some Perpetual Consequences of Linguistic Rules." *Journal of Verbal Behavior* 2, (1963), pp. 217–228.

This selection, by Ved Mehta, was abridged from a much lengthier article that appeared in *New Yorker* magazine, which in turn was taken from Mehta's book by the same title. The article was selected because it contains an explanation of transformational grammar by the master himself, Noam Chomsky, and because the way in which the material is presented—that is, through the interview technique—is helpful in clarifying some of the concepts of the grammar.

Mehta begins by briefly sketching a background of Chomsky's thinking both on grammar and language acquisition. In the interview, Chomsky explains his theory of grammar in practical terms, using sentence diagrams to explain his ideas, particularly with regard to the concepts of deep and surface structure. Chomsky summarizes his theory of transformational grammar: "Grammar is really in the mind—it is a fixed, finite set of internalized rules and conditions which associates the surface structures of sentences with particular meanings and makes it possible for the speaker of a language to generate an infinite number of sentences." It is the formalization of these rules and conditions that constitutes the content of transformational grammar that was presented previously in Jacobs' article and that will be presented in the selection by Ross and Ross.

Some excellent passages from the article—both pro and con—with regard to Chomsky and his theories are omitted here because of space limitations. Reading the original article in its entirety is recommended.

John Is Easy to Please

Ved Mehta

Linguists are stirring up quite a lot of intellectual dust just now with a theory of language known as transformational, or generative, grammar, which was first enunciated, in 1957, by Noam Chomsky, the leader of the linguistic vanguard, and which was recently denounced by Charles F. Hockett, a stalwart of the linguistic rearguard, as "a theory spawned by a generation of vipers." The two factions are polarized not only by rhetorical excess—Chomsky is a master of polemics in his own right—but also by actual issues, which are constantly being debated in the literature on the subject. Although Chomsky's two most influential books are *Syntactic Structures,* which his disciples call the Old Testament, and *Aspects of the Theory of Syntax,* which they call the New Testament, the clearest statement of the theory for someone unschooled in the technical jargon of transformational grammar is to be found in *Language and Mind,* an expanded version of three lectures that Chomsky, a professor of linguistics at the Massachusetts Institute of Technology, gave in 1967 at the University of California at Berkeley. In the book, Chomsky took specific examples of grammatical rules relating to English phonology and syntax, and tried to demonstrate that their application was subject to certain universal conditions. These conditions, he argued, were the principles of "universal grammar" and provided "a highly restrictive schema to which any human language must conform." He wrote, "The study of universal grammar, so understood, is a study of the nature of human intellectual capacities. It tries to formulate the necessary and sufficient conditions that a system must meet to qualify as a potential human language, conditions that are not accidentally true of the existing human languages, but that are rather rooted in the human 'language capacity,' and thus constitute the innate organization that determines what counts as linguistic experience and what knowledge of language arises on the basis of this experience." He claimed that the human mind was equipped at birth with a mental representation of the universal grammar, and that this grammar, by means of formal operations he called "transformations," enabled a speaker of any language to generate an indefinite series of sentences. Indeed, he argued, the human mind was uniquely equipped to learn "natural" languages, and a child would fail to learn, as a first language, either the language of another planet or an artificial language that did not meet the universal conditions. Unlike earlier students of language, who had been content merely to describe usage, Chomsky hoped to discover and catalogue the conditions that he believed underlay not just usage but the acquisition of language. Venturing into philosophy, he revived the classic rationalist notion—first stated by Descartes in the seventeenth century—that certain ideas were implanted in the mind as innate equipment. In fact, for the purposes of his argument, he adopted the Cartesian distinction between mind, the essence of which was understanding and will, and body, the essence of which was extension and motion, and contended that the central problem on which Cartesianism foundered (If mind and body were separate substances, how did they interact in man?) could be solved through the study of language, for the creative use of language, the ability to produce and understand sentences, was what most obviously distinguished man from animal.

Editor's Note: The author identifies philosophical differences between Chomsky's theory of language and the thinking of two contemporary philosophers, Hillary Putnam and Nelson Goodman. He describes arguments that ensued when Chomsky encountered Goodman and Putnam at scholarly conferences.

In an interview, Chomsky describes his early interest in and study of linguistics, including the influence of his mentor Zellig Harris. In a second interview, Chomsky begins to explain his theory of transformational grammar.

The entry under *labyrinth* in Webster's *New International Dictionary* (Second Edition) reads, in part:

> (lăb'ĭ'rĭnth), n. [L. *labyrinthus,* fr. Gr. *labyrinthos,* fr. *labrys* double ax, prob. of Carian origin. cf. *LABRYS.*] 1. an edifice or place full of intricate passageways which render it difficult to find the way from the interior to the entrance, or from the entrance to the central compartment; a maze; specif., in Greek myth, the labyrinth constructed by Daedalus for Minos, king of Crete, in which the Minotaur was confined.

The mythical labyrinth was, according to one authority, "so artfully contrived that whoever was enclosed in it could by no means find his way out unassisted," and another has written, "Once inside one would go endlessly along its twisting paths without ever finding the exit . . . . In whatever direction they ran, they, the victims, might be running straight to the monster; if they stood still he might at any moment emerge from the maze." As every schoolboy knows, these victims were Athenian youths and maidens sent as tribute to Crete, where they were fed to the Minotaur, who was half man and half bull. When the Athenian hero Theseus was sent to Crete as part of the tribute, Mino's daughter Ariadne fell in love with him and furnished him with a ball of thread to enable him to escape from the labyrinth. Theseus fastened one end of the thread to the inside of the door to the labyrinth and unwound the ball as he went along the twisted passages, until he came upon the Minotaur. He killed the Minotaur, and escaped from the labyrinth by following the thread back to the door.

After spending some time with Chomsky's works on linguistics, I discover that he has all the ingenuity of a Daedalus, so I take a big ball of thread with me when I go to meet him for the second time. I step through the door of his office and boldly ask him to explain transformational grammar.

"The traditional multivolume grammars that you find on the shelves of libraries present and classify precisely the examples that appear in them, and nothing else," he says. "But we transformationalists try to answer the mysterious and, I think, rather profound question: What qualities of intelligence does a human being possess that make it possible for him to use language creatively, to generate from the limited set of examples that he hears an infinite set of sentences? But perhaps the clearest way to explain the theory of transformational grammar is to show how transformations operate in sentences. Sentences consists of phrases of various types—noun phrases, verb phrases, adverbial phrases, and so on. OK? For purposes of analysis, every sentence can be enclosed within brackets, and its parts enclosed within smaller brackets and marked, and the parts of the parts enclosed within smaller brackets and marked, and so on. OK? You end up with a sentence that's properly bracketed, or parenthesized, in the technical sense that every left parenthesis is associated with a right parenthesis and the entire structure is exhausted at every stage of the analysis. Take the sentence 'John kept the car that was in the garage.' " (From my reading, I recognize the sentence as a variation of one of Chomsky's stock examples, "John kept the car in the garage.") "It consists of the noun phrase—in this case, really a noun—*John;* the verb *kept;* and the noun phrase *the car that was in the garage.* OK? The noun phrase *the car that was in the garage* consists, in turn, of the noun *car* and the sentence *that was in the garage;* the shorter sentence *that was in the garage* consists, in turn, of other phrases; and so on. OK? The whole sentence can be bracketed and labelled with abbreviations—sentence, noun phrase, noun, verb phrase, verb, article, and so on."

He diagrams the sentence on a sheet of paper:

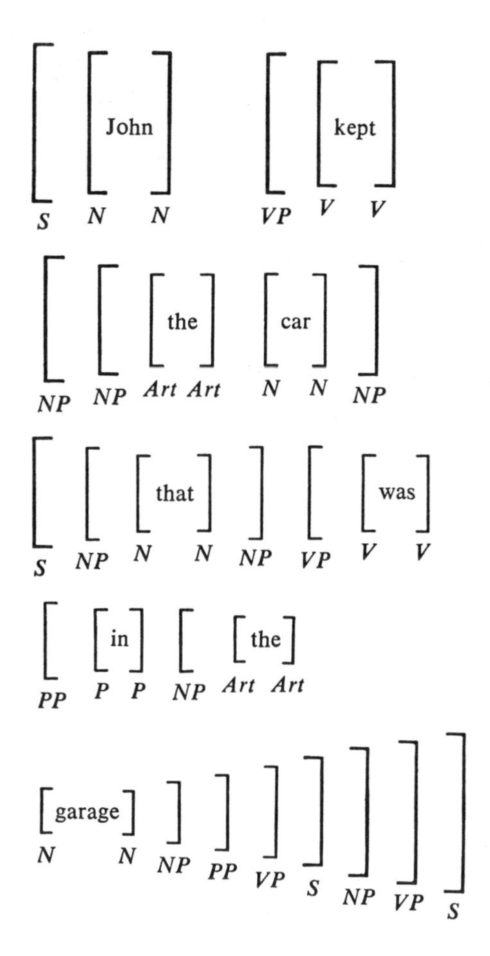

"Now, the fundamental idea of transformational grammar is that the bracketed and labelled representation of a sentence is its surface structure, and associated with each sentence is a long sequence of more and more abstract representations of the sentence—we transformationalists call them phrase markers—of which surface structure is only the first," he continues. "For example, underlying the surface structure of *John kept the car that was in the garage,* which might be represented by the phrase marker P_1, there would be, embedded and unspoken, a somewhat more abstract phrase marker, P_2, which would be converted into P_1 by what we call a *transformation,* transformation being our term for the operation by which less abstract phrase markers are generated from more abstract ones. And underlying P_2 would be a still more abstract phrase marker, P_3, which would be converted into P_2 by another transformation, and so on, back farther and farther, until you reach the most abstract phrase marker of all, which we call the deep structure of the sentence. Whereas the surface structure in general is not closely related to the meaning of the sentence, the deep structure appears to be closely related to meaning. OK?"

As Chomsky talks, he radiates feverish intensity. His cheeks become flushed, and his hands fly back and forth to underscore his points.

"Is it really the case that the meaning of the sentence is hidden in this complicated way?" I ask.

"Keep the old sentence, *John kept the car that was in the garage,* in the back of your mind for now and let me give you the simpler sentence, *John kept the car in the garage*, as an example of what I mean. OK? Notice that *John kept the car in the garage* is ambiguous—is open to two interpretations. Call them I_1 and I_2. I_1 would be exactly the same as *John kept the car that was in the garage;* you could paraphrase this interpretation as *It was the car in the garage that John kept.* I_2 would be *The car was kept in the garage by John*; you could paraphrase this interpretation as *It was in the garage that John kept the car.* Although you can't tell by the sound of the sentence which of the two interpretations is meant, the surface structure of the sentence is different for each interpretation. When we follow interpretation I_1, *It was the car in the garage that John kept,* we assume that the phrase *the car in the garage* is a unit, bracketed as a noun phrase."

He diagrams the phrase on the sheet of paper:

[the car in the garage]
NP NP

"But when we follow interpretation I_2, *It was in the garage that John kept the car,* then we assume that *the car in the garage* is not a unit, not a noun phrase," he continues. "Instead, *the car* is a full noun phrase—"

He diagrams:

[the car]
NP NP

"—and *in the garage* is an adverbial phrase—"

He diagrams:

[in the garage]
Adv P Adv P

"According to the interpretation I_1, *John kept the car in the garage* is an elliptical form of the explicit, and more abstract, sentence *John kept the car that was in the garage*," he continues. "The surface structure is generated from the more abstract sentence by the transformation that deletes the words *that was*. Ellipsis, a linguistic term that was in use long before the advent of transformational grammar, is one kind of operation that transforms one phrase marker into another. The abstract phrase marker *John kept the car that was in the garage* itself derives from a deeper, more explicit sentence—*John kept the car. The car was in the garage.*"

He diagrams:

[[John] [[kept] [[[the] [car]]
S N N PP P P NP NP Art Art N N NP

[[[the] [car]] [[was] [[in] [[the]
S NP Art Art N N NP NP V V PP P P NP Art Art

[garage]]]]]]]]
N N NP PP PP S NP NP S

I feel I am being drawn deeper and deeper into the intricacies of Chomsky's theory, but the explanation is so lucid (no doubt Chomsky has delivered it often) that I still have my bearings.

"This sentence brings us almost to the deep structure, which in the case we've been talking about, as it happens, is not very abstract," he goes on. "Now let's take a more complex example, the interrogative sentence *What did John keep the car in?* We transformationalists would argue that this sentence derives from an underlying, more abstract sentence, *John kept the car in the garage*—in which *the car* is the noun phrase and *in the garage* is an adverbial phrase—not by an operation of ellipsis this time but, rather, by the operations of substitution and prepositioning, which substitute *what* for *garage* and move *what* to the beginning of the sentence. These transformations yield the phrase *what John kept the car in,* which, in turn, is transformed by further operations into the sentence *What did John keep the car in*?"

I am beginning to lose my way. I ask him about the universal conditions that are supposed to govern transformations, and he tells me that although the sentence *John kept the car in the garage* is ambiguous, the question *What did John keep the car in*? is not ambiguous, for it is open to only one interpretation—It was in the garage that John kept the car.

"Why is it that the question is not ambiguous?" he asks rhetorically. "Well, we transformationalists would say that the question *What did John keep the car in?* is governed by a universal condition—undoubtedly a principle of universal grammar—that asserts that a noun phrase, here *the garage,* that is part of a larger noun phrase, here *the car in the garage,* cannot be extracted and moved. Thus, from the sentence *John kept the car that was in the garage* I cannot form the question *What did John keep the car that was in?* That would be impossible in any language. OK? When we take interpretation I_1 of the sentence *John kept the car in the garage,* in which *the car in the garage* is a noun phrase, we cannot extract the phrase *the garage* and put it in the front and form a question. But, as you noticed, when we take interpretation I_2, in which *in the garage* is an adverbial phrase, then we can substitute *what* for *the garage,* move *what* to the front of the sentence, and get *What did John keep the car in?* OK? This is an example of a rather nontrivial point—that in order to form questions the speaker of a language, in this case English, applies transformations such as the operations of substitution and prepositioning to mental representations of declarative sentences. Because these mental representations are a sequence of phrase markers, the speaker has to know, in order to produce and understand sentences, the underlying structures of the sentences, to which he is applying the transformations. He has to know, for example, whether the phrase marker to which he applies the transformation treated *the car in the garage* as a single noun phrase or whether it treated *the car* as a noun phrase and *in the garage* as an adverbial phrase."

"I don't quite grasp the distinction between the grammatical rules of transformation that you were speaking about before and these universal conditions," I say.

"An example of a grammatical rule of transformation would be the rule of question formation that I gave you," he says. "Let me clarify it further. Take the declarative sentence *John read the book.* If I want to form a question about the book, I move the phrase *the book* to the beginning of the sentence and prefix the questioning element *what* and I get *What book did John read?*"

"Don't you actually get *What the book did John read?*" I ask.

"That was a bad example, because it brings up complexities in the rule of question formation that I would just as soon not go into now," he says, and he presses on. "This grammatical rule of question formation can be applied to any noun phrase in the sentence. If I want to form a question about John, instead of the book, I say, *Who read the book?*"

"Actually, *Who John read the book?*" I ask.

"That was a bad example, too. But, to go on, all grammatical rules of transformation, like the rule of question formation, must meet certain universal conditions. One such universal condition, as you noticed, is that no grammatical rule of transformation can involve extracting a noun phrase from another noun phrase that properly includes it—*the car* from *the car in the garage.*"

I try to draw him away from examples by asking him how he regards the workings of these rules and conditions. "Surely they are not conscious?" I say.

"In the normal use of the language, we unconsciously and instantaneously make use of abstract representations," he says.

"If these rules and conditions are in fact unconsious, then why think of them in formal terms as structures—as mental representations?" I ask.

"Let me answer your question in this way," he says. "Take two examples somewhat more complex than the sentences we've been talking about: *John is eager to please* and *John is easy to please.* OK? I immediately recognize these sentences as the most famous examples of Chomsky's school. "We could assign to these two sentences their respective surface structures—a noun, *John,* followed by a verb, *is,* followed by a certain kind of adjective phrase, *eager to please* in one case, *easy to please* in the other. But the surface structures don't tell the whole story. If we say *John is eager to please, John* is the subject of *please*—John is doing the pleasing. We attribute to John the property of being eager to do something. Now, if we say *John is easy to please, John* is the direct object of *please.* We mean that pleasing John is easy and we attribute to the proposition *please John* the property of being easy. OK? Although the two sentences differ considerably in the grammatical relation between their parts—in what is predicated of what—these differences are not represented in their surface structures. In the case of *John is eager to please,* the surface structure and the deep structure are really identical—that *John* is the subject of *please* is already explicit in the surface structure. But in the case of *John is easy to please* the surface structure, *John is easy to please*, is quite different from the deep structure, *To please John is easy* or *For us to please John is easy*, and it requires a long sequence of operations to transform this deep structure into its surface structure. I won't try to explain all these transformations now, because they're a little too complicated. But in the deep structure of *John is easy to please* the verb-object relation between *to please* and *John* is explicit, whereas in the surface structure the relation is not explicit at all. It is possible, however, to conceive of a surface structure for this particular meaning—the meaning *To please John is easy*—in which the verb-object relationship between *John* and *to please* would be explicit. This would be true for the surface structure *To please John is easy.* To transform the deep structure *To please John is easy* into the surface structure *To please John is easy* involves only the simplest of operations."

"But in another language—say, in French or Latin—wouldn't the difference between what is predicated of what in *John is eager to please* and in *John is easy to please* be expressed by the case of the noun, or by the addition of a preposition?" I ask. "If so, then what you speak of as the contrast between the deep structures and the identity of the surface structures of these two sentences might be relevant only to English."

"Yes," he says. "In French or Latin, the surface structures of the two sentences would certainly not be identical, but the two surface structures would still show greater similarity to each other than the two deep structures would. OK? In French or Latin, these sentences would retain in their surface structures things like cases, which are a sort of residual deep structure. But in English they don't, so you get an amusing and striking example of sentences whose surface structures are identical but whose deep structures are radically different."

"But does the contrast between *John is eager to please* and *John is easy to please* actually matter to someone using English?" I ask.

"The real contrast between the two sentences shows up in the way in which we perform certain syntactic operations on them, like the operation of nominalization," he says. "If we have the sentence *John is weak,* we can perform the operation of nominalization and produce the noun phrase *John's weaknesses.* If we have *John is eager to please,* by the same operation we can produce the noun phrase *John's eagerness to please.* But if we perform the same operation on *John is easy to please,* we produce *John's easiness to please.* This is not a properly formed noun phrase. You can say *John's eagerness to please surprised me,* but you can't say *John's easiness to please surprised me.* If somebody said it, you would know what he meant, but you would also know that he didn't know how to speak English properly. Thus, the contrast between *John is eager to please* and *John is easy to please* appears as a difference in grammaticality when we perform the operation of nominalization. This simple example illustrates the fact that when we perform certain operations, we perform them not on actual sentences but on mental representations, on the sequences of abstract structures that underlie sentences. *For what we transformationalists are saying is that grammar is really in the mind—that it is a fixed, finite set of internalized rules and conditions which associates the surface structures of sentences with particular sounds and particular meanings and makes it possible for the speaker of a language to generate an infinite number of sentences.*"

Editor's Note: Italics in the preceding sentence are mine.

The interview continues with Chomsky briefly explaining his theory about the relation between sound and meaning in language. Turning to his theory of language acquisition, Chomsky says, "The infant must know the rules and conditions of grammar before he learns a language. . . . If we assume that any infant can learn any language—that no infant is genetically a speaker of a specific language—then every attribute we postulate in order to explain an infant's ability to learn one language must be true of any child's learning of any language, and so must be a universal condition of a universal grammar. Thus, on the basis of the evidence that we have from the study of a few languages, we can safely assume that for learning languages there must be a schematism in the mind—a physical mechanism in the brain—that is the same in every human being." (Chomsky's theory, you'll remember, was explained in an earlier selection: *Language Acquisition: Basic Issues,* part I, pp. 43–44.) Chomsky also goes on to answer critics' objections about the approach and the activities of the transformationalists, while expressing his objections to the structuralist approach to language study.

The article concludes with accounts of interviews with Charles Hockett, a well-known linguist and vocal critic of Chomsky, and with Roman Jakobson, "the elder statesman of linguistics," who speaks about some of the strengths and weaknesses of Chomsky's transformalist theory.

"Linguistics in the Elementary Classroom" is a clear and relatively complete summary of some of the "nuts and bolts" of transformational grammar. The selection was included at the strong suggestion of my students, who found it to be one of the more lucid and understandable presentations on the topic that they had encountered (apart from my lectures, of course!)

It is worthy of note that one of the authors is also coauthor of the Roberts English series and that the original publisher of the monograph (Harcourt, Brace, and Jovanovich) is also publisher of the Roberts series. Thus, you will find linguistics equated with transformational grammar and transformational grammar equated with that variety of the same which is found in the Roberts series. These facts notwithstanding, the selection does present many of the concepts of transformational grammar in terms that are clear and concise.

At the outset, Charles and Mary Ross sketch the background of the grammatical reformation in schools. They present the common parts of the grammar and include some parts not treated by earlier selections on the topic (namely modals and morphemes). The authors also briefly suggest applications and some of the practical values of teaching transformational grammar in the classroom.

Linguistics in the Elementary School Classroom

Charles S. Ross and Mary M. Ross

Many thoughtful elementary school teachers have very little sense of accomplishment in teaching English grammar because they suspect that traditional instruction in English grammar does little to improve the child's ability to express himself. Definitions, classification exercises, and usage drills do not seem to constitute a real subject matter, like the subject matter of mathematics or science. Teachers have been hoping that somehow there might emerge from the studies and writings of linguistic scholarship a reformation in the teaching of grammar: not just a "new grammar" but a way of teaching grammar that really would help teachers to help children speak, read, and write better.

The reformation which has emerged is in fact more thorough and broader than seemed likely even a few years ago. It involves the whole writing system: syntax (the study of the sentence) and phonology (the study of the relationship between sound and spelling). It aims to improve children's writing by teaching them how well-formed sentences are generated. It aims to improve children's ability to read by applying the principles by which they generate sentences to the interpretation of sentences written by others.

The stuff of which this reformation is made has been created for the most part in recent years by the scholars of the science of language—linguistics. These scholars have learned much from philosophers, logicians, psychologists. They have applied to the study of English the methods of inquiry which are being applied in their own fields by anthropologists, mathematicians, physicists. Objective inquiry has built up a body of new information about how the sound and writing systems of English work, and about the mechanisms by which an individual is able to generate an infinite number of well-formed sentences, many of them never before spoken or written by anyone else. It is this scholarship which provides for the teacher of English in the elementary grades a genuine subject matter which can be taught with satisfaction and a sense of accomplishment.

To this teacher perhaps the most challenging part of the emerging English program is the syntax, the study of the sentence. So it is some of the characteristics of the syntax that will be described here.

The Simple Sentence

Transformational grammar uses many of the familiar grammatical terms, but sometimes presents them differently—often with modified meanings. Of course, *sentence* is the first term of the new grammar. It is the first term introduced and the last one fully learned—for learning to understand the sentence is the objective of the whole study of syntax, and takes several years to accomplish.

In the new grammar, the child begins by dealing with many sentences of very simple structure. At first, the actual sentences are confined to unmodified affirmative statements. The underlying kernel structures *NP* and *VP* (noun phrase and verb phrase) are expressed in that order in the finished sentence:

The boy milked the cow.
Mr. White is a violinist.
They dashed upstairs.
Somebody broke a window.

Such sentences are called *simple sentences.*

Sentences like the following have the kernel structures *NP* and *VP,* but they are not simple sentences bcause these underlying structures have been expressed in a different order or have been added to or modified in some way:

Can Elsie cook?
John didn't leave.
Be good.

Sentences such as these are the result of changes called *transformations,* and therefore are *transforms.*

The first order of business in teaching the syntax is to familiarize the children with the structures that function as subject and predicate in simple sentences. In such sentences a noun phrase always comes first and always functions as subject. A verb phrase always comes next and always functions as predicate. Everything that is not the subject of a simple sentence is part of the predicate, so when the pupils can tell what the subject is, they can readily identify everything else as the predicate.

Determiners and Nouns

The term *noun*, like *sentence*, is not given a notional definition, such as "a noun is the name of a person, place or thing," nor is it given a temporary "term holder" designation such as *naming word*. Instead, *noun* is introduced as a term, and children learn to recognize nouns in several ways. One way is through experience with numerous examples. Another is by position of the word in the sentence. Still another is by recognizing that nouns follow words such as *the a (n), some, these, many*. Words of this kind are called *determiners*. The pupil learns that a determiner usually signals that a noun will follow and tells something about the noun.

An important part of the syntax in contemporary grammar is semantics—the study of meanings. For example, the meanings of the determiners is an important part of the study of noun phrases. The determiner *a* in "A dog bit Hilda" means *one*. But in "A horse likes oats," the determiner *a* doesn't mean one at all. This sentence means the same thing as "Horses like oats." Other determiners—*the*, *some*, and the "null" (or missing) determiners in noun phrases such as "horses" or "mud"—have their own semantic aspects, and are related systematically to the others in the group.

The Noun Phrase

Four kinds of words or groups of words function as subject in a kernel structure:

Determiner + common noun	(*The boy* milked the cow.)
Proper noun	(*Mr. White* is a violinist.)
Personal pronoun	(*They* walked to school.)
Indefinite pronoun	(*Everyone* seemed friendly.)

Each of these kinds of subject is called a noun phrase, even though it may be a single word. Noun phrase is the name for a structure, but not for a word class. *Noun* and *personal pronoun* are examples of names of word classes. A noun phrase such as *he,* which is a member of the personal pronoun word class, can take the place of another noun phrase:

The boy milked the cow. → *He* milked the cow.

The arrow → is the rewrite symbol, showing in this case that the first sentence is rewritten with a different noun phrase as subject. Notice that the pronoun does not take the place of the noun *boy,* but of the complete noun phrase, *The boy.*

Verbs and the Word *Be*

In a simple sentence, the first word of the predicate is usually a verb or a form of the word *be—am, is, are, was,* or *were.* The word *be* and its forms do not behave in the way verbs do, so it seems most effective in teaching not to call *be* a verb, but to consider it a class by itself. This makes it possible to simplify the treatment of the syntax considerably.

One obvious example of differences between *be* and verbs is the number of tense forms: three for *be,* two for verbs in the present tense; two for *be,* one for verbs in the past tense. Another is the requirement that *be* must be followed by a complement, whereas a verb may or may not have a complement:

He is a *soldier.*	(a noun phrase)
She is *pretty.*	(an adjective)
They are *in the boat.*	(an adverbial of place)

The word *be* seems to function as a kind of tense-carrying dummy, rather than as a verb, in English. A foreigner learning English tends to dispense with *be* entirely: "He soldier," "She pretty," "They in the boat."

Tense

One of the ways in which generative transformational grammar makes the study of English more rational and understandable is its treatment of tense.

Every predicate must have one word in it that expresses present or past tense. This tense-carrying word will always be the first word in the predicate of a simple sentence.

In the new grammar, *tense* is used in the normal linguistic sense: distinctions of time shown inflectionally by suffixes. Combinations of words such as *will go* are not included as tenses. In the sentence "John will go tomorrow," the first word in the predicate is *will,* so *will* expresses the tense. The form *will* is the present tense of the modal *will.* (The past tense is *would.*) So this sentence is in the present tense. In "John goes tomorrow," it is *goes*, a present tense form of the verb *go*, that expresses tense, so again, the tense is present. In "John has gone," it is *has*, a present tense form of *have* that expresses tense, and the tense therefore is present.

It is clear then that tense, though related to time, is simply the form of whatever word expresses tense in a particular sentence. In a simple sentence the word that expresses tense must be a verb, *be*, *have*, or a modal.

Languages differ in the number of tenses—that is, in the different forms which express tense—that they have. English has two. Latin has six; modern Italian has five. The reason English has been said to have six tenses in certain school grammars is that Latin had six tenses.

In transformational grammar, then, there are only two tenses: *present* and *past*. In a simple sentence the tense, present or past, is always shown by the first word of the predicate:

They *are* hungry.	(present)
They *were* hungry.	(past)
They *want* some food.	(present)
They *wanted* some food.	(past)
They *have* wanted some food.	(present)
They *had* wanted some food.	(past)
They *may* want some food.	(present)
They *might* want some food.	(past)

Simple Form and *S* Form of Verbs

Transformational grammar makes the student conscious of the actual working of his language. For example, all English verbs in the present tense have two forms: the simple form (*walk*, *see*) and the *s* form (*walks*, *sees*). When the subject of a sentence is singular, the *s* form of the verb is used:

The boy *walks*. The dog *sees* the squirrel.

The *s* form of the verb may end in the sound /s/* as in *walks*; or /z/ as in *jobs*; or as a separate syllable /ə-z/ as in *judges*. But whatever sound it has, it is always spelled with *s* or *es*.

When the subject is plural the simple form of the verb is used:

The boys *walk*. The dogs *see* the squirrel.

---

* It is necessary to make a distinction in linguistic writing between names of sounds and the letters used to spell the sounds. Symbols printed between slanted lines, such as /s/, refer to sounds rather than to letters.

Notice that the verbs are not considered to be singular or plural, as they are in traditional grammar. They merely correspond in form to the requirements of the subject.

Modals

There are five modals in English. Their present tense forms are *may*, *can*, *will*, *shall*, *must*. Four of the modals—may, can, will, and shall—have past tense forms: might, could, would, should. The modal *must* has no past tense form—only a present tense form. Of course, these tense forms of modals—present and past—convey a wide variety of time meanings.

Morphemes

The new grammar makes use of the concept of the morpheme to help pupils understand the structure of English. A morpheme is a single piece of meaning expressed by a word or part of a word. For instance, the word *boy* is a single piece of meaning—a male child. The plural suffix *s* also represents a morpheme—the meaning plural. So *boys* is two morphemes: *boy* + plural. *Boy's* as in *boy's coat* is also two morphemes: *boy* + possessive.

Here are some examples of words that represent one, two, and three morphemes:

One	Two	Three
boy	*boys* (boy + plural)	*boys'* (boy + plural + possessive)
lady	*ladies* (lady + plural)	*ladies'* (lady + plural + possessive)
man	*men* (man + plural)	*men's* (man + plural + possessive)

We add morphemes to verbs and adjectives as well as to nouns. One morpheme that is added to verbs and *be* is *tense*:

present + *walk* → *walk* or *walks*
past + *walk* → *walked*
present + *be* → *am*, *is* or *are*
past + *be* → *was* or *were*

Which form is taken by the present tense of the verb or *be*, and the past tense of *be*, depends on the subject.

Another morpheme that is added to verbs and to *be* is *ing*:

ing + *walk* → *walking*
ing + *be* → *being*

Traditionally, the *ing* form was called the *present participle.* But in the new grammar the first word of the predicate, not the *ing* form of the verb, expresses tense:

He *is* walking.	(present)
She *was* being tiresome.	(past)

So it would be confusing and pointless to call the *ing* form of the "present" participle or the "present" anything, and it is much less ambiguous merely to call it the "*ing* form."

Still another morpheme besides tense and *ing* that is added to verbs and to *be* is the morpheme *participle*, abbreviated *part.* The participle form is the form of the verb we use after *have*: have *looked*, have *grown.* This form was traditionally called the past participle. But it does not really indicate tense. The participle *grown* in "will have grown," for example, certainly does not suggest past. In the new grammar, the tense of "will have grown" is present and is expressed by the modal *will.* It is once again less ambiguous to drop the "past" and merely call *grown* the participle form of the verb *grow.*

Morpheme Strings

Transformational grammar puts morphemes together in *strings* to show the structure of sentences. In the strings of morphemes that follow, the morphemes of *tense* (present or past), *ing*, and *part*, apply to what comes after them.

In the following morpheme string, the morpheme *pres.* (present) applies to the verb *seem*:

the + *girl* + pres. | *seem* + *hungry*

The student sees that the subject is the singular noun phrase *the girl*, the first word of the predicate is the present tense form of the verb *seem* that goes with the singular subject, and the last word is *hungry.* So he translates the morpheme string into this sentence:

The girl seems hungry.

Notice the great emphasis upon the concord of the subject and verb and the highlighting of sentence structure that exercises of this kind provide.

In the following morpheme string the tense is *past*, the first word of the predicate is *be*, and the subject is *plural*:

the + *boy* + plural + past + *be* + *late*

Here the student must choose the past tense form of *be* that goes with a plural subject, *the boys*. He translates the morpheme string into the following sentence:

The boys were late.

By following clear rules objectively, the student has an opportunity to work out for himself the grammatical form of this sentence, rather than merely to repeat the sentence as part of a "correct usage" drill.

The strings of morphemes can be made more and more complex, of course, as the student grows in his capacity to deal with structural interrelationships. This morpheme string contains a *be* + *ing*:

they + pres. + *be* + *ing* + *swim* + *in* + *the* + *pond*

The noun phrase *they* is the subject; the present tense form of *be* that goes with *they* is *are*; when *ing* is added to *swim*, the word *swimming* results. So the morpheme string yields this sentence:

They are swimming in the pond.

The following string contains *have* + *part.*

the + *woman* + plural + past + *have* + part. + *be* + *busy*

Woman + plural is *women*, so the subject is *women*; the past tense form of *have* is *had*; the participle form of *be* is *been*. So the morpheme string yields this sentence:

The women had been busy.

Transformations

All of the grammar that has been summarized up to this point, and a great deal more which has been omitted because it is for the most part familiar, deals with simple sentences. It is amazing to see how much syntax is to be learned by a study of the simple, uncomplicated, affirmative statement in the new grammar.

However, the thorough, careful background in the underlying structure of the simple sentence is merely a foundation for the part of the program to come. Most of the sentences we say and write are much more complicated in structure than noun phrase + verb phrase. Even yes/no questions such as "Did you finish the work?", negative statements such as "You didn't finish the work," and commands such as "Finish the work" are more complicated in structure than simple sentences. Sentences such as "The men who were here fixed the furnace and put in a new water heater" are, of course, more complicated still. All of these sentences result from changes in kernel structures called *transformations*.

The study of transformations and their contribution to greater maturity in composition and reading is the culmination of a course in the new grammar.

Questions, negative statements, and commands involve only one noun phrase and one verb phrase, although structures within them are changed in order, added to, or deleted. Such transformations are called *single-base* because only one set of kernel structures is affected by the changes that produce them. Students typically have little difficulty in generating these types of transforms. However, single-base transformations reveal source mechanisms that are very general in English, and show beyond question the underlying orderliness of English grammar.

Transformations that involve two or more simple sentences are not more complex than the single-base types. These involve combining two or more sets of kernel structures that might have been expressed as separate sentences, but in fact come out as one. Such transformations are called *double-base*. It is by giving students conscious mastery over mechanisms for generating such sentences that we apply the grammar to writing or speaking, and to reading as well. One such double-base transformation that is very useful is called the *relative clause* transformation. In this transformation we rewrite one sentence, called the *insert sentence*, as a noun phrase expanded by a relative clause; then we replace a noun phrase in the other sentence, called the *matrix sentence*, with this expanded noun phrase.

Here is one way to present this transformation, step-by-step. We may begin with either the insert or the matrix sentence. Suppose we begin with the insert. The sentence is rewritten as a noun phrase expanded by a relative clause:

insert sentence: The mechanic was on duty.
noun phrase + rel. clause: The mechanic who was on duty

Now we rewrite the matrix sentence, dropping the noun phrase that the expanded noun phrase is to replace, and marking the position for the insert with the symbol *NP*:

matrix sentence: Mr. Willis distrusted the mechanic.
matrix with symbol: Mr. Willis distrusted + *NP*

Finally we replace the *NP* in the matrix with the expanded noun phrase from the insert, producing what is called the *result sentence*, or the *transform*:

transform: Mr. Willis distrusted the mechanic who was on duty.

Now, if we wish, we may delete the relative pronoun and *be* from any relative clause in which a form of *be* shows the tense. This gives up the following:

Mr. Willis distrusted the mechanic on duty.

Notice that this deletion works with *be* sentences, not with sentences in which a verb carried the tense—one more instance of the unique character of the word *be* in English.

The transformation illustrated above converted the insert sentence into a noun phrase expanded by a relative clause. The following is called the *subordinating transformation.* One word that can be used as a *subordinator* is the word *that.* We can make any sentence at all into a subordinate clause by putting *that* in front of it:

insert sentence: The school house burned.
subordinate clause: that the school house burned

We now insert the subordinate clause in a matrix sentence, first rewriting the matrix and using the symbol *S* to show where the insert sentence is to go:
matrix sentence: An event shocked everybody. → *S* + shocked everybody.

Finally, we replace that symbol *S* in the matrix with the subordinate clause:

transform: That the school house burned shocked everybody.

In sentences such as the transform above, the subordinate clause is actually a noun clause that functions as subject of the sentence. In everyday English, we put the subordinate clause last and begin the sentence with *it.* This called the *it transformation*:

it transformation: It shocked everybody that the schoolhouse burned.

There are, of course, many different kinds of transformations to be experienced as the student progresses in transformational grammar. These and other grammatical experiences in such a program give the student a consciousness of growing power in expression.

Applying Transformations

As the pupil learns transformations such as the four that have been used as examples, he can be helped to apply them both in reading and in writing.

In reading, a knowledge of transformations makes it possible to analyze a complex sentence, isolating the set of simple sentences that make it up. Here is an example of a complex sentence that can be analyzed by means of the four transformations that we have discussed: the relative clause transformation, the deletion transformation, the subordinate clause transformation, and the *it* transformation.

> Complex Sentence: It was obvious that the fire which had started below decks would spread to the planes on the flight deck.
> Simpler Sentences from the Complex Sentence: Something was obvious. The fire would spread to the planes. The fire had started below decks. The planes were on the flight deck.

The opposite process, synthesis, can be used effectively to increase maturity of written expression, once the students have learned some of the double-base transformations. Here is an example in which a group of simple sentences can be synthesized into a single more complex sentence by using three of the same four transformations: relative clause, subordinate clause, and *it*.

> Simpler Sentences: An event seemed likely. The storm would spoil the picnic. The storm was brewing.
> Process of Synthesis: We substitute the symbol *S* in the first of the simpler sentences to show that the insert is to go where "an event" now appears.

S + seemed likely

We change the second of the simpler sentences into a subordinate clause, using *that*.

that the storm would spoil the picnic

We transform the third sentence into a noun phrase expanded by a relative clause using *which* because we don't want to repeat the word *that*.

The storm which was brewing

We put all this together into a single sentence as follows.

> That the storm which was brewing would spoil the picnic seemed likely.

Finally we apply the *it* transformation.

> It seemed likely that the storm which was brewing would spoil the picnic.

Exercises as complex as the one above, of course, are for older students who have become familiar with the mechanisms of transformations. But even as early as the third grade, children can synthesize sentences such as "Alice washed the dishes" and "Alice made the beds" by compounding the predicates: "Alice washed the dishes and made the beds." Such simple exercises in synthesis at the presystematic level of instruction are no less effective because they are experimental and intuitive.

Writers, of course, do not synthesize their sentences in a step-by-step, conscious series of transformations. They grasp the possibilities because they are experienced writers—the synthesis is intuitive. Nevertheless, synthesis actually takes place. The evidence indicates that raising the use of transformation to a conscious level helps pupils write more maturely at an earlier age. Solving problems of composition by applying grammatical principles should be part of every English program.

Conclusion

What may this new English mean for the student? The student who follows such a program will give concentrated attention over eight or ten crucial years to the nature of expression, the structure of simple and complex sentences, and the morphemes that make up the structure. He will come directly face to face with the sound and spelling system of the English language, and find that truly it is a system, not a mere collection of irrational orthographic customs.

For the teacher, the new English promises great rewards because it provides a true subject matter. Teaching English as a discipline that has its own sequences, its own content and clearly defined goals will mean for many a new opportunity and a new satisfaction.

As the title suggests, the following article has a practical orientation, yet it includes a sound theoretical base for understanding and teaching transformational grammar. Zidonis sees the major responsibility of the language teacher as "interpreting for our students the insights into language currently being made by linguists." He focuses on the role of discovery in a three-step approach normally followed by linguists: "(1) careful observation of language data, (2) a rendering of this observation into rule-like definitions, and (3) checking the rules against more complicated data to see whether revisions need to be made."

Then he suggests practical examples of how these procedures can be carried out, illustrating from students' everyday speech. He examines some of the benefits or reasons for studying transformational grammar in the classroom, and concludes by identifying strategies that are used by some educators to keep transformational grammar out of the curriculum.

Incorporating Transformational Grammar into the English Curriculum

Frank J. Zidonis

Perhaps our major responsibility as teachers of language is to interpret for our students the insights into language currently being made by linguists. Unless we make use of this discipline in our classroom instruction, we risk shutting our students off from a rich source of meaningful inquiry. I think it is a fair judgment to make that typical school lessons in language are not generally characterized by a spirit of inquiry. Grammatical units—when they are even attempted by the English teacher today—are invested with an aura of certitude that belies the rich complexity of the language they purport to describe. We have for years been disillusioned by our students' confusion over the traditional definitions of parts of speech and functional use of sentence elements, a confusion that is seldom cleared up by subsequent reviews. We usually infer that there is something amiss with the student who fails to grasp the description of his language as the school grammar presents it, and that there is nothing deficient in the school grammar itself.

None of us today of course can take refuge in the kind of linguistic security that this closed view of language once afforded. Recent work in linguistic grammars has pointed up the many deficiencies of the school grammar. Probably the most glaring deficiency lay in the very semblance of completeness and accuracy that the school grammar was made to convey to our students. This deception was perpetrated upon them unwittingly, for we lacked the critical techniques for evaluating a grammar:

we did not really think seriously about what a grammar was to accomplish nor how it was to accomplish its end. We were quite outside the discipline in which we should have been operating, a discipline being in essence a method of inquiry.

The act of discovery, the sense of adventure, the satisfaction of original observation—all these are too often elements missing in our classrooms. We need to become involved with our students in making serious inquiry into the facts of the language we use and into attempts to explain those facts. Such inquiry will cover a range of problems extending from the effective use of metaphor down to the formation of the passive transformation rule. Nor should we pretend that every linguistic problem has a solution at the present time—an attempt simply to describe the ordinary determiner system of English should prove humbling enough. Rather, we should adopt an open-minded attitude toward language study in our classrooms, one characterized possibly by a three step approach: (1) careful observation of language data, (2) a rendering of this observation into rule-like descriptions, and (3) checking the rules against more complicated data to see whether revisions need to be made.

Let me illustrate this procedure. Suppose that the facts to be carefully observed by the class involve studying the behavioral effects in various sentences of the negative word *not* and its contraction, *n't*. Attention to the details of English use reveals quite quickly that the placement rule for *not* works differently from the one for its contraction. We do have the sentence,

Won't you try harder next time?

but not its uncontracted counterpart,

Will not you try harder next time?

In the uncontracted version, *not* must be shifted after *you*, to produce

Will you not try harder next time?

The second stage of the proposed procedure challenges the class to develop rules by which the acceptable sentences are produced and the unacceptable ones blocked. Finally, the rules developed are applied to a wider range of more complicated sentences to determine whether they hold up as they have been written. If the rules do not hold up, of course, they need to be revised, if possible.

Once inquiry into a discipline is undertaken, I think there are numerous side effects that take place—most of them, if not all, for the good. Students working with the placement rule for *not*, for example, can apply other transformations at the same time. Such experimentation often reveals the importance of the order which the rules of a grammar must follow. Suppose that in the data for the *not* placement rule we had included the sentence,

Mary does not understand the lesson.

What is the passive form for this sentence? The grammatical problem involved here is that of dealing with the form *does.* This element has entered the sentence as a result of the process that places *not* in its proper position. The passive transformation needs to be applied before the placement rule for *not* is applied, producing then the form,

The lesson is not understood by Mary.

Thus, the three-step procedure suggested here is a way of solving the sorts of problems that the grammar itself is able to pose, for a discipline, in addition to being a way of knowing, or perhaps *because* it is a way of knowing, is also a way of asking questions. The intellectual process that the student is being asked to reconstruct is much like the one that the linguist follows: (1) the careful observation of behavioral changes in real sentences; (2) an attempt to account for these changes by constructing rules—in effect the formulation of a hypothesis; and (3) the verification of the hypothetical formulation by its applicability to other linguistic data—that is, by its ability to predict the grammaticality of other structures in the language. This is, in short, the process of theory construction and validation. And it is in this sense that I take Jerome Bruner's observation to be valid:

> Intellectual activity anywhere is the same, whether at the frontier of knowledge or in a third-grade classroom. What a scientist does at his desk or in his laboratory, what a literary critic does in reading a poem, are of the same order as what anybody else does when he is engaged in like activities—if he is to achieve understanding. The difference is in degree, not in kind.[1]

We must still decide whether a transformational grammar should be studied in the English classroom. What benefits would our students derive from such study? We lament the fact that we in English seem to be singled out from the school subjects and asked to meet certain pragmatic tests; but we are in fact singled out, and so we ought to have developed a more convincing rationale for ourselves than we have heretofore: Valor must sometimes be the better part of discretion. In this connection, I am sure that we have all had occasion to cite some of the pertinent research evidence from our field regarding especially the teaching of grammar and its possible effect on composition. I have many times heard people make confident summaries of such research and draw inescapable conclusions proving the unrelatedness of grammatical study

[1] *The Process of Education.* Cambridge: Harvard University Press, 1960, p. 14.

for compositional skills. A serious examination of the research design in such studies, in the manner of Lumsdaine in the *Gage Handbook of Research on Teaching*,[2] supports another sort of conclusion, however: a diminishing respect for the kinds of studies that constitute research in our field. The use of grammar in the English curriculum remains, I believe, an open question so far as research is concerned.

Examining the content of the discipline seems to me to be a more fruitful way to decide upon uses of transformational grammar. The preliminary task that the curriculum maker needs to complete would be to examine the structure of a transformational grammar to identify the key concepts this structure contains and to establish the relations that exist among them. That English, any natural language, is systematic and therefore characterizable by a system of rules seems incontrovertible. As Chomsky points out,

> The central fact to which any significant linguistic theory must address itself is this: a mature speaker can produce a new sentence of his language on the appropriate occasion, and other speakers can understand it immediately, though it is equally new to them. . . . On the basis of a limited experience with the data of speech, each normal human has developed for himself a thorough competence in his native language. This competence can be represented, to an as yet undetermined extent, as a system of rules that we can call the grammar of his language.[3]

Now a grammar can concentrate on sentences in several ways. It can consider the sentence primarily as a sequence of sounds or characters—that is, the *form* of the sentence, or utterance, is all important. Of course, this is the stated concern—and limitation—of the structural linguist. Or a grammar can consider the sentence as the expression of a thought and try to discover how it is that a sentence expresses its thought. To some extent the traditional grammarian has been interested in this problem. A third approach, that of the transformationalist, is an expanded combination of the first two approaches. Thus a grammar might undertake to explain (1) how a sentence expresses its meaning, (2) how the sentence assumes the form it has, and (3) how its meaning and form are related. That the meaning and form of a sentence are often quite different is clear from the fact that there are sentences which we can understand only by supplying some "missing elements." Any imperative sentence in English, for example, omits the elements *you* and *will*, as in the sentence,

---

[2] Chicago: Rand McNally & Company, 1963. See in particular the problems of statistical interpretation, pp. 664–67.

[3] Noam Chomsky. "Current Issues in Linguistic Theory." *The Structure of Language*. Jerry A. Fodor and Jerrold J. Katz, eds. Englewood Cliffs, N. J.: Prentice-Hall, 1964, 50–51.

Close the door.

School grammars, incidentally, omit mention of the missing modal *will* in these cases, although we intuitively know that it belongs there when we add the tag question,

Close the door, *will* you?

Or, with the negative tag,

Close the door, *won't* you?

Consider, next, the instances in which the form—the surface structure—of the sentence does not necessarily reflect the relationships that exist among the various elements of the sentence. In such cases, we need to pierce through the surface structure of the sentence if we are to understand it. The instances I have in mind are perfectly straightforward sentences, well-formed, and not ambiguous. To understand them, however, and we understand them effortlessly, we have learned to supply certain elements and to rearrange certain others. Take, for example, the sentence,

The checkered flag signaled the end of the race.

What do we understand the subject of this sentence really to be? Ostensibly, it is *flag*. But would we want to ascribe a subject-predicate relationship to *flag* and *signaled* in this sentence? I think not, especially when we compare it with the subject-predicate relationship in the sentence,

An official signaled the end of the race with a checkered flag.

Here, it seems clear, *official* and *signaled* are related as subject and predicate, whereas the phrase *with a checkered flag* appears as an instrumental adverb. Is there much difference between the two sentences, finally? Or do we not in fact interpret the first one much as we do the latter one? In both sentences, it seems, *flag* performs an adverbial function, even though it appears as the ostensible subject in the first.

In the terms of transformational grammar, we might say that to understand a sentence, we must know what the *deep structure* of the sentence is—that is, we must perceive what the underlying organization of the sentence is. This underlying organization, the way the elements of the sentence are related, moreover, is often obscured by the final form the sentence takes, that is to say, by its surface structure.

The transformational model of generative grammar consists of two major components. The first is a set of Base Rules that produce the *deep structure* of a sentence, which reveals how the various elements of the sentence are grammatically related to one another. It is the deep structure that enables us to impose a semantic interpretation upon the sentence. The second component is a set of Transformational Rules that act upon the deep structure to provide the *surface structure* of the sentence, the actual sounds we utter or the characters we see in print.

This relationship between deep structure and surface structure appears to be a concept of central importance in the structure of a transformational grammar of English. Other important relationships are those between grammatical and deviant sentences; competence and performance; acceptable and unacceptable; and grammatical, deviant, acceptable, and unacceptable sentences. The explanatory power of the relationship between deep structure and surface structure is suggested in the following schema, which provides another way of considering the entire language-arts curriculum.

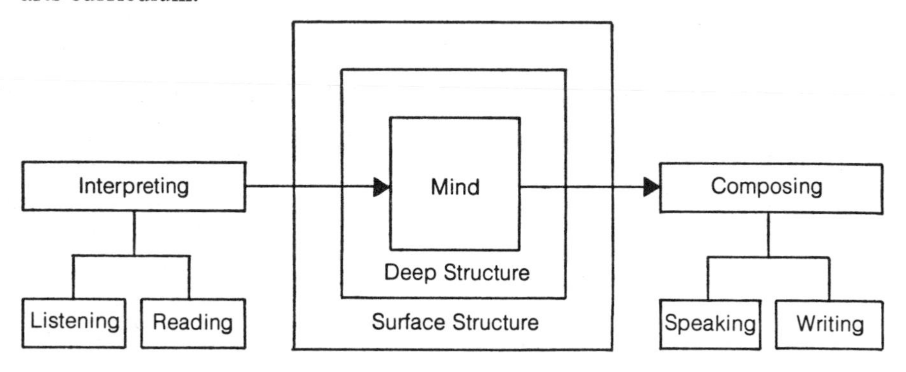

The schema identifies two basic skills in the English program; interpreting and composing. Interpreting involves the ability to decipher from the surface structure present what the deep structure is in order to impose the semantic interpretation upon it. Since the surface structure can be ambiguous, recovering the deep structure is not always simple. In composing, the path is reversed and goes from deep structure to surface structure. Under *interpreting* skills we would group *listening* and *reading*; under *composing, speaking*, and *writing.*

I should like to dwell finally on a not entirely facetious review of strategies I have encountered being used by teachers in the field to maintain their professional stance and, at the same time, remarkably, to maintain the *status quo.* In a spirit of camaraderie, I offer these ploys to those who are not going to change instruction in any way but who could use a professional reason for not doing so.

Strategy A. "I have always been interested in practical aids for helping my students write better. If transformational grammar provides such help, I might try it. But, after all, the author of *Beowulf*, Chaucer, Shakespeare, Milton, Dickens, and others, didn't study transformational theory and they wrote fairly well." If delivered dramatically enough, you can reach a note of irony, or even sarcasm, with the words *fairly well* so sharp as to devastate your transformational opponent. Of course, as grammar is discussed herein, everyone can be said to have internalized a transformational grammar.

Strategy B. Whereas Strategy A is an aggressive one, basically questioning the need for transformational study at all, Strategy B is ideal for the person comfortable with traditional materials as they are presented in the popular language arts series. It goes like this: "In all these competing systems of grammatical analysis, I find that there is a heavy reliance on new terminology. Our students could easily become submerged in a morass of conflicting terms, notions, and procedures. They ought to have a solid basis in conventional grammatical study to provide them with a framework for studying the new grammar." Notice this teacher can now reasonably continue laying that solid basis of traditional terminology again.

Strategy C. Perhaps the most professional-sounding position to take is the one embodied here. This position reflects well on the open-mindedness of the teacher and shows him to be among the more sophisticated. It is very briefly stated, one sentence sufficing: "The evidence isn't all in, yet." Unfortunately, none of us will be around when all the evidence is in, hence, there is little point in commenting on this classic delaying tactic of the conservative curriculum coordinator.

Strategy D. The general theme of the final strategy runs something like this: "Language is beautiful. Why can't we accept it in all its beauty instead of picking it to pieces and then reassembling it. I'm afraid that a rigorous study of our language will simply result in shutting us off from the beauty of English—like missing the forest because of the trees."

Objections made against a rigorous study of language are much like those levied against the literary critic who advocates close reading of the text. The fear is that, if made rigorous, such study is no longer enjoyable. Let me close with a thought from Robert Penn Warren on this possibility:

> I know perfectly well that there are some readers of poetry who object to this process. They say that it is a profanation, that they simply want to enjoy the poem. And we can be comforted by the fact that the poem, if it is a true poem, will, like the baby's poor kitty-cat, survive all the pinching and prodding and squeezing which love will lavish upon it. It will have nine lives too. Further, and more importantly, the perfect intuitive and immediate grasp of a poem in the totality of its meaning and structure—the thing we desire—may come late rather than early—on the fiftieth reading rather than on the first.[4]

---

[4] "The Themes of Robert Frost," in *Selected Essays*. New York: Random House, 1958, page 119.

The final selection in part II is a delightfully written but rather jaundiced view of the new grammar seen from many perspectives. Sledd identifies views and trends in the teaching of grammar. He presents the older view ("a mysterious and exasperating subject"), the climb-on-the-linguistics-bandwagon view, the baffled view, and the cynical view of new grammar. He looks at the effect that new grammar is having (or might have) on college and university English departments, teachers, professional organizations, publishing houses, and the College Entrance Examining Board, and at the effect that these agencies are having on new grammar. Despite a skeptical tone throughout, Sledd seems to reveal a ray of hope at the end of the article with his two final views. He is particularly critical of college English departments, more hopeful for schools.

While at times the tone of what Sledd has to say seems tongue-in-cheek and facetious, the intent is undoubtedly very serious, with implications for all of us.

Snafu, Fubar, or Brave New World? National Trends in the Teaching of Grammar

James Sledd

"This is a 'golden age' for the English profession."
—NCTE blurb

Wee mynde not the stinke yf wee haue the chynke.
—Elizabethan proverb

"Ahab must come to gripes with the whale."
—English major

1. *The popular view.* When Americans think of the teaching of grammar, they think of English grammar as traditionally taught by teachers of English—a mysterious and exasperating subject, but allegedly useful to students and citizens who hope to speak and write correctly or to learn a foreign language. Grammar is English grammar, it is applied grammar, and English departments are responsible for teaching it. It is not a serious intellectual inquiry or a proper study for well-adjusted males.

To some extent, those familiar connotations have changed in recent years. The general public has grown vaguely conscious of something called linguistics, which has bred something called the new grammar, which commands a certain amount of wary, awed respect, like the new math; but among the less sophisticated there is also a good deal of feeling that though linguists can be tolerated as unamiably eccentric academics, they are suspiciously clever, incapable of using English properly, and just possibly subversive.

2. *Bull market in linguistics.* Though this popular view is one determinant of present trends in teaching, it is otherwise only deviously related to present realities: ignorant misunderstanding must be assumed but need not be discussed as the public stage for every venture in democratic education. Actually the study of grammar and particularly English grammar, is today not just respectable intellectually but more lively, more important, and more attractive to more people than it has been for a long time. Linguists, philosophers, mathematicians, assorted scientists, and educational theorists not uncommonly argue its intrinsic importance to their studies and to the proper study of mankind; and the demands for applications of grammatical knowledge are multifarious. The old cry of status-seekers for guides to correctness is now the least of many voices. Business and industry want a certain number of linguistic technologists; educators and politicians want teachers of the world's most popular language to foreigners at home and abroad; the poor and ignorant at home must learn to read, write, and sometimes speak some kind of standard English if they are not to become the inflammable waste of a society which needs no unskilled labor; the schools and colleges must turn out thousands of literate middle-class underlings to feed our omnivorous machines; and increasing numbers of genuinely expert linguists will be needed to do some part of the thinking and high-level teaching that may keep the whole operation from collapse. Pure and applied linguistics is now a booming, clamorous business.

3. *The problem of English departments.* Miss Bessie Jones, assistant professor of emeritus English in Purity State College, is utterly baffled by new clamor and new grammar alike. She disapproves of both, and she is not alone. Departments of English dignify her timid aversion with orations against the sciences, which become tolerable only when the National Science Foundation must be used as a political lever to set up a National Humanities Foundation. Since somebody once said that linguistics is or might become or hopes to be scientific, one very noticeable trend in the nation's grammatical instruction is for the serious study and teaching of the mother tongue to be edged out of departments of English, which keep their stray linguists mainly because an ark which did not have one pair of every species would be non-U. Five years ago an eminent linguist proposed that departments of foreign languages take over the teaching of English grammar too.

It might not be done worse by German or French than it is done by English now. Certainly in the schools and even to some extent in the colleges and universities, one still looks to English departments for English grammarians; but sometimes one does not find them, and when one does find them in the higher institutions, they are likely to be unhappy, mediocre, and obstreperous. They are so because their original training was not the best (since they got it in English departments) and because they now have to live among literary colleagues who dislike and disprize the teaching of composition and grammar, the preparation of teachers, the multiplication of linguists, and the people variously responsible for these afflictions. Obstreperous mediocrities are not the best leaders in a crisis.

Yet the mediocre grammarians in English departments, it might be argued, are sinned against as vigorously as they sin. Present company and other exceptions duly excepted, college professors of English literature have done as much to bring on our golden age. The literary professors as a group are not notably constructive citizens. In fact, too many of them dislike almost everything about the world they live on except English literature, high salaries, low teaching loads, and government grants. They dislike linguistics because they dislike science, and in particular they dislike the name of service departments, as if *Ich dien* were a plebeian motto. The problem of unserviceable English departments, as their literary members see it, is thus to find a politic way of doing as much as they can for themselves and literature and no more than they have to do for literacy. They use the freshman course (once a course in composition) as an instrument of reproduction, the means of supporting the graduate students who teach it, and they equip the teachers whom they send into the schools with their own prejudices and not much else. The study of grammar and composition is not likely to become a serious concern in a college English department unless the government offers to subsidize it.

4. *A brazen judgment on the golden age.* Distressed by debt and this state of affairs, a happily obstreperous grammarian in an English department recently described the golden age in his branch of the profession as snafu, susfu, and perhaps fubar. That was two years and more ago, but no retraction has yet appeared of the ten following summary statements:

(1) that nobody is satisfied with our teaching of English grammar, (2) that there is, however, no general agreement on what is wrong or what we should do about it, (3) that departments of English and schools of education refuse to train prospective teachers adequately for their work in grammar and composition, (4) that we must therefore abandon hope for an adequate supply of really competent teachers, (5) that the untrained teachers whom we are turning out face a peculiarly confused and confusing situation in the field of English linguistics, (6) that the confusion is increased by the controversies about the purposes and values of grammatical instruction, (7) that suitable textbooks and teaching materials are available neither for structural nor for transformational grammar, (8) that all forms of modern grammar are now under violent attack by intellectual bookburners, (9) that the American public will never pay for the kind of teaching it says it wants, and finally (10) that the struggling apprentice teacher cannot expect much help or guidance from professional societies, foundations, or governmental agencies. We are in a bad way, and things are not likely to get much better.

If these things are true, then efforts to improve the teaching of English grammar in this country and to extend its applications must not be limited to English departments only, which indeed (in colleges and universities) are the chief obstacles to progress; and a survey or recent expedients, though it may begin with English departments, must not be limited to their undertakings. The college professors of English, an unkind obstreperosity might say, have sounded like brass and tinkled their begging-bells but have abstained from any excesses of good works.

5. *Diversionary tactics I: The talkathon.* The less said the better about the fashionable attempts to define the field of English. English as an academic subject is a historical accident, and none the worse for that; but linguistically inclined individuals (in search of the womb and unit) have chosen to find the essence of the subject in language, literarily inclined individuals have found it in literature, and committees on basic issues have proposed to build ideally cumulative and sequential curricula in their fundamental liberal discipline on puzzling enumerations like "writing, rhetoric, criticism, linguistics, and the history of the language," from which all intelligible distinctions have been banished. A second trend in the teaching of grammar may therefore be identified as the wasting of time in selfish and superficial talk instead of getting on with the job.

6. *Diversionary tactics II: Let George do it.* A third trend has been the movement by the colleges and universities to pass the buck of grammar and composition to the schools. Majors and graduates in English, we are told by eminent professors thereof, do write abominably and do corrupt their freshman students, whom the professors refuse to teach; but the the colleges and universities can do little to change this situation, since bad linguistic habits are fixed beyond correction by the time a student has finished school. The colleges and universities will be doing their full duty if they train the schools' prospective teachers. The school-teachers must then teach schoolboys to read and write better than the professors, going "beyond simple *literacy* and *correctness* to teach *effectiveness* in writing and *subtlety* in literary analysis."

Nobody believes such things are possible, of course; but even if they were, the colleges and universities have yet to show their willingness to train teachers. English majors are too often unprofessional refuges for little boys who want Culture and little girls who want little boys, but the same department whose major is a disgrace and whose apprentice teachers learn nothing about their language, its use, or the teaching of either will eagerly grasp at funds for an institute to retrain the practising teachers whom the department left untrained when they were apprentices. Hastily planned and inadequately staffed, the ubiquitous institutes must undo four years' damage in eight weeks. They would be justified as devices for keeping originally well-trained teachers alert and currently informed in changing fields, but in present circumstances the money which is spent on institutes would be better spent in improving undergraduate curricula and teaching.

7. *Experiment in the schools.* More hopeful trends in the teaching of grammar are apparent in the schools than in the colleges, at least where English departments are concerned. In 1964 the NCTE, in which schoolteachers are strongly represented, rebuked the more prestigous MLA for its attitude toward the teaching of composition, which the NCTE considers "the continuing responsibility of all levels of our educational system"; and a number of good public and private schools are continuing or launching hopeful experiments in the teaching of modern grammars. One salutary though embarrassing consequence will be that even larger numbers of college students will find their lower-division courses inferior to their high-school work. Perhaps the best schools may soon offer institutes for college teachers.

Experiments with new grammars in the schools would be less hazardous if the study of English grammar were itself more settled. At least four different grammatical systems, each with its own variants, are presently competing for pedagogic favor—the traditional schoolroom grammar; the scholarly nonstructural grammar of men like Jespersen, Curme, and Long; the American structural grammar of such linguists as Trager, Smith, Fries, and their disciples; and the transformational grammar of Noam Chomsky and his group at M.I.T. The last five years have seen increasing interest in transformational doctrine, which is making its way into more and more of the less glacial curricula and which has now been popularized in several textbooks for schools and colleges; but both curricula and textbooks are likely to be put out of date when they appear, since the basic doctrine itself has been subject and will continue to be subject to frequent and extensive revision. If the new math is already giving way to newer math while conservatives complain that the new itself was hastily inaugurated without adequate preparation of teachers, one can see the possibility of a similar situation in English linguistics (includng English grammar). A linguistic scholar who wants to remain a scholar may find himself compelled to take frequent leaves and to mantain at least a loose attachment to some research team; school grammarians too will need periodic leaves or subsidized refresher courses; and good textbooks are likely to be the work of multiple authors, multiply subsidized, with frequent revisions and whole batteries of teaching aids, audiovisual and other. The demands of the future are frightening when one remembers present failure: most present teachers of English are unprepared to teach even the oldest grammar well; the available new textbooks are not only out of date when they are published but are generally mediocre; and the whole situation is enormously complicated by the simultaneous necessity of fitting the presently unemployable for useful citizenship in a world dominated by great cities and runaway technology.

Meanwhile college English departments snort with the Seven Sleepers.

8. *Commercial publishing, or Bughouse Square.* Like the schools, commercial publishers are less somnolent, though as puzzled as everyone else by current trends. To exist, the publishers must please the market, particularly the market of the schools and that of the proliferating junior colleges, where teachers, standards, and clear purposes are in short supply and the one certainty seems to be that teen-agers must be kept off the streets and the labor-market for two more years. Since most administrators and old-line teachers will not risk the new grammars, there is a good deal of standpatism in recent textbooks, though even the most conservative textbookators are likely to tack on an inaccurate chapter or two about structural or transformational grammar; but a policy of stand-pat infuriates the highly vocal reformers. Unfortunately for the publishers' peace of mind, the reformers do not agree among themselves. Some are linguists who cannot write and who know nothing about teaching English composition and grammar; others are English teachers with limited knowledge of linguistics; and while both groups are voluble in rash claims and bitter condemnation of traditionalists, they propose to teach a number of different grammars for a number of different reasons. In their debates, the old controversy about the relevance of grammar to composition has been revived, and while some speak mainly for grammar as intrinsically valuable, others prefer to agree that its irrelevance to composition was never really proved and that transformational grammar, whose devotees are often peculiarly inept in writing, will turn youngsters into stylists and teachers into sophisticated analysts of style. Perhaps it may be so; but an understandable wariness is observable among the publishers. They seem to talk a good deal about teams of writers from linguistics and English, from schools and colleges, who together might produce salable eclectic or transitional grammars. There is much to be said for such schemes, though an eclectic grammar may be an inconsistent mishmash and at best will add still another system to those presently in competition.

9. *The College Entrance Examination Board.* The great service now rendered by commercial publishers is the obvious result of economic competition: since they will publish any grammar which they think is good enough to sell to any substantial segment of the market, they maintain a public platform on which any competent grammarian of any stripe can have his say. Despite the contempt of intellectuals for the marketplace, that service may be greater than those rendered by agencies which seek more actively to direct present trends in the teaching of grammar. Notable among these is the College Entrance Examination Board, with its Commission on English. Its institutes have been highly praised but have perhaps confused more teachers of grammar than they have genuinely enlightened, and the Board's examinations (some of them fondly known as

"the cutting edge of curricula change") have so far done nothing remarkable to improve the study and teaching of the English language in our schools. One hopes that the current revision of the examinations will make them more effective.

10. *The architects of the Great Society.* The success of the new government-sponsored institutes in English will be more easily judged in the winter than it can be predicted in the spring of 1965. They have been planned in frantic haste, and there will apparently be considerably more of them than there are competent grammarians, so that not much should be expected when mediocre staffs attempt to execute rash plans; but the institutes will perhaps be as useful as much busy research work for Project English has been. One cannot imagine that that other instrument of academic bureaucrats and bureaucratic academics, the proposed National Humanities Foundation, will dirty its hands with the teaching of the English language. It will be too busy appointing committees, carpeting offices, and sharing with our fellow-countrymen "whatever understanding can be attained by fallible humanity of such enduring values as justice, freedom, virtue, beauty, and truth." Like Curriculum Centers, however, the Foundation will derive great prestige from these amiable activities.

In so imperfect a world, less spiritual agencies of government are likely to be more significant for grammarians and their pupils. Governmental concern for the teaching of English as a second language will continue to produce some visible results, like courses in languages and linguistics for members of the Peace Corps or elementary textbooks in English for foreign students; and city, state, and federal governments have at least begun serious practical and theoretical work on the problems of English-teaching to poor and ignorant minorities. The possibilities for good and evil in this enterprise are presently incalculable. Little will have been accomplished if the main result is the conversion of lower-class monsters to middle-class monsters, the culturally deprived to the culturally depraved; but at least the dream is alive of opening a way to some measure of freedom, through real literacy, for multitudes who say they want to be free. Though the inseparable connection of literacy with freedom has scarcely been established, English teachers who are willing to sacrifice themselves for others have some excuse for talking about a golden age.

11. *Landscape in dust storm.* An unheroic and unromantic pedagogue will emerge from a survey of national trends in the teaching of grammar with the less optimistic feeling that he has tried to summarize a windmill, which creates some turbulence but only goes round and round. He will feel a prevalent sense of urgency, or crisis, of possibilities for achievement in a larger world than English grammarians have been accumstomed to; but he will also feel a sense of confused frustration. Is a knowledge of English grammar to be sought and conveyed as an intrinsically valuable part of

the knowledge of man, is it a means to the more mundane end of proficiency in the use of English, or is it both—or neither? If it is both, which aspect of the subject should be emphasized by educators, and how should either value be ranked, in the English department to which the pedagogue belongs, in comparison to the values of English literature, which is certainly essential to the life of the academic spirit and the continued employment of professors of English? Which of the many systems of English grammar deserves the pedagogue's allegiance? How can the pedagogue find time to achieve or maintain some mastery of the subject, and when, where, how, and to whom should he teach it or urge that it be taught?

Real social pressures are more likely than theory to answer these questions for him, if ever they are answered; and meanwhile the pedagogue will laugh or grieve, according to his temperament, as he contemplates a splendid exemplification of the affluent society's most firmly conditioned reflex: in times of crisis we appoint committees, issue directives, deny our personal responsibilities, and appropriate large sums of government money (in various senses of that verb). In the teaching of English grammar in the last ten years, we have made more noise than progress.

12. *Politic, cautious, and meticulous.* The main reason has been unwillingness to come to gripes with the Great Whale, the English departments—the largest humanistic departments—in our colleges and universities. English departments are dominated by professors of literature—some of them (it is impertinent to say) men of great learning, wisdom, and integrity, but others, less exalted souls who make it their prime function to teach the next generation of perturbed spirits to teach the next that a laboratory is the devil's workshop but that literature can do everything the devout still hope for from religion. Such men know little of English linguistics and want their student to learn no more, with the result, as Professor Prokosch told the MLA in 1937, that "the teaching of the structure of the language of our country is in the great majority of even our best universities badly neglected, or almost entirely disregarded." Naturally, then, since English departments train English teachers, "many English teachers in American elementary and high schools are not qualified to teach their native language." Until they are, the teaching of grammar will get no better fast.

Even now, to be sure, some useful things can be and are being done. Since present teachers must go on teaching daily with present textbooks and materials, probably "the best most schools can do is to teach a good traditional grammar or a scholarly nonstructural one like Perrin's." They should teach grammar systematically, both for itself and as a help in teaching the use of English, because a language is a system and cannot be taught as anything else. The better schools "might consider the introduction of special courses in the English language for college-bound students of superior ability." Some of the best schools are already doing more—choosing the best available grammar, subsidizing the training or retraining of their teachers, preparing their own teaching materials, and devising, for a four-year high-school program, at least an introduction to the principal fields of English linguistics. The open-door policy of commercial publishers guarantees publication of materials from such advanced programs, or from any other source, whenever they are available.

The great stumbling-block remains the college and university English department, where the dominant literary faction contemplates its own wisdom and virtue in frightened, superior alienation. Such people do not welcome criticism or even tolerate it unless they have to, and since they are powerful in the academic establishment, only the imprudent or the comfortably secure will tell them that they must make a choice. They will not serve the best interests of the literature to which their principal allegiance is rightly due if they try to serve literature alone. An example of selfish detachment from the needs of their society is a strong counter-argument to their claims that literature as they teach it makes men wise and good, and as written literature has never been of great value to the illiterate, so verbally oriented literary criticism cannot enlighten the linguistically obtuse. America can get along without the "presentational knowledge" that "life is a mystery calling to a mystery." It cannot get along if its college graduates cannot write and if its high-school graduates have the abilities of fourth-graders.

To be blunt: Either the English departments will work (or accept) a revolution and give far more time and energy than they give now to the teaching of the English language and of English composition and to the preparation of teachers; or they will remain a dowdy sanctuary for a vestigial priesthood, slowly declining into sterility and irrelevance. There is little chance of a revolution unless external pressure—economic pressure—is applied. If the country wants better teaching of the English language and its use we must have a much larger supply of competent teachers: only teachers can improve teaching. English departments on their own initiative will not furnish that supply, and attempts to bribe them with government grants will not succeed: grants will be used, by the establishment, to consolidate the old regime. Deprivation is the only means of persuasion that remains. Until English departments lose their budgets if they do not teach the language and its use and train teachers properly, the great national trend in the teaching of English grammar will be to go from bad to worse.

Postscript

Whether or not you buy one brand of new grammar or another lock, stock, and barrel, there is a lot in new grammar that can be adopted and adapted for teaching language arts to pupils at any level.

Pupils Have Grammar

Whenever they speak language, your pupils exhibit their knowledge of grammar. Start off by letting them know how much they know. Write each of the following eight words on separate pieces of paper and place them in a box: go, day, boys, school, every, and, to, girls. Have one pupil draw the slips of paper from the box at random and place them in the order in which they were drawn. The resulting string of words will probably not make sense (unless your luck that day is incredible, at which point you should run out and buy a ticket on the Irish Sweepstakes). The first time I tried this with children, the resulting "sentence" was: To boys every day girls and go school. Now have the children rearrange the words in various ways to make a sentence that is grammatical—that conforms to the syntactic patterns of English. (Boys and girls go to school every day. Girls and boys go to school every day.) Pretty soon, your class will run out of possibilities. (Every day school girls go to boys, may be suggested, but this leaves out and.) This type of activity develops the awareness of language structure, that words are not strung together like beads on a string but rather they fit together in an ordered way. And pupils already know the pattern of the puzzle; they know the grammar of the language.

Now make six separate lists of words according to their classes (or parts of speech if you prefer)—words that pattern such as: the, boy, went, quickly, to, good. Write each word on a slip of paper or index card. You may want to put the words into six separate boxes or color code them according to word class. Have groups of pupils draw these words and rearrange them, putting them into "slots" to see which words go together to make sentences in an order that fits the grammar of our language.

Incidentally, I've seen remedial reading teachers use exercises similar to this. The words on index cards are used to develop word recognition skills and rearranging them helps comprehension.

Parts of Speech

When (or if at all) parts of speech should be taught is a debatable issue. The controversy was well summed up in an experience that I had working with a language arts curriculum committee. While we were trying to decide where to put parts of speech in the curriculum, a third grade teacher at one end of the long table said, "I don't care if my pupils know how to define an adjective, just so long as they can use many adjectives well in their writing." Her seventh grade colleague at the other end of the table pounded his fist and replied, "Well I'm sick to death of having to teach parts of speech in junior high school. I expect pupils to know what an adjective is when they graduate from elementary school." Linguistics doesn't provide resolutions to debates like this, for as Kenneth Goodman said in his article in part I, "A language curriculum cannot be built without dealing with linguistic matters, just as a bridge cannot be built by engineers without dealing with the laws of physics. But knowing the laws of physics does not determine how the bridge may be built, or where, or when, or in fact whether it should be built at all."

But even as this debate rages, most teachers continue to teach the parts of speech, if only because they are required to do so. Here's where the structuralist's techniques for identifying parts of speech by their structural markers are useful. Write the first stanza of Lewis Carroll's *Jabberwocky* on the board or on an overhead transparency:

> 'Twas brillig, and the slithy toves
> Did gyre and gimble in the wabe;
> All mimsy were the borogoves,
> And the mome raths outgrabe.

Most students find this poem rather interesting, even if nothing more is done with it.

Underline those words that are part of our lexicon ('Twas, and, the, did, in, all, were). Now try to identify the parts of speech of the nonsense words by their structural markers. Which structural elements hold this nonsense together? *Toves* and *wabe* can be seen as nouns, *gyre* and *gimble* as verbs, and *slithy* as an adjective because of their positions in the sentence, by the affixes that are used with some of them, and by the function words that accompany them (*the* in the case of the nouns and *did* in the case of the verbs). *The slithy toves did gyre and gimble in the wabe* fits a grammatical sentence pattern with which all pupils are familiar (The grouchy men did grumble and complain in the bar. or The happy kids did run and jump in the field.)

Moreover, if we were to rearrange some of these structural elements (for example: the slithy tove did gyrs and gimbls) it wouldn't sound just right. It would violate the grammar of English and thus disturb our "built-in sense of grammaticalness." This type of activity can be used to call pupils' attention to agreement between nouns and verbs.

Use the Jabberwocky frame:

'Twas __________ and the __________ __________
Did __________ and __________ in the __________;
All __________ were the __________,
And the __________ __________ __________

to have your pupils write their own poems. The results might be something like:

'Twas raining and the slippery eels
Did slither and slide in the mud.
All chilly were the fishermen,
And the wise fish understood.

Corny? See what your class can do with it!

Another more conventional way of introducing parts of speech is to use the frame: The __________ boy *ran* down the __________ street. What words fit into the first blank to describe the boy? The second blank to describe the street? What words can be used in place of *run*? When lists have been made, let the students write their own sentences using the words they have listed and others they can think of. This not only uses the concept of verbs and adjectives, but it also develops pupils' skill in descriptive writing. Using this exercise, one of my pupils produced the sentence: The fat boy squeezed down the narrow street. An interesting and rather humorous word picture!

Sentence Patterns

From the kind of activities described above, it is an easy jump to the study of sentence patterns. Maybe a bulletin-board display of common sentence patterns (found on pages 114 and 154 of this book; a more complete list can be found in structural grammar texts) would make a good introduction.

N V	Men cried. Women screamed.
N V N	John loves Mary. The clown did a somersault.
N V N N	He gave his neighbor a punch. She threw him a kiss.
N V Adj	My teacher is great. This book seems boring.
N V Adv	They worked hard. My friends arrived early.

(Notice that what we know as pronouns fit into the noun class.) From their own writing, your students can expand the list of patterns and examples.

The next step might be to expand the various word groups. The noun *men* can be expanded to: The big strong men with tears in their eyes. Your pupils can elaborate further, using adjectives and prepositional phrases, beginning with one-word modifiers and expanding from there. Lefevre gives an example of this kind of sentence expansion on pages 154–55.

Have your students check their own writing. Which sentence patterns are prevalent? Have them listen to a tape recording of a segment of their conversations. What sentence patterns are prevalent there? What are the differences evidenced between their speech and their writing?

Try giving your class practice in manipulating basic sentence patterns to produce negative statements, questions, and passive sentences. Take, for example, the very simple N V N pattern. What possibilities are there for questions here? How is this pattern made negative? Students will soon discover the rules in many of these language structures.

In manipulating these and similar sentence patterns your pupils will also discover that different members of the same word class behave differently. For example, in making the sentence *The boy hit the ball* passive, we say *The ball was hit by the boy.* But the sentence *The book cost five dollars* can't be reordered in the same way; we don't say *Five dollars was cost by the book.* This can lead to a discussion of verbs (transitive, intransitive, linking, the verbs *to be, to do,* as well as auxiliary verbs); of nouns (mass nouns and count nouns), and of other parts of speech or word classes. *The beautiful girl* means *The girl is beautiful,* but does *The drinking fountain* mean *The fountain is drinking?* This kind of activity can lead to a greater awareness of how our language operates.

Making Sentences Grow

Starting with basic sentences represented by the patterns in the previous section (which transformationalists used to refer to as *kernels*) your class can examine and apply procedures for making their sentences grow. The mark of a good writer is skill in combining more and more basic sentences in various ways. I would suspect that the gains in sentence construction reported in the research on teaching transformational grammar in the classroom can be traced directly to pupils' improving their skill in sentence-combining transformations. Take the series of simple sentences shown here:

> The crowd was large.
> The game was in the bottom of the ninth inning.
> The score was tied.

Harry hit a home run.
Our team won the game.
The crowd was happy.
The crowd cheered.

Depending on the grade level of your pupils, you might want to start with fewer sentences or expand the list to twelve or fourteen smaller sentences.

One way of combining any or all of these seven sentences into one large one is through coordination. (The crowd was large and it was the bottom of the ninth inning and the score was tied and . . . .). Another way is through modification. (The crowd which was large and the game which was in the bottom of the ninth inning . . .). Still another way is subordination (When the crowd was large and when the game was in the bottom of the ninth inning and when . . .). We can recognize all of these sentences as the products of a rather immature writer. The mature writer will use a combination of coordination, modification, subordination, and other linguistic devices to make these seven little sentences into one big one.

Have your students try it. There is no one single formula by which all must be combined to come up with the "right answer" for the final product. (The large and happy crowd cheered when, in the bottom of the ninth inning, Harry hit a home run to break a tie and win the game for our team. *or* In the bottom of the ninth with the score tied, Harry's home run won the game for our team, and the large, happy crowd cheered.) There are many possibilities. In fact, it has been said that one of the distinguishing features of new grammar (compared to traditional grammar) is that it focuses on possibilities rather than prohibitions in language matters. Transformational grammar contains explicit rules on how to make larger and more complex sentences out of simpler ones. Good writers use these rules intuitively; the grammar describes what the good writer does when he uses these devices.

Structural Ambiguities

Over the years, structural ambiguities have given composition teachers a few smiles and many tears in what W. Nelson Francis calls "mingled delight and despair."

While eating our lunch, the plane took off.
Keep your hand off the wall because it's filthy.
Serve prunes thoroughly stewed.

What happens in examples like these is that there is a conflict between form and meaning; that is, either the words in the sentence seem to suggest one meaning while the sense of the sentence suggests something else, or the words in the sentence are so ordered that the meaning is unclear. While linguistics per se will not eliminate dangling participles or misplaced modifiers in pupils' writing, a heightened consciousness of the structural features of the language will likely lead to a greater awareness of possibilities for incongruities in language, ambiguities that result from the way in which words are arranged. (Fries identifies some of these possibilities in *The Structure of English*, as does Norman Stageberg in "Some Structural Ambiguities" in *The English Journal*, November 1958.) A good starting point for eliminating or at least reducing these structural ambiguities might be the analysis of the students' own writing. The aim here is to improve students' clarity of expression, to make their sentences clearer vehicles of thought.

Discovering Standards of Usage

What do you want for your students, good grammar or good taste? They probably already have good grammar in the sense of language structure, but they may need to become more aware of good taste in language matters. Good taste refers to usage, the attitudes that speakers have toward different aspects of their language. While these attitudes extend beyond grammar to matters of phonology and lexicology, we'll limit our consideration to grammatical form.

Maybe a good starting point would be a discussion of just what "good English" is. This opens the door to questioning the very foundation upon which a large part of our professional activity has conventionally been based, but this is what linguists have been doing for years (which is maybe why they have met so much resistance and hostility from some educational quarters). *Good* is a value-laden term and the search for the answer(s) to "What is good English?" will likely send students looking in different directions to find the answer to the related question "Good according to who(m)?"

Try using a list with expressions such as:

He *don't* listen.
George *doesn't* have *no* money.
I *ain't* going out tonight.
If I *was* you, I'd do my homework.
Drive *slow*.
The exam really wasn't really *all that* hard.
Who did you give the book *to*?
It's *me*.
Everybody in the cafeteria ate *their* lunch.
Winston tastes good *like* a cigarette should.

Each of these expressions violates some rule of traditional grammar in the italicized words. You might want to include expressions prevalent in the language of your own students.

For each item on your inquiry form, ask the students to indicate whether the expression is Good English, or Bad English. Include a provision for Don't Know or Not Sure. Discuss the results and reasons for their choices. Your class might want to administer this form to their parents or other members of their community as part of a class project.

Standards of usage differ from one situation to another. Take an expression such as: Me and Charlie is friends (or if you want to stay "closer to home:" I plan to boldly ask her to go out) and ask the students to tell you who would probably be disturbed by these expressions and who wouldn't. They might want to list situations where it may be *safe* to use these expressions (in the bowling alley with friends, for example) and where it wouldn't be so safe (in a job interview).

What do these types of activities accomplish? First, they allow students to use discovery techniques about their language—and this is at the heart of the linguistic process. Also, students learn that there are value judgements about the many ways of using language and that it may behoove them to learn the appropriate form of language to use when these values are at stake. They may even learn where these judgements come from. And finally, they may leave your English class with something more than a lifelong fear of grammatical errors and with confidence in their ability to use the form of language that will fit the many situations in which they may find themselves.

Conclusion

These are but a few of the applications that can be drawn from new grammar in teaching language arts. Many of them are not unique to new grammar; some teachers have been doing things like this for years. The idea behind them all is to build on the extensive intuitive knowledge that students already have about their language, in order to refine, expand, extend, or otherwise enrich this knowledge; to make language arts instruction a more lively enterprise in the classroom; and to fulfill the major responsibility that Zidonis identifies for teachers—"to interpret for our students the insights into language currently being made by linguists."

One More Step

Questions and activities for further learning.

1. Gleason, Francis, Zidonis, Sledd, and others take pot-shots and level serious accusations at the current abuses, shortcomings, and faults of

language arts—particularly grammar—teaching. Make a list of these criticisms and the ways in which linguistics—particularly new grammar—might help overcome some of the problems identified. What are the faults, abuses, and dangers inherent in the linguistic approach?

2. H. A. Gleason writes, " . . . the current teaching of grammar is actively hostile. Not only does it contribute nothing to the announced objectives of English teaching, but it goes a long way toward rendering the whole ineffective." Do you agree with his statement? Do you agree with his suggested solutions? Think of ways in which Gleason's solutions might be put to work in your own school.
3. Over twenty years ago, W. Nelson Francis wrote, "It is now as unrealistic to teach 'traditional' grammar of English as it is to teach 'traditional' (pre-Darwinian) biology or 'traditional' (four-element) chemistry. Yet nearly all certified teachers of English on all levels are doing so." To what extent is this criticism valid today? How can this persistence of traditional grammar be explained?
4. After clearing in your mind the difference between grammar and usage (pages 112–113), make a list of the traditional grammar rules that have little application in the everyday language of native speakers of modern American English.
5. Make a notebook or folder on those parts of the content of transformational grammar that have direct application and use in your own language arts teaching.

(lĭng gwĭs′tĭks)

Part III

Linguistics and Reading

Introduction

Reading is a process of dealing with language in its printed form. As such, it is a language activity, one of the language arts, and is thus within the purview of the linguist.

When linguists brought their thinking to bear on reading instruction, schoolmen listened for a number of reasons. For one thing, reading is the number one curriculum concern of educators (and of parents too). It is at the center of the curriculum in the early grades and an important part or need in the curriculum of all grades. Virtually every teacher in the elementary grades teaches reading, and pupils need reading skills in all subjects at all levels. More research has been done on reading than on any other subject in the curriculum. More has been written, more conferences held, more materials have been producd, more approaches tried, and more national interest has been expressed about reading than about any other aspect of the school's instructional program.

Despite all this widespread attention to the matter, our success in teaching children how to read has fallen far short of spectacular. While most children do learn to read at some time in their school lives, too many don't achieve the level of reading skill that they are capable of reaching. Still more never discover the joy of reading nor do they ever read except when they absolutely have to. The millions of illiterates in our society have become a blot on our national consciousness.

And then came the linguists. They brought with them the prestige of recognized scholarship and an aura of respect generated by the very nature of their discipline. The popularity of linguistics in teaching reading was both rapid and widespread. The "linguistic approach" joined the parade of look-say, phonics, individualized, language experience, i/t/a, color coded approaches, and other methods of teaching beginning reading. An assortment of new "linguistics materials" flooded the market. Publishers of existing materials added the name of a linguistic advisor to their team of authors and some even added the linguistic label to their materials without making any changes whatsoever. Linguistics quickly became what Wolfram calls "a marketable item" in reading instruction.

Many teachers saw linguistics as the total answer to their problems in teaching reading (which, of course, it is not). Others saw linguistics as nothing more than new wine in old bottles. But much of what the linguists have to say about reading makes a lot of sense and it does have application in teaching children how to read.

What Do Linguists Say About Reading?

Not all linguists agree on how the results of their specialty ought to be applied in teaching reading. There is, however, some common ground, a core of information about language that they agree upon. When this core of information is applied to teaching reading, the result is said to be the *linguistic approach.*

One thing that all linguists agree upon is the primacy of spoken language, that speech is the first form of language and that the vast majority of children already use spoken language by the time they are expected to learn to read.

Another area of consensus among linguists is the alphabetic nature of our writing system; that is, the individual sounds in our language are represented in writing by individual letters (called *graphemes*). Bloomfield expresses it in this way: "Writing is merely an attempt, more or less systematic, at making permanent visual records of language utterances . . . In alphabetic writing each character represents a *unit speech-sound*" (or phoneme). Thus, say the linguists, the primary job of the reading teacher is to help children to attach the language sound (which they already know) to the symbol that is used to represent that sound in writing. Bloomfield: "In order to read alphabetic writing, one must have an ingrained habit of producing the sounds of one's language when one sees the written marks which conventionally represent the phonemes . . . It is this habit which we must set up for the child who is to acquire the art of reading." Fries: "To read any writing efficiently, one must develop high speed recognition responses to the graphic signs as representations of significant language parts. English writing, although there are some uses of word writing, is alphabetic."

A third area of agreement among linguists is that the phoneme-grapheme correspondence in English is fairly regular. In a perfectly regular alphabetic language, there would be an exact one-to-one correspondence between sounds and symbols; that is, one symbol would represent only one sound all the time. No reading teacher needs to be told that English is not perfectly regular. We have different sounds represented by the same symbol (as the *a* in *fat, fate,* and *father*) and the same sound represented by different symbols (as the /iy/ or "long e" sound in *meat, feet,* and *Pete*). Because of these sound-symbol inconsistencies, it became popular to teach children to read by using whole words. Although Bloomfield called the sound-symbol relationship "extremely imperfect," later research and language analysis, notably by Paul Hanna and others,[1]

---

[1] Paul R. Hanna et al, *Phoneme-Grapheme Correspondence as Cues to Spelling Improvement.* Washington, D. C.: U. S. Government Printing Office, U. S. Department of Health Education and Welfare, U. S. Office of Education, 1966.

has shown that English orthography is actually more regular than it is irregular. As many as four-fifths of our most frequently used words are spelled according to a regular and consistent relationship between sounds and symbols. This is not to say that over 80 percent of English words have a perfect one-to-one sound-symbol correspondence, but that the majority of our words are spelled according to an observable system governing this phoneme-grapheme relationship. Linguistic research has shown that our sound-symbol relationship is more regular than we had realized, and certainly not so irregular that we must forego the alphabetic principle altogether in teaching reading.

Putting these three factors together—the primacy of speech, the alphabetic nature of our language, and the sound-symbol regularity—gives the first recognizable feature of the linguistic approach; that is, the patterned nature of the words in materials for teaching beginning reading. This type of writing has been typified by the Seuss-like "The fat cat sat on the mat," and parodied by sentences such as "Flick the tick off the chick with a thick stick, Nick." In order to understand the rationale for this type of writing, one must understand the concept of vocabulary control.

By the time they begin to learn to read, children have already learned to understand and use many thousands of words in their speaking and listening vocabularies. (One researcher found the number to be 26,000 words by first grade.) However, in preparing materials designed to teach children to read their language, only certain of these words are selected to be presented in print. The selection of these words is known as *vocabulary control.* In beginning reading materials in the conventional sight method or look-say approach, this selection was controlled on a meaning frequency basis; that is, words were selected because they were already familiar to the child as part of his daily oral-aural vocabulary. Thus, we find words such as: mother, father, run, jump, dog, cat, and so on, in preprimers and primers of basal series. These words are repeated over and over in the hope that children will learn to recognize them in print. The language-experience approach uses words that the child dictates, so vocabulary control is exercised not by a textbook author but by the child himself.

What is the basis of vocabulary control in the linguistic approach? Sound-symbol regularity. Words are presented in which the symbols represent one and only one speech sound. The idea is to provide systematic exposure to the most frequent and regular sound-symbol patterns in our language, usually beginning with three-letter words in which the vowel sound is short. When the most regular and consistent sound-symbol relationships have been mastered by the child, words containing less regularity between the letters and the sounds they represent are introduced in a controlled and structured way.

Linguists aim at reducing inconsistencies in beginning reading materials. To illustrate using a rather simplified example, let's compare two sentences. The sentence—Stop and go, mother—typifies the type of sentence found in conventional beginning basals. All the words are familiar to the young child, but look at the vowel *o*: it is used three times to represent three different sounds. Now take the sentence—Stop on a log—which, although it is not exactly patterned, is typical of what might be found in a linguistic series. In this sentence, the vowel *o* is also used three times but each time it represents the same language sound. This vocabulary control on the basis of sound-symbol regularity explains why we find sentences such as—The fat cat had a nap—in linguistic readers. Some words that are essential to making sentences need to be taught by the sight method (words such as *of* which is sounded /uv/ or *was* which is sounded /wəz/ or /wɔz/) but the major focus of instruction is on the regularly patterned words.

This rationale for vocabulary control in linguistic materials is often misunderstood by teachers. At least one teacher I know was in the habit of teaching patterned words (*hop, mop, top,* and the like) in her linguistic series in the same repetitious way she had always taught words in the sight approach. Another teacher friend once approached me with the expression "the tan fan" and said, "Wouldn't it have made more sense to use *brown* instead of *tan?* After all, the children are more likely to be familiar with *brown* than *tan.*" She had missed the point of the reason for using *tan* instead of *brown.*

This, then, is the first and most apparent characteristic of the linguistic approach to reading: beginning materials containing words that are controlled to assure regularity and consistency between the letters used and the sounds those letters represent, and an early emphasis on teaching children to decode or to unlock the sound letter relationships of their language.

There are other aspects of the linguistic approach to reading that receive different emphases in the several linguistic programs on the market today.[2] These characteristics are neither common to all linguistic programs, nor are they unique to the linguistic approach alone. Some linguistic programs insist on children learning the alphabet by rote prior to formal contact with printed words; others start right out with reading words. Some include nonsense words (*fab, baf, lig,* and others) as a useful step to later word analysis. Two series use no pictures whatsoever, concentrating only on language clues; others use stick figure drawings; still others use full color illustrations. Some use conventional reader level-designations (1^1, 1^2, 2^1,

---

[2] A good review of linguistic programs currently being used in schools can be found in *Approaches to Beginning Reading* by Robert C. Aukerman. New York: John Wiley and Sons, 1971, pp. 141-227.

2^2, and so on) while others don't. In most linguistic programs, early oral reading is emphasized as a check on mastery of basic decoding skills that have been taught. Most linguistic reading materials try to reflect the natural language patterns of children (compared to the traditional *Oh, Oh! Look, look. See, see.*) One series uses the principle of programmed learning. Each linguistic program includes its own unique features. In all of the linguistic series, different language elements are introduced at different times. Also, it should be noted that many programs not classified as linguistic include some features of language emphasized by the linguist.

What about Comprehension?

So far, we have been dealing with the decoding aspects of language, but what about comprehension, which to most teachers and reading experts is the ultimate goal of reading?

The linguist, even the structural linguist with his emphasis on decoding regular words, does not ignore meaning in language. "In the teaching of reading," Fries says, "even from the beginning there must be complete meaning responses, not only to words but to these words in full sentences, and to these sentences in sequences of sentences." With the linguists' early emphasis on decoding in the beginning stages of reading, comprehension did not receive the attention it had received in conventional meaning-emphasis programs. Comprehension was seen as the second step to the reading process, one that followed after the decoding process had been applied in reading printed material. As decording was seen from a phonological base, meaning came to be seen from a syntactical base. The order and relations of words in a sentence provided the basis for reading comprehension. (To repeat an earlier example, *John ate the fish* has a very different meaning than *The fish ate John,* even though the words themselves are the same.) The role of pitch, stress, and juncture in comprehension was highlighted. These aspects are covered in the article by Lefevre that follows.

Chomsky and the transformationalists have brought a new dimension to reading comprehension with the concept of deep structure and surface structure. Reading comprehension is seen to come not from individual words themselves nor only from the way in which these words are arranged. Rather, understanding is derived from an awareness of the elements and relationships underlying any written sentence. Thus, even though the form and arrangement of words in the sentences *John threw the ball* and *The ball was thrown by John* are different, the underlying meaning (deep structure) of both sentences is the same. Reading comprehension, then, comes from understanding or grasping the deep structure of sentences in the language. In two articles that follow, Wardhaugh touches on this matter ("The importance of such a linguistic theory for an understanding of comprehension surely cannot be overestimated.") and Simons bases his whole concept of comprehension (including his means for measuring it) on the theory of surface and deep structure.

Reading and Dialect

The subject of dialect has long been of prime concern to the linguist. It has also been an area of concern (and often confusion) for the reading teacher. Teachers are often faced with the job of teaching children to read with a set of materials in which the language bears little resemblance —phonologically or grammatically—to the language that their pupils use. What, then, can the linguist offer the teacher in the way of helping her do a better job of teaching reading to children who speak a nonstandard dialect?

The linguist can offer an awareness and understanding of dialect. Dialect exists in speech but, with the possible exception of those materials that are written in "eye dialect," written language follows a standard, dialect-free form. The word *car*, for example, is written c-a-r, but it is pronounced differently in Boston than in New York, Dallas, or Kansas City, not to mention the way it is said in London, Melbourne, Dublin, and other areas of the English-speaking world. Any standard written English text can be read in any number of dialects.

Another fact that the linguist points to is the legitimacy of the child's dialect as a language form. The text says, "Jane and Sally were together." The child reads, "Jane and Sally was together." What the child is doing in this case is translating the written form into the dialect equivalent in his own language. This type of phenomenon in reading is what Kenneth Goodman has referred to as a *miscue,* not a *mistake* in the traditional sense of the word.

Perhaps the greatest contribution that the linguist can make to the matter of dialect and reading rests in the identification of the specific features of the dialect that a child speaks. Linguists identify and describe features of dialect very precisely. It is important for teachers to understand at which points the child's dialect interferes with his reading and understanding of standard printed English, which "mispronunciations" are the result of dialect differences, and which are the result of reading errors. Some promising research on this topic is currently being carried out by Dr. Kenneth Johnson at the University of California at Berkeley.

Most of what has been written about dialect and reading (including the two articles on the topic that are included in this anthology) relate to what is called Negro-American dialect. This is so, largely because a great deal of linguistic research and analysis has been done on this dialect and because of the generally low reading scores in urban centers that have a heavy concentration of black Americans. A lot of what has been written about Negro-American dialect, however, can also be applied to teaching children who speak other dialects of nonstandard English—children on Indian reservations, rural whites in Appalachia, Chicanos in the Southwest, to name a few. Phonological, grammatical, and lexical features differ from dialect to dialect, but linguists can offer insight into the dialect of any group of children, highlight the legitimacy of their dialect, and point to conflict points between the dialect they speak and the standard written English found in their reading texts.

Several solutions have been proposed for helping children who speak nonstandard dialects in their attempts to learn to read standard English. Of the alternatives that Wolfram suggests, the fourth (revising reading materials to include nonstandard dialect features in beginning reading materials for children) has attracted both professional and public attention. (See "Black English," *Time*, August 7, 1972, page 46). A number of dialect or "ghetto readers" have been written. While the intent of these materials is sound—to create materials that will help the child bridge the gap between his spoken dialect and standard written English—it is fair to point out (as Wolfram has done) that many parents and community leaders see such materials as a racist attempt to preserve a form of language that sets the child apart from standard speakers and thus to maintain another basis of discrimination against the black child. Thus, the social and political ramifications of dialect readers overshadow the supposed educatonal advantages of these materials.

One thing the linguist *can't* offer the teacher in this respect is a single answer to resolve the question of how to best teach reading to children who speak a nonstandard dialect. Wolfram's article in this part of the text is testimony to the widespread (and at times volatile) debate on the whole question.

Linguistics and Literature

The central concern of the linguist is language and since language is the medium of literature, the linguist's concern extends into this latter field as well. Literature is also a topic of more than passing concern to reading and English teachers at all levels. The findings of the linguists can hardly be avoided in the study of literature and the linguists' techniques can lead pupils to a greater appreciation of, and insight into, literary works.

The sound of language is the major tool of the poet. The linguist is interested not only in how the poet uses sounds at the end of lines to make them rhyme, but also in how he uses sounds within each line itself. The linguist is also interested in the rhythm and melody of language, as Lefevre points out later. He is interested too in literature as syntax. The poet, playwright, essayist, novelist, and other literary artist manipulates sentences and sentence patterns to create the effect that he wants in his writing. Syntactic analysis can be part of stylistics, as Gleason pointed out in his article in part II. The skilled writer also chooses words and arranges sentences to create the mood and effect he desires in his writing. All of these language features and devices that the writer uses are in the purview of the linguist. As Wardhaugh says, "Linguists are indeed conducting research which is relevant to an understanding of poetic and literary style, and some of this research is proving to be most revealing." More and more of the techniques that the linguist uses are bound to be found in literature texts of the future.

Spelling, Too

Passing reference is made here to spelling for two reasons. First, most language teachers are just as concerned with pupils' ability (or inability) to spell as they are with pupils' reading skills. Second, a lot of what has been said about linguistics and reading can be said about linguistics and spelling as well. There are differences, of course between reading and spelling. For one thing, spelling requires production, while reading involves recognition of written language units. Spelling involves the production of one letter at a time in single words; reading deals mostly with groups of letters in meaning-bearing patterns. These differences notwithstanding, spelling involves many of the same skills we use when we read. In reading, we go from print to sound to meaning in decoding language; in spelling we take much the same route in the opposite direction, going from meaning to sound to writing in encoding language. Here, indeed, is common ground.

Despite our oft-spoken concern about spelling, rarely do we teach it in any formal way. What we usually do is present pupils with a list of words (often out of context and with no immediate functional application) and have them study and memorize them. Sometimes we include exercises designed to provide related practice and/or additional reinforcement, but we don't teach the subskills of spelling as we teach the subskills of reading, even though spelling skills can be identified.

One of these skills is the application of the sound-symbol relationship in encoding language. English is an alphabetic language. Whether we are encoding or decoding it, written symbols (graphemes) are used to represent basic speech sounds (phonemes). This phoneme-grapheme correspondence is fairly regular, which suggests the presentation at the same time, of spelling words that follow a consistent pattern. In traditional spelling programs, words such as *today, rain,* and *same,* in which the same vowel sound is represented in writing in three different ways (*ay, ai,* and *a*), are presented in the same lesson. Similarly, I've seen a lesson contain *room, book,* and *door,* three words in which the same double vowel represents three different speech sounds. In spelling programs that are linguistically based, words in which a letter or combination of letters representing a consistent sound-spelling pattern (*hill, bill,* and *fill* or *fame, came,* and *same*) are presented together. Once the more simple and consistent patterns have been mastered, other regular patterns are introduced and exceptions are taught as such. Thus, a linguistic spelling program, like a linguistic reading program, is built on the regularity that exists in our language.

A person's ability to spell will also be abetted by his awareness of prefixes, suffixes, and roots. The linguist calls these language units morphemes and they are usually taught in the reading program under the banner of structural analysis. The historical linguist can shed light on why certain words are spelled the way they are: the *k* in *knee,* for example, or the Greek-looking *psy* in *psychology.*

For anybody interested in the topic of linguistics and spelling (or just plain spelling without the linguistics for that matter), *Spelling: Structure and Strategies* by Paul R. Hanna, Richard E. Hodges, and Jean Hanna is a highly recommended reference.

The Old Question

We come again to the old practical question: Is the linguistic approach to reading any better than other approaches that have been tried in the past? Will linguistics help our pupils meet more success in learning to read? Individual independent research studies comparing the linguistic approach with some other method or combination of methods usually reveal either an edge for linguistics or no significant difference. Studies along these lines have been done by Davis,[3] Dolan,[4] Sabaroff[5], and others.

In trying to answer the question: How good is the linguistic approach in comparison with other approaches?—two rather large-scale research efforts are particularly worthy of note. Jeanne Chall reviewed research studies done on beginning reading instruction between 1912 and 1965. In

---

[3] D. C. Davis, "Phonemic Structural Approaches to Initial Reading Instruction." *Elementary English* 41 (March, 1964): 218–223.

[4] Sr. Mary Edward Dolan, "A Modified Linguistic versus A Composite Basal Reading Program." *The Reading Teacher* 17 (April, 1964): 511–515.

[5] Rose E. Sabaroff, "Improving Achievement in Beginning Reading: A Linguistic Approach." *The Reading Teacher* 23 (March, 1970): 523–527.

carefully analyzing this mass of research, Chall found that some code emphasis—that is, attention to the decoding process with words controlled on the basis of sound-letter relationships—in the beginning stages of reading instruction was likely to produce better results.[6] This code emphasis is not unique to linguistics, however; it is also characteristic of a systematic phonics approach to beginning reading.

In the early 1960s the U.S. Office of Education sponsored a national study of first-grade reading instruction. The linguistic approach, along with other approaches, was measured against the basal approach to determine which of these many approaches produced superior spelling and reading achievement at the end of the first grade. The most common finding in the linguistic versus basal comparison: no significant difference between treatments. The linguistic group achieved better scores on tests of word recognition; the basal group showed somewhat greater speed and accuracy in reading; there were no differences in comprehension. The project also included studies of a phonic/linguistic approach (Lippincott program) compared to more traditional basal materials. In these studies, the phonic/linguistic program tended to show superior results in tests of word reading, paragraph meaning, spelling, and word-study skills, with no significant differences in the areas of rate or accuracy of reading. But the overall conclusion of the whole project was that no approach was found to be uniquely effective.[7]

Since the conventional basal approach was the constant in all the twenty-seven research studies conducted as part of the project, no comparisons of the linguistic approach versus other newer approaches (language experience, i/t/a, etc.) were made.

Thus, after all this research, we are left with the same major conclusion that we had before linguistics came along—that there is no one best way to teach reading. What, then, are the advantages of linguistics in reading?

Apart from the values identified by Jones and West in their articles in this section, linguistics and the linguistic approach do have something to offer in reading instruction. Linguistics offers an effective approach to word-study skills which, the national first-grade study concluded, must be emphasized and taught systematically regardless of the method used. We have known for a long time that different children learn in different ways. The linguistic approach offers another alternative to teaching children who fail with more conventional approaches, an alternative that many teachers have used to achieve successful results. Linguistics provides the teacher with another string to her bow, another dimension that might

---

[6] Jeanne Chall, *Learning to Read, The Great Debate.* New York: McGraw-Hill, 1967.

[7] Guy L. Bond and Robert Dykstra, "The Cooperative Research Program in First-Grade Reading Instruction." *Reading Research Quarterly* 2 (Summer 1967): 5–141.

be added to the eclectic approach we so often hear about. Linguists are not reading specialists (although some have set themselves up as such), but they do have something to say about language. Linguistics is not the whole answer to reading instruction but it does have something to contribute.

Of course one of the problems in determining the effectiveness of a linguistic approach is the fact that it is not a single unitary method. There are lots of principles about language that have to be built into any reading instruction program and when all is said and done, the teacher is faced with the job of determining just what is meant by the "linguistic approach." Is it the *Can the man fan Dan* type of materials characteristic of the structural ilk of men like Bloomfield and Fries? Or is it a linguistic approach that focuses more on sentence patterns, similar to the one that Lefevre describes? Or is it a program that builds on the language concepts put forth by the transformationalists, like the one that Simons employs? Or is it a hybrid of many of these factors built into the reading program?

However one defines a linguistic approach to reading, linguistic science offers both teachers and students insights into the language that they are dealing with. How effective instruction will be when teachers put all this knowledge to work still largely remains to be seen.

Leonard Bloomfield is known as the Father of American Linguistics, and the publication of his famous book, *Language*, in 1933 is said to mark the beginning of the linguistics era in the United States.

Bloomfield's "Linguistics and Reading" signaled the beginning of the linguists' attention to reading instruction. Bloomfield set out to "outline the main facts about reading which are known to the linguists." In the article he describes the alphabetic nature of the English writing system in some detail. He criticizes the phonics and word methods of teaching reading that were popular at (and since) that time, as well as the sentence method. He then gives a basic outline of his own approach, which consisted of letter recognition as the first step, followed by left-to-right scanning, and then the use of words in which the sound-symbol relationships are consistent, beginning with two- and three-letter words (including nonsense syllables) and progressing to less regular words.

After Bloomfield's death, his work in reading instruction was carried on by Clarence Barnhart, and the continuation of this work resulted in two publications that went a long way toward bringing the linguistic approach to practical reality. One publication was the book *Let's Read, a Linguistic Approach* (Detroit: Wayne State University Press, 1961) and the other was a series of linguistic readers *Let's Read: A Linguistic Approach* (Bronxville, N.Y.: Clarence L. Barnhart, Inc., 1963).

Linguistics and Reading

Leonard Bloomfield

Any large gain in the speed and effectiveness of reading instruction in our schools would bring great advantage to the community. Saving years of every child's school time, it would open the way for other improvements in education. To the writer of this essay it seems very likely that such a gain could be effected with small trouble beyond what is involved in the discarding of a few long-established prejudices.

As to motivation and as to most aspects of classroom procedure, our reading methods have been admirably developed; the time should be ripe for the application, in the schoolroom, of the facts about reading which today are recognized by all professed students of language. A procedure which takes account of these facts, when tried out with individual children, has proved very successful. Trial in the classroom can be made only with the cooperation of schoolmen. It has been begun on a small scale; the present writer would be glad indeed if this essay should lead teachers and school authorities to cooperate in such attempts.

In this essay I shall outline the main facts about reading which are known to linguists. These facts will here be set forth somewhat dogmatically, since space forbids an account of how they were discovered; such an account would have to tell a large part of the history of linguistic science during the last hundred years.[1]

The art of writing is not a part of language, but rather a comparatively modern invention for recording and broadcasting what is spoken; it is comparable, in a way, with the phonograph or with such a recent invention as the radio. Every human society that has come within our ken possesses a fully developed language, but, until recently, only a few communities have practised writing. Until one or two centuries ago, moreover, in communities like our own, which practised writing, this art was carried on only by a very small minority of the population.

Writing is merely an attempt, more or less systematic, at making permanent visual records of language utterances. It is evident, of course, that by learning to read and write, the individual greatly extends his linguistic horizon and that such developments as the growth of his vocabulary are from then on largely tied up with his reading. Nevertheless, it is a great mistake to confuse the acquisition of literacy with the acquisition of speech: the two processes are entirely different.

Writing seems in every instance to have grown out of *picturing.* Picturing (or *picture writing*) consists in drawing pictures to represent a message. The elements in the pictures, such as figures of different animals, are conventionalized, so that one need not depend too much on draughtmanship.[2]

The important feature of picture writing is that it is not based upon language at all. A reader who knows the conventions by which the pictures are drawn, can read the message even if he does not understand the language which the writer speaks. If the reader knows that the picture of an animal with a big tail means a beaver, he can get this part of the message, even though he does not know how the word for a beaver would sound in the writer's language. In fact, he can read the picture correctly, even if he does not know what language the writer speaks. Without going too far into the psychology of the thing, we may say that the reader does not get the speech-sounds (the words or sentences) which the writer might use in conversation, but he gets the practical content (the "idea") which in conversation he would have got from hearing those speech-sounds.

The second main type of writing is *word-writing.* In word writing each

---

[1] This history is very interestingly presented in H. Pederson's *Linguistic science in the nineteenth century*, translated by J. Spargo, Cambridge, Massachusetts, 1931.

[2] The best examples are to be found in G. Mallery's study, published in the fourth and tenth Annual Reports of the Bureau of American Ethnology, Smithsonian Institution, Washington, 1886 and 1893.

word is represented by a conventional sign, and these signs are arranged in the same order as the words in speech. Chinese writing is the most perfect system of this kind. There is a conventional character for every word in the language. Each character represents some one Chinese word. As the vocabulary of a literate person runs to about twenty thousand words, this means that in order to read even moderately well, one must know thousands of characters. Learning to read Chinese is a difficult task, and if the Chinese reader does not keep in practice, he is likely to lose his fluency.

It is probable that word writing grew out of picture writing; at any rate, in the systems known to us, some of the characters resemble conventionalized pictures. However, the difference between these two kinds of writing is far more important for our purpose than any historical connection. The characters of word writing are attached to words, and not to "ideas." In picture writing you could not distinguish such near-synonyms as, say, *horse, nag, steed,* but in word writing each one of these words would be represented by a different character. In picture writing very many words cannot be represented at all—words like *and, or, but, if, because, is, was,* and abstract words like *kindness, knowledge, please, care* —but in word writing each word has a conventional symbol of its own.

We ourselves use word writing in a very limited way in our numerals, and in signs like &, +, −, =, and the like. The symbol 5, for instance, by an arbitrary convention, represents the word *five,* and there is no question of spelling or sound involved here: the symbol is arbitrarily assigned to the word. The characteristic feature of word writing, from the point of view of people who are used to alphabetic writing, is that the characters, like 5 or 7, do not indicate the separate sounds which make up the word, but that each character, as a whole, indicates a word, as a whole. Viewing it practically, from the standpoint of the teacher and pupil, we may say that there is no spelling: the written sign for each of the words (four, seven, and so on) has to be learned by itself. You either know that the character 7 represents the word *seven,* or you don't know it; there is no way of figuring it out on the basis of sounds or letters, and there is no way of figuring out the value of an unfamiliar character.

Word writing has one great advantage: since a character says nothing about the sound of the word, the same characters can be used for writing different languages. For instance, our numeral digits (which, as we have seen, form a small system of word writing) are used by many nations, although the corresponding words have entirely different sounds.

The third main type of writing is *alphabetic writing.* In alphabetic writing each character represents a *unit speech-sound.* The literate Chinese, with his system of word writing, has to memorize thousands of characters—one for every word in his language—whereas, with an alphabetic system, the literate person needs to know a few dozen characters—one for each unit speech-sound of his language. In order to understand the nature of alphabetic writing we need to know only what is meant by the term *unit speech-sound,* or, as the linguists call it, by the term *phoneme.*

The existence of unit speech-sounds or phonemes is one of the discoveries of the language study of the last hundred years. A short speech,—say, a sentence,—in any language consists of an unbroken succession of all sorts of sounds. Systematic study has shown, however, that in every language the meaning of words is attached to certain characteristic features of sound. These features are very stable and their number ranges anywhere from fifteen to around fifty, differing for different languages. These features are the unit speech-sounds or phonemes. Each word consists of a fixed combination of phonemes. Therefore, if we have a written character for each phoneme of a language, the sum total of characters will range anywhere from fifteen to fifty, and with these characters we shall be able to write down any word of that language.

The existence of phonemes and the identity of each individual phoneme are by no means obvious: it took several generations of study before linguists became fully aware of this important feature of human speech. It is remarkable that long before scientific students of language had made this discovery, there had arisen a system of alphabetic writing,—a system in which each character represented a phoneme. It seems that alphabetic writing developed out of word writing, and that this remarkable development has taken place only once in the history of mankind,—somewhere between 2000 and 1000 B.C. at the eastern end of the Mediterranean, with Egyptians, the Semitic-speaking peoples (such as the Phoenicians), and the Greeks, successively playing the principle role. All forms of alphabetic writing, then, are offshoots of a single original system. The details of this origin, and of the later history, so far as we can get at them, are of great interest, but would carry us too far afield. It is important for us to know that alphabetic writing was not invented at one stroke, as a finished system, but that it grew gradually and, one could almost say, by a series of accidents, out of a system of word writing. Neither then nor at any time since was there any body of experts who understood the system of phonemes and regulated the habits of writing. Among modern nations, some have almost perfect alphabetic systems, such as the Spanish, Bohemian, and Finnish systems of writing, but others have relatively imperfect systems, such as the Italian, Dutch, or German, and still others, have extremely imperfect and arbitrary systems, such as the modern Greek, the French, and the English.

We can illustrate the nature of alphabetic writing by means of English examples, for, in spite of its many imperfections, our system of writing is in origin and in its main features alphabetic. This is proved by the simple fact that we can write all English words by means of only twenty-six characters, whereas a system of word writing would demand many thousands. As an illustration we may take the written representation of the word *pin.* It consists of three characters, and each of these three represents a single phoneme. If anyone told us to use these three characters to represent the word *needle,* we should find the suggestion absurd, because these characters do not *fit the sound* of the word *needle.* That is, each of three characters, *pin,* is used conventionally to represent a unit *sound* of our language. This appears plainly if we compare the written symbols for other words, such as *pig, pit* or *bin, din,* or *pan, pun,* or if we reverse the order of the letters and read *nip.*

The alphabetic nature of our writing appears most plainly of all, however, when we put together a combination of letters that does not make a word and yet find ourselves clearly guided to the utterance of English speech-sounds; thus, nobody will have trouble in reading such nonsense-syllables as *nin, nip, lib.*

If our system of writing were perfectly alphabetic, then anyone who knew the value of each letter could read or write any word. In reading, he would simply pronounce the phonemes indicated by the letters, and in writing he would put down the appropriate letter for each phoneme. The fact that we actually can do both of these things in the case of nonsense words, such as *nin,* or *nip,* shows that our system of writing is alphabetic.

In order to read alphabetic writing one must have an ingrained habit of producing the sounds of one's language when one sees the written marks which conventionally represent the phonemes. A well-trained reader, of course, for the most part reads silently, but we shall do better for the present to ignore this, especially as we know that the child learns first to read aloud.

The accomplished reader of English, then, has an over-practiced and ingrained habit of uttering one sound of the English language when he sees the letter *p,* another sound when he sees the letter *i,* another when he sees the letter *n,* and so on. In this way, he utters the conventionally accepted word when he sees a combination of letters like *pin, nip, pit, tip,* and, what is more, all readers will agree as to the sounds they utter when they see unconventional combinations, such as *pid, nin, pim.* It is this habit which we must set up in the child who is to acquire the art of reading. If we pursue any other course, we are merely delaying him until he acquires this habit in spite of our bad guidance.

English writing is alphabetic, but not perfectly so. For many words we have a conventional rule of writing which does not agree with the sound of the word. Take, for instance, the two words which are pronounced *nit.* One is actually spelled *nit,* but the other is spelled *knit,* with the extra letter *k* at the beginning, a letter which ordinarily represents one of the phonemes of our language.

Now someone may ask whether the spelling of *knit* with *k* does not serve to distinguish this word from *nit* "the egg of a louse." Of course it does, and this is exactly where our writing lapses from the alphabetic principle back into the older scheme of word writing. Alphabetic writing, which indicates all the significant speech-sounds of each word, is just as clear as actual speech, which means that it is clear enough. Word writing, on the other hand, provides a separate character for every word, regardless of its sound, and at the cost of tremendous labor to everyone who learns to read and write. Our spelling the verb *knit* with the extra *k* (and the noun *nit* without this extra *k*) is a step in the direction of word writing. This convention goes a little way toward giving us a special picture for the verb *knit,* as opposed to its homonym, and it does this at the cost of a certain amount of labor, since the reader must learn to ignore initial *k* before *n,* and the writer must learn where to place it and where not to place it. It is none the less important to see that in its basic character our system of writing is alphabetic—witness merely the fact that we get along with twenty-six characters instead of twenty-six thousand.

The letters of the alphabet are signs which direct us to produce sounds of our language. A confused and vague appreciation of this fact has given rise to the so-called "phonic" methods of teaching children to read. These methods suffer from several serious faults.

The inventors of these methods confuse writing with speech. They plan the work as though the child were being taught to pronounce—that is, as if the child were being taught to speak. They give advice about phonetics, about clear utterance, and other matters of this sort. This confuses the issue. Alphabetic writing merely directs the reader to produce certain speech-sounds. A person who cannot produce these sounds, cannot get the message of a piece of alphabetic writing. If a child has not learned to utter the speech-sounds of our language, the only sensible course is to postpone reading until he has learned to speak. As a matter of fact, nearly all six-year-old children have long ago learned to speak their native language; they have no need whatever of the drill which is given by phonic methods.

The second error of the phonic methods is that of isolating the speech-sounds. The authors of these methods tell us to show the child a letter, say *t,* and to make him react by uttering the (*t*) sound. This sound is to be uttered either all by itself or else with an obscure vowel sound after it. Now, English-speaking people, children or adults, are not accustomed to make that kind of noise. The sound (*t*) does not occur alone in English utterance; neither does the sound (*t*) followed by an obscure vowel sound. If we insist on making the child perform unaccustomed feats with his vocal organs, we are bound to confuse his response to the printed signs. In any language, most phonemes do not occur by themselves, in isolated utterance, and even most of the successions of phonemes which one could theoretically devise, are never so uttered. We must not complicate our task by unusual demands on the child's power of pronouncing. To be sure, we intend to apply phonetics to our reading instruction, but this does not mean that we are going to try to teach phonetics to young children. In the absurdity of trying this we see the greatest fault of the so-called phonic methods.

In spite of the special methods, such as the phonic method, which have been advocated at various times, the actual instruction in our schools consists almost entirely of something much simpler, which we may call the *word-method.* The word-method teaches the child to utter a word when he sees the printed symbols for this word; it does not pretend to any phonetic breaking-up of the word. The child learns the printed symbols, to be sure, by "spelling" the word,—that is by naming, in proper succession, the letters that make up the written representation of the word, as *see-aye-tee*: *cat,* and so on. No attempt is made, however, to take advantage of the alphabetic principle. If one examines the primers and first readers which exemplify the various methods that have been advocated, one is struck by the fact that the differences are very slight: the great bulk of the work is word-learning. The authors are so saturated with this, the conventional method, that they carry their innovations only a very short way; they evidently lack the linguistic knowledge that would enable them to grade the matter according to relations between sound and spelling. It is safe to say that nearly all of us were taught to read by the word-method.

The word-method proceeds as though our writing were word-writing. Every word has to be learned as an arbitrary unit; this task is simplified only by the fact that all these word-characters are made up out of twenty-six constituent units, the letters. In order to read a new word, the child must learn the new word-character; he can best do this by memorizing the letters which make up this new word-character, but these letters are arbitrarily presented and have nothing to do with the sound of the word.

The most serious drawback of all the English reading instruction known to me, regardless of the special method that is in each case advocated, is the drawback of the word-method. The written forms for words are presented to the child in an order which conceals the alphabetic principle. For instance, if near the beginning of instruction, we present the words *get* and *gem,* we cannot expect the child to develop any fixed and fluent response to the sight of the letter *g.* If we talk to him about the "hard" and "soft" sounds of the letter *g,* we shall only confuse him the more. The irregularities of our spelling—that is, its deviations from the alphabetic principle—demand careful handling if they are not to confuse the child and to delay his acquisition of the alphabetic habit.

Our teaching ought to distinguish, then, between *regular* spellings, which involve only the alphabetic principle, and *irregular* spellings, which depart from this principle, and it ought to classify the irregular spellings according to the various types of deviation from the alphabetic principle. We must train the child to respond vocally to the sight of letters, and this can be done by presenting regular spellings; we must train him, also, to make exceptional vocal responses to irregular spellings, and this can be done by presenting systematically the various types of irregular spelling. For instance, we must train the child to respond by the *k*-sound to the sight of the letter *k* in words like *kiss, kid, kin, kit,* but we must also train him not to try to pronounce a *k*-sound when he sees the written *k* in the words like *knit, knife, knee, knight.*

The knowledge required to make this classification is not very profound. Although this knowledge is easily gained, persons who lack it are likely to make troublesome mistakes. The author of a text-book and the class-room teacher does not need a profound knowledge of phonetics; he needs only to realize that information on this subject is available and that he need not grope about in the dark.

Although the various methods that have been advanced are, in practice, only slight adaptations of the universal method of word-reading, it will be worth our while to glance at one of them which has some vogue, namely the *sentence method* or *ideational reading.* This method attempts to train the child to get the "idea" or content directly from the printed page.

When a literate adult reads, he passes his eyes rapidly over the printed text, and, scarcely noticing the individual words or letters, grasps the content of what he has read. This appears plainly in the fact that we do not often notice the misprints on the page we are reading. The literate adult now observes the laborious reading of the child, who stumbles along and spells out the words and in the end fails to grasp the content of what he has read. The adult concludes that the child is going at the thing in a wrong way and should be taught to seize the "ideas" instead of watching the individual letters.

The trouble with the child, however, is simply that he lacks the long practice which enables the adult to read rapidly; the child puzzles out the words so slowly that he has forgotten the beginning of the sentence before he reaches the end; consequently he cannot grasp the content. The adult's reading is so highly practiced and so free from difficulty that he does not realize any transition between his glance at the page and his acceptance of the content. Therefore he makes the mistake of thinking that no such transition takes place,—that he gets the "ideas" directly from the printed signs.

This mistake is all the more natural because the adult reads silently; since he does not utter any speech-sounds, he concludes that speech-sounds play no part in the process of reading and that the printed marks lead directly to ideas. Nothing could be farther from the truth.

The child does his first reading out loud. Then, under the instruction or example of his elders, he economizes by reading in a whisper. Soon he reduces this to scarcely audible movements of speech; later these become entirely inaudible. Many adults who are not very literate, move their lips while reading. The fully literate person has succeeded in reducing these speech-movements to the point where they are not even visible. That is, he has developed a system of internal substitute movements which serve him, for private purposes, such as thinking and silent reading, in place of audible speech-sounds. When the literate adult reads very carefully,—as, when he is reading poetry or difficult scientific matter or a text in a foreign language,—he actually goes through this process of internal speech; his conventional way of reporting this is that he internally pronounces or "hears himself say" the words of the text. The highly skilled reader has trained himself beyond this: he can actually shunt out some of the internal speech-movements and respond to a text without seizing every word. If you ask him to read aloud, he will often replace words or phrases of the printed text by equivalent ones; he has seized only the high spots of the printed text. Now this highly skilled adult has forgotten the earlier stages of his own development and wants the child to jump directly from an illiterate state to that of an over-trained reader.

It is true, of course, that many children in the upper grades—and even, for that matter, many postgraduate students in the university—fail to seize the content of what they read. It was this unfortunate situation which led to the invention of ideational methods in reading instruction. This however, meant confusing two entirely different things. So much can be said however; the child who fails to grasp the content of what he reads is usually a poor reader in the mechanical sense. He fails to grasp the content because he is too busy with the letters. The cure for this is not to be sought in ideational methods, but in better training at the stage where the letters are being associated with sounds.

The extreme type of ideational method is the so-called "nonoral" method, where children are required not to pronounce words but to respond directly to the content. They are shown a printed sentence such as *Skip round the room,* and the correct answer is not to say anything, but to perform the indicated act. Nothing could be less in accord with the nature of our system of writing or with the reading process such as, in the end, it must be acquired.

The stories in a child's first reader are of little use, because the child is too busy with the mechanics of reading to get anything of the content. He gets the content when the teacher reads the story out loud and, later on, when he has mastered all the words in the story, he can get it for himself, but during the actual process of learning to read the words he does not concern himself with the content. This does not mean that we must forego the use of sentences and connected stories but it does mean that these are not essential to the first steps. We need not fear to use disconnected words and even senseless syllables, and, above all, we must not for the sake of a story, upset the child's scarcely formed habits by presenting him with irregularities of spelling for which he is not prepared. Purely formal exercises that would be irksome to an adult are not irksome to a child, provided he sees himself gaining in power. In the early stages of reading, a nonsense syllable like *nin* will give pleasure to the child who finds himself able to read it, whereas at the same stage a word of irregular spelling, such as *gem*, even if introduced in a story, will discourage the child and delay the sureness of his reactions.

There is always something artificial about reducing a problem to simple mechanical terms, but the whole history of science shows that simple mechanical terms are the only terms in which our limited human capacity can solve a problem. The lesser variables have to wait until the main outline has been ascertained, and this is true even when these lesser variables are the very things that make our problem worth solving. The authors of books on reading methods devote much space to telling why reading is worth while. The authors of these books would have done far better to stress the fact that the practical and cultural values of reading can play no part in the elementary stages. The only practical value of responding correctly to the letters of the alphabet lies in the messages which reach us through the written or printed page, but we cannot expect the child to listen to these messages when he has only begun to respond correctly to the sight of the letters. If we insist upon his listening, we merely delay the fundamental response.

If you want to play the piano with feeling and expression, you must master the keyboard and learn to use your fingers on it. The chief source of difficulty in getting the content of reading is imperfect mastery of the mechanics of reading.

Space forbids our giving more than a meager outline of a system of reading instruction based upon the facts which have been set forth on the preceding pages.

The first step, which may be divorced from all subsequent ones, is the recognition of the letters. We say that the child *recognizes* a letter when he can, upon request, make some specific response to it. One could, for instance, train him to whistle when he saw an A, to clap his hands when he saw a B, to stamp his foot when saw a C, and so on. The conventional responses to the sight of the letters are their names, *aye*, *bee*, *cee*, *dee*, and so on, down to *zee* (which in England is called *zed*). There is not the slightest reason for using any other responses.

It is an open question whether all the letters, small and capital (in printed form, of course) should be taught before reading begins.

At the preprimer stage the habit of left-to-right scanning should be developed by means of appropriate exercises, which may well afford, at the same time, an introduction to the letters and the numeral digits.

Our first reading material must show each letter in only one phonetic value; thus, if we have words with *g* in the value that it has in *get*, *got*, *gun*, our first material must not contain words like *gem*, where the same letter has a different value; similarly, if we have words like *cat*, *can*, *cot*, our first material must not contain words like *cent*. Our first material should contain no words with silent letters, (such as *knit* or *gnat*) and none with double letters, either in the value of single sounds (as in *add*, *bell*) or in special values (as in *see*, *too*), and none with combinations of letters having a special value (as *th* in *thin* or *ea* in *bean*). The letter *x* cannot be used, because it represents two phonemes (*ks* or *gz*), and the letter *q* cannot be used, because it occurs only in connection with an unusual value of the letter *u* (for *w*).

Our first reading material will consist of two-letter and three-letter words in which the letters have the sound-values assigned at the outset. Since the vowel letters are the ones which, later on, will present the greatest difficulty, we shall do best to divide this material into five groups, according to the vowel letter.

The work of this first stage is all-important and should be continued until the pupils are very thoroughly trained. Nonsense syllables, such as *bam*, *bap*, *mim*, *mip*, should be included. Words unfamiliar to the child, such as perhaps *van*, *vat*, should not be avoided; they should be treated as nonsense syllables or, if there is time, accompanied by a very brief explanation of their meaning.

Short sentences of the type *Nat had a bat* can be used at this stage.

The second stage takes up regular spellings in which double consonants and other digraphs appear in consistent uses, for example: *ll* as in *well*, *th* as in *thin*, *sh* as in *shin*, *ch* as in *chin*, *ee* as in *see*, *ea* as in *sea*, *oa* as in *road*, *oo* as in *spoon*. If a very few words of irregular spelling are introduced at this stage (for example, *is*, *was*, *the*), it is possible to devise connected reading of reasonably varied content.

The third stage takes up words whose spellings may be called semi-irregular, for example the type of *line*, *shine*, *mile*, *while* or the type of *bone*, *stone*, *hole*, *pole*. At this stage, also, two-syllable words whose spelling is consistent with the other materials, can be taken in: *winter*, *summer*, *butter*, *sister*, (but not, for instance, *father*, *mother*, *brother*). A small set of the commonest irregular words (pronouns, forms of the verbs *be*, *have*, *do*, and *go*) is included because it enables us to give extended readings of connected text.

The last stage takes up irregularly spelled words, such as *father*, *mother*, *night*, *all*, *rough*, *cough*, *though*. It is only here that the question of reading vocabulary need be considered. In the first three stages an individual word (apart from the small stock of irregular ones that have been taken in) offers no problem: all that is needed is the habit of connecting letters with sounds. At those stages, unfamiliar words like *van, moot, mote,* afford good practice precisely because they are unfamiliar, and the same can be said of nonsense syllables. At the fourth and last stage, however, each word, being entirely irregular in shape, is a separate item to be memorized. At this last stage, accordingly, we use only familiar words which are needed for reading.

No matter how well we plan in other respects, our teaching will yield inferior results so long as the material which we present is clumsily chosen. Only if we choose our material in accordance with the nature of English writing will the classroom procedure which we have so carefully developed, produce proper results. The children will learn to read in a much shorter time, and they will read more accurately, more smoothly, and with better understanding of the content.

Like Bloomfield, Charles Fries was a noted linguist interested in the application of linguistics to reading instruction. Fries' theory of reading is fully explained in his widely known book, *Linguistics and Reading,* and applied in the *Merrill Linguistic Readers,* of which Fries is the senior author.

His article that follows presents briefly the basis of his theory: "To read any writing effectively, one must develop highspeed recognition responses to the graphic signs as representations of significant language parts. . . . The spelling-pattern approach to the teaching of reading develops the relation between the word-patterns (as sequences of phoneme contrasts) and spelling-patterns (as sequences of grapheme contrasts)." Fries also acknowledges the importance of comprehension in reading.

In addition to Fries' basic theory, the article contains some interesting history of efforts to reform English orthography, a brief definition of linguistics, and a short account of the work of the linguist.

Linguistics and the Teaching of Reading

Charles C. Fries

The discussions in English concerning the methods and materials for the teaching of reading began at least four hundred years ago. John Hart finished the writing of his *The Opening of the Unreasonable Writing of Our Inglish Toung* in 1551.

> For even so I have opened the vices and faultes of our writing: which cause it to be tedious, and long in learnying: and I learned hard, and evill to read. . . . And then have I sought the meanes (herin writen) by the which we may use a certaine, good and easi writing, onli following our pronunciation; and keping the letters in their auncient, Simple and Singular powers.

Hart ends his discussion with an offer to teach several "reasonable" but totally illiterate men to read in one month.

> I therefore profer myself to instrust thre, fower, or more, souch reasonable men as never knew letter, within the space of one moneth . . . so as they shalbe hable to read perfectli any inglish sentence and matter, which shalbe writen or printed, with souch letters and in souch an ordre sett, as this treatise hath taught.

Hart's *Orthographie* of 1569 developed much more completely the principles set forth in his manuscript of 1551 and proposed the use of an "augmented" Roman alphabet as a consistent spelling of the "sounds."

Hart's final book was published in 1570, *A Methode or comfortable beginning for all unlearned whereby they may bee taught to read English, in a very short time, with pleasure.* John Hart's book of 1570 was the first book in English, so far as I know, to present a textbook from which to teach beginning reading using an alphabet based upon the principle of using "as many letters in our writing" as there are "voices" or sounds in our "speaking." To do so Hart made what amounted to a phonemic analysis of English speech, an analysis that sheds considerable light upon the pronunciation of English at the time of Shakespeare's birth. In other words, we have in Hart's *Methode* of 1570 the first attempt to apply to the problem of teaching reading the best linguistic knowledge of that day.

William Bullokar in 1585 published a "reading" text of *Aesops Fables in tru Orthography with Grammar nots.*

Charls Butler* in 1634 says of his "alphabet" that "with its use the learners attein unto a more perfect and reddy reading in one year, than otherwise they have doon in three."

Alexander J. Ellis, well known by linguistic scholars dealing with the history of the English language for his great work on *Early English Pronunciation* (1867–1889), in his little book *The Alphabet of Nature* (1845) lists twenty-seven others who had devised special "phonetic alphabets" for the teaching of reading. Among these twenty-seven were Benjamin Franklin with his *New Alphabet and Reformed Mode of Spelling* in 1768, and Brigham Young in 1845 with his *Desert Alphabet for Teaching Reading.*

In 1842 Isaac Pitman, who in 1837 had produced a successful system of shorthand called *Phonography,* with the assistance of Alexander J. Ellis, developed his *Phonotopy,* a "phonetic print" through which to teach children to read. Phonotopy preserved all the letters of the Romanic alphabet which could be used to advantage but added "seventeen new letters . . . for those sounds of the English which were generally designated by combinations of letters in the Romanic print," and thus "a fixed character for every sound." This "augmented Roman alphabet" was tried in the schools of England and in those of America as a "new method" for beginning reading.

Reports of the use of this "phonetic-alphabet" and of the "phonetic books" as initial steps in the teaching of reading appeared in *The Massachusetts Teacher,* VI (1853): 25–28, and in the *Journal of the Proceedings of the National Educational Association,* 1873: 207–219. George L. Farnham, a school superintendent conscientiously devoted to the search for methods that would procure the most efficient reading, reported upon his five-year trial of the "phonetic system" in the preface of his little book, *The Sentence Method of Teaching Reading, Writing, and Spelling,* 1881.

The earliest contributions to the teaching of reading from the application of "linguistic" knowledge came from John Hart in the sixteenth century

---

* The spelling of his first name is the one he insisted upon during his life.

and from those who followed his leadership during the next three hundred years. These men attempted to develop and use an alphabet based upon the conventional Roman alphabet (omitting the *c*, *x*, and *q* as superfluous) but supplemented by approximately a dozen new letters, so that the first stages of the learning process could be simplified by having materials in which the single letters had a one for one correspondence with single sounds. This approach attempted to solve the problems created by English conventional spelling by substituting for that spelling a more "consistent" and "simpler" alphabet.

On the whole, only a few of the new alphabets thus created were developed by those having sufficient linguistic knowledge to make a satisfactory and helpful analysis of the English sound system. Fewer still gave any attention to the problems of passing from the reading of materials spelled with the new alphabets to the reading of materials spelled conventionally. Farnham says of his pupils, after five years of trial of such "phonetic readers," that "few of them became good spellers" and that "the two systems of analysis . . . had so little in common that permanent confusion was produced in the mind."

Those trained in linguistics have, however, continued to study the problems of the English sound system, the relation of the sound system to the graphic representation of that system in our conventional spelling, and the development of the language ability of children. Very few materials have been explored for practical help with problems of the teaching of reading. Concerning the nature of alphabetic writing in contrast with other systems, there is, for example, the basic structural approach by I. J. Gelb, *The Study of Writing* (Chicago, 1952). A more technical approach is given by C. F. Voegelin and F. M. Voegelin, "Typological Classification of Systems with Included, Excluded, and Self-Sufficient Alphabets," in *Anthropological Linguistics*, III (January 1961): 59–96.

For a very brief and rather nontechnical statement of the sound system of American English, see chapter II of C. C. Fries, *Teaching and Learning English as a Foreign Language* (University of Michigan Press, 1945).

For statements concerning English spelling as graphically representing English phonemes, see Robert A. Hall, *Sound and Spelling in English* (Philadelphia: Chilton, 1961); Eleanor Higginbottom, University College, London, "A Study of the Representation of English Vowel Phonemes in the Orthography," *Language and Speech*, III (April–June 1962), 67–117; Paul L. Garvin and Edith Crowell Trager, *The Conversion of Phonetic into Orthographic English: A Machine-Translation Approach to the Problem* (Canoga Park, California: Thompson Ramo Woolbridge, November 1963).

For the descriptive analysis of the language of children, see Ruth Hirsch Weir, *Language in the Crib* (The Hague: Mouton, 1962). See also the good bibliography of *Language in the Crib* for other studies covering the child's language development.

The linguistic studies listed here do not themselves seek to apply to the teaching of reading the results they present. Linguistics or linguistic science consists of a body of verified and verifiable knowledge concerning the nature and functioning of human language that has been won by the devoted labors of a host of scholars over many years. This knowledge is cumulative, building upon the past and constantly growing. Like all science it is impersonal. It does not depend upon nor does it accept the private theories of individuals. Only those generalizations concerning the relations of linguistic phenomena that arise out of evidence verifiable by all qualified workers in the field—evidence that has been collected and evaluated in accord with rigorous procedures and techniques—became part of this body of knowledge.

The linguist, as a linguist, thus has a special competence in a particular limited field—a competence in a special body of knowledge. We cannot assume that the well-trained linguist merely by virtue of the fact that he is a linguist is competent to deal with the applications of his science to and of the problems of teaching. I believe, as with other sciences, the engineering applications of the linguists' special knowledge require an *additional* special competence, which includes an understanding of the particular problems of the field of application and the status of the struggles to solve them.

In the great body of accumulated knowledge that constitutes the substance of linguistic science there is much that needs to be patiently and vigorously explored in order to find its significance when brought to bear upon the complex persistent problems of teaching every boy and girl who can "talk" to read. Linguistics has more to offer than the repeating of the work of John Hart and Charls Butler and A. J. Ellis in making another phonemic alphabet and in trying again to ignore the special difficulties of modern English spelling. It has much more to offer than another "back to phonics" program. But what it has to offer is not a ready-made, complete, new set of teaching devices or plans or methods that will make highly successful the classroom use of the common materials of the word-method or of the common materials of the phonics programs.

What linguistics has to offer consists primarily of the principles of

(1) a new and different approach to evaluating the language achievement of the pupils who are to be taught to read;

(2) a new and different statement of the process and progress of reading achievement in terms of the language development of the pupils;

(3) a new understanding of the basic relation of modern English spelling to the phonemic patterns of modern English words.

Brief comments on these principles must suffice here.

(1) The linguist competent to deal with the application of his special knowledge, in analyzing and describing with some precision the language achievement of the child as he enters the reading program, is not "word-centered" in his approach. His primary consideration is not the number of vocabulary items for which the child "knows" a meaning. Size of vocabulary has certainly some significance. But the range of the child's responses to the various contrastive functioning units, the phonemes, that English uses to separate and identify the lexical items, certainly holds much greater significance. Of equally high significance are the child's responses to the whole range of contrastive markers that identify the basic structures to which grammatical meanings are attached.

(2) In respect to the process and progress of reading achievement the linguist raises the following question. Given a child who has learned to understand certain stories told to him, or read to him, just what must that child learn now in order to add to his present language ability to understand the stories you tell him the ability to understand the same stories through his own reading? Reading ability and reading progress must always be measured against language ability and language progress.

(3) The purpose of all the basic writing systems of the languages of the world is to provide a graphic code through which one who has learned the code of the language signals and the code of the writing can interpret the written materials in terms of the language they represent. To read any writing efficiently, one must develop high speed recognition responses to the graphic signs as representations of significant language parts. English writing, although there are some uses of word writing and some syllabic writing, is alphabetic.

Apart from the highly sophisticated *phonetic* (not phonemic) alphabets, like the more than four hundred signs accepted for the International Phonetic Alphabet, alphabet writing, as generally used, does not attempt to provide a guide to the pronunciation. In general, the pronunciation has provided something of a guide for the alphabetic writing.

In the history of English writing, however, a basic change occurred during the first part of the Early Modern English period, 1450 to 1550. This change put English spelling considerably out of line with the spelling of the other languages that use the Roman alphabet, and also considerably out of line with the spelling of the other stages of the English language.

The "sounds" changed (a phonemic redistribution), but the old spellings remained. A new *principle* of redistribution became dominant. The spelling patterns that developed historically pulled exceptions into conformity. The actual basis of the representation changed from items of graphemes to patterns of graphemes.

The spelling-pattern approach to the teaching of reading develops the relation between the word-patterns (as sequences of phoneme contrasts) and spelling-patterns (as sequences of grapheme contrasts), but it differs fundamentally from any of the types of "phonics." It uses whole words but it differs in basic principles from any of the common word-methods. Nor is the spelling pattern approach to be equated with the use of "word families." The spelling-pattern approach reveals much more regularity in the spelling of present-day English than we could see formerly when spellings were measured by the ideal of "item" correspondence and "item" distribution.

Linguistics does not ignore meaning of any kind. It insists that statements about the signals of meaning to be *scientific* must be made in physical terms, but it does not deny that practical language deals with a complex range of various kinds of meanings which must be understood. In the teaching of reading, even from the very beginning there must be complete meaning responses, not only to words but to these words in full sentences, and to these sentences in sequences of sentences. The cumulative comprehension of the meanings in the sequences of sentences must become so complete that the pupil can, as he goes along, supply those portions of the language signals (intonation, stress, pause) which the bundles of spelling-patterns do not represent.

Lefevre presents a different view of linguistics and reading than that presented in the two previous articles. He begins with a criticism of the theories of Bloomfield and Fries as being too narrow a view of the reading process.

Lefevre sees reading as a language-related process. His approach goes beyond words and puts the primary emphasis on sentence patterns rather than on word patterns. He also concerns himself with structural devices "between and among sentences," leading to paragraphs and longer reading selections. He applies linguistics to the reading of literature as well. Lefevre gives a great deal of attention to the role of intonation (pitch, stress, and juncture) in both reading and literature.

His theory is presented more fully in his book, *Linguistics and the Teaching of Reading* (New York: McGraw-Hill, 1964). His more recent book *Linguistics, English, and the Language Arts* has already been cited as being a particularly practical reference for teachers who want to use linguistics in the classroom.

A Comprehensive Linguistic Approach to Reading

Carl A. Lefevre

I

Introduction: The Need for a Synthesis of Linguistic Approaches

We often hear such questions as these: What do you think of the linguistic approach to reading? Just what is the linguistic approach to reading anyhow?

Such questions are off point because at present no single linguistic approach merits the use of the noun marker or determiner *the*, which would signify the one and only. Bloomfield and Fries have given their names to spelling and word methods of teaching beginning reading, and despite all denials, reading teachers will consider both methods as part of phonic word analysis because both deal with relationships of sound and spelling; they do not even venture into *structural* word analysis. The veneration that these men have earned by their other work in linguistics hardly justifies the use of the exclusive term, "the linguistic approach," to designate their narrow methods. Possibly no single method ever will deserve it.

This is true for a number of reasons. Primarily, our present knowledge is so far from closed that it is commonly said to be exploding; this is true in linguistics as in other disciplines. Moreover, in no age has progress been achieved through blind or myopic imitation of what has already been done. Quite the contrary. Modern linguistics is both a revolution in and a continuation of the study of language. When we break eggs to make our omelet, we do not lose the eggs.

What must inevitably come, in my opinion, is a synthesis of linguistic approaches to reading: a synthesis developed, controlled, and corrected by means of an interdisciplinary attack on reading problems, bringing to bear all pertinent knowledge; a synthesis in line with the best experience of teachers of reading and the English language arts, and in line with the best experimentation these teachers are capable of. Such a synthesis must move far beyond spelling and word attack and into reading processes at the sentence level *even in beginning reading*; eventually it should range into problems of reading extended discourse, not only of exposition but the many forms of literature. This is something of what is meant by "a comprehensive linguistic approach to reading."

II

Linguistic Phonics: Phonemes and Spelling

Leonard Bloomfield. If Leonard Bloomfield's son when he entered school had not encountered a "far-out" exponent of the kind of phonics Bloomfield derided as "the hiss and groan method" of teaching reading, the development of linguistics applied to reading might have been quite different. As it was, Bloomfield invented an approach to beginning reading that limits instruction during a long introductory period to a rigid alphabetical principle—single phoneme by single letter—applied to a language whose spelling is notoriously inconsistent with its phonemes. It is hard not to feel that Bloomfield's method was the result of an impassioned effort to straighten out some of the worst kinks of bonehead phonics. However it was, his introductory method featured such so-called sentences as "A man ran a tan van," and "Can a fat man pat a cat?"

Unfortunately, this kind of ingenious but un-English material not only bears the great name of Bloomfield, but it has been hailed as "*the* linguistic method of teaching reading." Bloomfield's followers among linguists are too many to be counted; his work has been the source of numerous graduate theses; the imitative materials based upon it are too numerous to be cited. All this is a bit like "The Emperor's New Clothes."

C. C. Fries. Recently C. C. Fries, the present dean of American linguists, has presented an extension of the Bloomfield method of teaching beginning reading. If the Bloomfield method is a spelling approach at the level of single letters and phonemes—and it is—the Fries method is a spelling approach at the level of one-syllable words. Fries himself admits that it is a specialized word method; it generates such un-English sentences as these, presented all in capital letters: "PAT A FAT CAT" and "A CAT BATS AT A RAT." It is difficult to detect any qualitative difference between Bloomfield's "Can a fat man pat a cat?" and Fries' "A CAT BATS AT A RAT." It is the misfortune of both methods to present, among *the very first lessons in reading*, tongue twisters and jawbreakers far removed from the language of children.

I understand, however, that Mrs. Rosemary Wilson and her associates in consultation with Fries, are making adaptations and additions in classroom experiments with these materials.

Some important distinctions. We seem to have been so blinded by our ritual thinking of handwriting and print as spelling that we have come almost to equate both writing and reading with spelling, though we know better. Correct spelling has become a shibboleth, even in the very beginning stages of teaching reading and writing: too many children have a traumatic fear of misspelling. (The elimination of this fear is no doubt an important reason for whatever successes may rightfully be claimed for *i/t/a,* along with the *i/t/a* emphasis on *writing.*)

Let us make some important comparisons and contrasts among the operations of *spelling*, *writing*, and *reading.* As linguistic operations, spelling and writing are active in a sense that reading is not. Spelling requires recognizing and producing single letters and single words; writing, however, requires the creation of meaning-bearing patterns of words using the sentence as the basic building block of composition. Thus we see that writing, not spelling, is seriously concerned with communication. Now consider reading: reading involves no active production of letters, words, or sentences at all; what reading requires is recognition and interpretation of the graphic counterparts of entire spoken utterances as unitary meaning-bearing patterns; *this is reading comprehension.* These considerations may help us to evaluate the role of spelling in reading and in reading instruction.

Sooner or later all the letters in all the words, and all the words laid end to end, line after line, and page after page, must reach not from here to eternity in the child's eyes; all words must pattern themselves into sentences. The sentence is the fundamental unit both for written composition and for reading comprehension; with patience and skill, sentences may indeed be skillfully put together in interesting ways to compose all the larger language constructs—but not in the primary grades. The first lesson is that each sentence begins with a capital letter and usually ends with a period. Let the children take it from there, with no more initial emphasis on spelling than the reading process itself requires.

III

Reading in Terms of the Requirements of the English Language System

Reading as a language-related process. Because our writing system ultimately represents the spoken language, any attempt at a *direct* interpretation of the graphic symbols laid out in neat rows on the printed page is not the best approach to reading. We must go first from writing to sound, and then from sound to message; even the most rapid reading probably involves both steps in virtually simultaneous succession. Written and printed communications not only can be read aloud, but when they are read visually, or "silently" as we say significantly, the mental ear still picks up, be it ever so fleetingly, the sound track of the same utterances in speech. It is this echo of the sound of speech, more than mere punctuation, that groups and orders English words into meaning-bearing patterns. When the pattern does not come off right, we go back and reread until it "sounds right."

The process of going from print to sound to meaning is rather more than what is often meant by so-called inner speech, suggesting stammering, inefficient comprehension. It involves the process of thought itself, "a silent flow of words," as Sapir phrased it. Or in Vigotsky's penetrating statement, remarkably pertinent to reading comprehension: "Thought is not expressed in words, but comes into existence through them." Thus, to approach visual reading as the direct interpretation of a set of graphic symbols, like the Morse code in print, would be quite superficial, and very seriously misleading. What is needed now in reading is an approach in depth, an approach to, and through, the basic language itself.

Since writing and print represent graphic counterparts of spoken language patterns, the natural and best way to read is precisely in those terms. English language patterns have been described by linguists as composed not only of the basic individual sounds—*phonemes*; not only of the basic meaning units, words and word parts—*morphemes*; but normally of sentences, which in turn have components that may be arranged in an infinite variety of patterns and orders—*syntax*. Beyond this trilevel structure, the sounds of language, and this is true of English in a very significant way, include the overall melodies and rhythms of patterns longer and more complex than words, phrases, and clauses. In beginning reading these patterns would be sentences predominantly.

Reading sentence patterns. Introductory treatments of descriptive and structural linguistics usually suggest common English kernel sentences, note some of the possibilities of expansion, substitutions, and inversions, and give an indications of passive and other transformations. In his method of "sector analysis," Robert Allen is developing an interesting approach to reading and writing sentences by analyzing the important sentence parts. My own book, *Linguistics and the Teaching of Reading* (McGraw-Hill, 1964) is the first work to attempt a comprehensive application of linguistic data to reading and writing processes with primary emphasis on the sentence. This is an introductory book, of course, and makes no attempt to be comprehensive. *Writing by Patterns*, a collaboration of Helen and Carl Lefevre, is a work text that applies structural grammar to writing problems in grades 11–14, depending on the students' needs; much of the material is applicable to reading, and the two are treated somewhat as cross related. (This book was published in April, 1965 by Alfred A. Knopf.)

The great virtue of descriptive and structural grammar is its objectivity, its clear focus on the structure of the code as the means of carrying the message. This virtue is not found in the recent transformational and generative grammars, which, under the banner of "deep grammar," enter the subjective realm of the message. They also admittedly hark back to traditional grammar and school grammar. While these new-old grammars represent a legitimate effort to penetrate the relatively unknown area between language structure and psychological meaning, they will not necessarily help the native English speaker read and write his language. No one any longer defends the old grammars on these grounds.

Transformational or generative grammar attempts to formulate all the "rules" according to which it is assumed the native speaker can invent new sentences of his own and interpret new sentences invented by others. It is questionable whether these subjective, "internalized" rules will prove helpful in teaching native speakers to read and write, however, because teachers and pupils alike possess native linguistic intuition and intelligence enabling them to invent and interpret new sentences unconsciously, without recourse to rules for invention and interpretation. For teaching the skills of literacy, it hardly seems necessary to codify native linguistic intuition and intelligence. On the contrary, these invaluable traits should be exercised freely and creatively, rather than self-consciously analyzed. On the other hand, a clear, objective consciousness of the structural patterns themselves and their common transformations, available through study of structural grammar, can improve the pupil's understanding of his language as a code, and hence liberate his creative energies to develop his skills of literacy.

Reading paragraphs and extended passages of exposition. Up to now, linguistic analysis of reading problems has been largely confined to structures below the level of syntax: phonemes and morphemes. We have seen, however, that applications of syntactical data have already begun to yield some results, and it seems probable that similar and related data and principles can be extended into the analytical readings of longer passages. Making this extension is an important next stage in linguistics and in English linguistics applied to teaching the skills of literacy. Some work has already been done and more is in progress.

So far as I know, Zellig Harris was the first modern linguist to make a tentative entry into rigorous "discourse analysis"; his student and colleague, Noam Chomsky, has given some further consideration to this topic. Current applications of Kenneth Pike's "tagmemics" and experimental investigations by some of his students into extended language patterns and forms give promise of producing interesting new insights into the structure of both expository prose and literature. It seems possible that tagmemics may have the potential of relating language patterns to particle, wave, and field theories.

An obvious first consideration in analyzing the "organic" structure of well-written paragraphs is the use of structural joints and connective tissue not only *within* sentences, but *between* and *among* sentences. For example: simple pronoun references, both to the usual persons and to "things" and abstractions; similarly noun references; similarly by structural extension references by means of other word-form classes, such as verb cross references by means of derivational prefixes and suffixes added to the same base.

Also, referring ahead or back to a noun, an adjective, or an adverb having the same base; parallel syntactical patterns including elliptical constructions that constitute structural references to each other; the use of all structure words, such as the coordinating conjunctions, *and*, *but*, *for*, *nor*, *or*, *yet*, *so*; and especially the subordinating conjunctions, such as *although*, *because*, *however*, *moreover*, *nevertheless*, *since*—the whole set; and the correlatives, such as *if . . . then*, *not only . . . but also*, *while ...still*, and so on through the list. These are some of the syntactical devices that extend into paragraph construction and into longer passages of well-knit prose.

Reading literature as syntax. Structural resources of English such as we have just been considering in expository passages also lend themselves admirably to imaginative writing. Creative writers are fertile in their producton of structural inventions and manipulations of language patterns; an extended treatment would require detailed discussion of many points of linguistic interest in literature that can only be mentioned here, however.

For example, what I call structural puns, the unconventional substitution of a member of one word class for another, such as a noun for a verb, and then using grammatical inflections with the substituted word (Ciardi, Keats, Wordsworth); unusually long and involved sentence patterns running to many lines (Browning, Chaucer, Faulkner, Shelley, Steinbeck); extended syntactical patterns treated as sentences, but are "fragments" according to school grammar (Blake, Coleridge, Dickens, Keats, Shelley, Whitman, Wordsworth); myriad special sentence patterns, apostrophes, commands, inversions, prayers, wishes, apposition, compounding of elements, ellipses, parallelism of ellipses, parallelism of certain word forms, or of word groups and clusters, phrases, clauses (writers far, far too numerous to mention).

The point in a discussion of reading is that to fully comprehend literacy passages having unusual, or as often as not unique structure, the reader must absorb the entire meaning-bearing patterns as a whole. He may do this either by an automatic, unconscious, and intuitive process which is the fruit of long experience, or he may do it by means of a direct analysis of each author's peculiar and characteristic uses of language resources. Direct linguistic analysis is an excellent means of breaking an author's code and so involving pupils in an appreciative study of literature in their early and formative years. In time they should automatically respond to the meaning-bearing structures as wholes, each one having its overriding intonation pattern, or tune; in this respect, literary passages are comparable to the phrasing of music, building toward larger movements.

IV

Reading in Terms of Intonation: Requirements and Options

Intonation in visual, or silent, reading. The English graphic system partially represents the important sounds of the language system far beyond the representation of phonemes by graphemes, beyond the representation of morphemes by spelling, even beyond the representation of sentence patterns by capitalization, word order, and punctuation. The *part* in the term *partially* stands for intonation, both in single elements and in overall patterns of the melodies and rhythms of English.

Merely to pronounce words having two or more syllables requires correct accent; in linguistic parlance, *accent* is called *stress* and is defined as "loudness"; stress is a very important grammatical and syntactical feature of intonation. "He puts the emphas′is on the wrong syllab′le" is a hoary linguistic joke that makes the point. Putting the emphas′is on the wrong syllab′le betrays the speaker as either nonnative or a half-educated fool, the latter being a lot more fun.

The difference between *con′tract* and *contract′* distinguishes noun from verb in a whole set of contrasting pairs. This grammatically important distinction is not signaled by any specific feature of the writing system; only the distribution of such words in larger patterns gives the clue. And yet no literate native speaker of English misses the point. The same use of stress difference also distinguishes a set of pairs of nouns and verb-adverb groups, as in *set′ up* and *set up′*, and still another set, pairs of compound nouns and noun groups, as in *black′ board* and *black board.*

Many, though not all, punctuation marks correspond to decisive points of intonation in equivalent spoken language patterns. The period always, and the semicolon usually, are signals for a special way of dropping the voice, indicating that the preceding meaning-bearing pattern has been completed; conversely, the absence of a period normally indicates that the voice should *not* be allowed to drop in the end-signaling way between the opening capital letter and the closing semicolon or period. Persons who use this "fade-fall terminal" within sentences in oral reading are reading either by single words—word calling—or by fragmentary word groups that do not bear meaning. This kind of reading, all too common in the elementary school, destroys the unity of the unitary meaning-bearing pattern. It is a dangerous practice, because, unchecked, it may lead to a habitual internalized word-and-fragment-seeing procedure in silent reading, deadly to reading comprehension.

The fade-fall terminal also occurs at the end of many questions in English, notwithstanding the popular falsehood, "A question always ends with a rising inflection." For example: Who won the game? Where are the keys? Who was it? A rising inflection on these questions changes their meaning completely, the point being that the difference between a fade-fall and a fade-rise terminal in such questions is the only structural signal we have for a qualitative difference of intent. There is no graphic symbol for it at all. The fade-fall terminal would be the high-frequency choice in such questions.

The rising inflection may be used to terminate other questions also: Where did you say my notebook is? Did you tell me that this is your car?—The one hard rule for the fade-rise terminal to signal a question in English applies to statements converted to questions solely by this terminal. It is often used ironically in such questions as "You call this a ball game?" The rising inflection is the only spoken signal we have that this is a question rather than a statement.

A rising tone is commonly used within sentences where commas occur and usually in counting and in listing: one, two, three, four, five; wood, glue, nails, cloth, paint. The fade-fall is used only at the end of the last item.

The foregoing comments are concerned only with gross obligatory features of English intonation, those features that native speakers normally produce with intuitive ease and that foreigners find extremely difficult to master. In primary teaching of reading to children who are native speakers, all we have to do is see to it that they read orally (in order to hear silently with the mental ear) intonation patterns that are indigenous to their speech communities. This is all we have to do about intonation—but it is exceedingly important that we do it unfailingly and very well.

Intonation in oral reading and interpretation. Many linguists designate all that we call "tone of voice" as *paralanguage*; it includes such effects as whining, laughing or crying while talking, or talking with overtones suggestive of these; talking with relish or gusto; talking with distaste or disgust; using rasping, whispering, oversoft, or overloud tones; and all like effects. Paralanguage is often referred to as an "over-lay" of subjective interpretive characteristics on the basic code pattern required for communication; the point is that every speaker must use the required features of the language code but he may exercise various intonational options as well. His options must never violate the code, however, except for a deliberate communicative purpose.

Some linguists designate as *kinesics* all those nonlingual actions that accompany speech, often more important in communication than all that could possibly be communicated by the bare linguistic structures themselves. *Kinesics* includes all bodily gestures, nudges, nods, shrugs, finger, hand, and arm signals; facial gestures such as winks, smiles, sneers and leers—the whole gamut of expressive actions, so important in acting and interpretation.

All these rich resources of human communication should be brought to bear on the oral reading of literature, for the sheer joy of it, but also in order to develop associations that may carry over into the individual pupil's visual or silent reading of literature.

Oral reading with expression is interpretive reading that builds upon but far outreaches obligatory intonation features and patterns; with sufficient practice oral reading can develop into a fine art, closely allied with acting. So long as the interpreter observes the requirements of the intonation system, he is limited only by the dictates of good taste and judgment. Keen interest in both written composition and in silent reading can be stimulated by the teacher's skillful involvement of the children's creative imagination and vivacity in oral interpretation.

Reading literature as language and form. Sensitivity to the nuances of language, appreciation of dialects, access to poetry, responsiveness to the forms of literature—all can best be cultivated on the basis of *the whole sound of the piece* when well read aloud. Not every reader need be an artist in oral interpretation—a producer; every child has his own potential, however, worthy of a little classroom attention. Surely every child should have many opportunities to hear and attend to good oral interpretations of literature—to be a consumer. If the child has the authentic sound in his ear, his eye then in silent reading can help his mental ear tune in on the mnemonic sound track by association with other pieces; but if he has never had the authentic sound in his ear, his mental ear will be deaf to the graphic presentation, no matter how beautifully done.

Professional readings, movie, television and radio presentations, are all excellent sources of enrichment, but the audiovisual device of choice is the classroom teacher, or a parent, in everyday, seemingly casual interpretative readings. No one loves literature because he was assigned to love it; no one can possibly feel in his heart that it is great, just on his teacher's say-so. The best approach, not only to drama and fiction, but above all to poetry, is to hear it live and flowing sweetly on the tongue. A parent at home or a teacher in the schoolroom is not an artist way off somewhere on a high pedestal, but someone you know and can touch.

The arbitrary division of poems into lines, and rigid notions of meter, present problems that often baffle and finally discourage the young hopeful trying to appreciate poetry. The line of verse is a visual rather than an auditory unit; even when an elaborate rhyme scheme is followed, the echoing of the rhyme is contained within meaning-bearing structures. Stanzas and other verse forms are overlaid, often very skillfully, on English syntax. In poetry as in prose the good old sentence is still the basic building block of English. Nothing is more destructive of good verse than a ding-dong metrical reading, line by line, with a fade-fall terminal at the end of every line. (A mechanically repeated fade-rise terminal would be no better.) Every sentence should be read as a sentence, with syntactical terminals where they belong according to English syntax—not according to lines, or to rhymes.

Any attempt to read English poems with a uniform two-stress meter is fordoomed and absolutely fatal to poetry, because English is a four-stress language. This four-stress system itself is a structural part of the language system as a whole, not an interpretive option of the speaker or oral reader; the interpreter does have options but his options fall within the English four-stress system. This stress system and the meter of any poem can be reconciled if the presumed two stresses of the meter are regarded as relative rather than absolute stresses. That is, certain stresses are regularly heavier than the others, but the heavy stresses are not equally heavy.

For an example, let's take a look at Stevenson's *Requiem*, a simple poem in two stanzas, having an *a a a b*, *c c c b* rhyme scheme. The *a* and *c* lines have four beats, or heavy stresses, each; they begin and end with a beat. The *b* lines begin with two weak stresses (the equivalent in certain respects on one heavy stress or beat), and then have three more beats. Taking the fade-fall terminals as the chief clues, the poem is written in four sentences: (1) lines 1–2; (2) lines 3–4; (3) lines 5–6; (4) lines 7–8. Visually, the second stanza is punctuated as a single sentence with a colon at the end of the first line.

The poem is presented here twice: first marked for a uniform two-stress metrical rendition; second, marked with suggestions for a reading that observes the meter, but follows the four-stress system. The stress notations are: ⁄ for heavy stress; ^ for medium stress; ∖ for light stress; ◡ for weak stress. Instead of two stresses, one strong and one weak, we use heavy, medium, and light for strong, reserving the weak stress of the four-stress system for the weak stress in the two-stress metrical reading. Thus we preserve the contrasts of the meter without killing the poem.

Requiem

Under the wide and starry sky
Dig the grave and let me lie;
Glad did I live and gladly die,
And I laid me down with a will.
This be the verse you grave for me:
Here he lies where he longed to be:
Home is the sailor, home from the sea,
And the hunter home from the hill.

Requiem

Under the wide and starry sky
Dig the grave and let me lie;
Glad did I live and gladly die,
And I laid me down with a will.
This be the verse you grave for me:
Here he lies where he longed to be:
Home is the sailor, home from the sea,
And the hunter home from the hill.

The mistaken effort to achieve equality of beat and uniformity of meter throughout this or any poem cannot help but produce a metronomic, rocking-horse effect. The deadly soporiferous sequel is too well known. Children don't naturally hate poetry; they love it. But given too much poetry read in a rocking-horse jog, they will either learn to ignore it if they are normal, or kill it with kindness if they are teacher's pets. A few will go to college and major in English in spite of all.

A final point. Longer language constructs, such as poems, essays, sonnets, short stories—especially those literary forms that can be read at one sitting, as Poe suggested for the proper length for a short story—probably have overall melodic and rhythmic contours, embracing all components into an organic form so as to create a sense of completion when the piece has run its course. That is, the various forms of writing, particularly creative writing, are not static forms, but intricate linguistic processes, events patterned through time. The graphic form of these processes or events is the permanently organized embodiment of the writer's original creative experience: this I take to be the essence of literary form. In performing the piece, as it were, either silently or orally, the reader recreates for himself the writer's experience in the form he has shaped it to, but with appropriate nuances and overtones of the reader's own.

In all this, literary forms resemble songs or sonatas; longer works may well resemble concertos, symphonies, operas. This is not mere imagery. Musical notation and all the forms of music have developed within cultures of men who speak; the analogies and interrelationships of speech and song, of language and longer forms of music, make a fascinating subject for study.

Unlike the three previous selections, Herbert D. Simons' article is concerned only with the matter of how linguistics can contribute to the area of reading comprehension. Simons' article is based on linguistic theory and psycholinguistic research on the topic of surface structure ("the superficial structural relations") and deep structure ("the underlying structural relations") of sentences originally set forth by Chomsky.

His opening distinction between the product and the process of comprehension is an important one. In his new perspective, the author uses the old *John is eager to please* and *John is easy to please,* to explain the concepts of deep and surface structure, citing research on the concepts. He then presents his own theory of measuring comprehension by the recovery of deep structure. He concludes by suggesting directions for further research along these lines.

The section in which Simons reviews research related to the various major approaches to reading comprehension had to be edited out for reasons of space limitation. This section is valuable for anyone interested in insights into comprehension exercises and tests found in standard reading materials. Reading the original article in its entirety is recommended.

Reading Comprehension: The Need for a New Perspective

Herbert D. Simons

In 1917 Thorndike described reading comprehension as: . . . a very complex procedure, involving a weighing of each of many elements in a sentence, their organization in the proper relations to one another, the selection of certain of their connotations and the rejection of others, and the cooperation of many forces to produce the final response.

In spite of a vast literature produced on reading comprehension over the past fifty years. Thorndike's description still almost exhausts the accumulated knowledge of this fundamental intellectual process. The workings of the mind during reading comprehension remain a great and profound mystery.

In this article, past research in reading comprehension is first reviewed and then criticized for not providing an explanation of the basic processes in reading comprehension. The thesis presented is that the inability of research to reveal the processes in comprehension is due to the research not being based on theory.[1] Finally, a new approach to comprehension research, based on linguistic theory, is suggested.

---

[1] The term theory as it is used here will refer to a group of hypotheses about a topic that meets these minimum requirements:

It is important, before beginning the discussion of reading comprehension, to distinguish between the products and processes of comprehension. The comprehension process is the mental operations that take place in the reader's head while he is reading. These operations are generally not observable and not open to introspection. On the other hand, the products of the comprehension process are the behaviors produced after comprehension has taken place, such as answers to test questions.

Since the comprehension process is inaccessible to direct observation, research designed to shed light on it is limited to dealing with its products or behaviors. Therefore, any covert mental process such as comprehension is studied by looking at the behaviors associated with it and on the basis of these behaviors the characteristics of the process are inferred. Most of the research reviewed has necessarily used the approach of measuring or describing the product, and then inferring the process. The research reviewed here is evaluated by the degree to which it is successful in inferring a description of the comprehension process.

This paper maintains that theory based research is necessary if basic psychological processes are ever to be understood. Theory-based research has the advantage of helping to provide a principled way of separating relevant from irrelevant facts, of determining appropriate behavioral criteria, and suggesting important hypotheses that can be subjected to empirical test. Also, theory based research allows empirical research to be conducted on a rational and systematic basis.

Research into basic psychological processes can lead to the improvement of instruction. Process-oriented research is motivated by the assumption that the effectiveness of an instructional technique is in part dependent on the extent to which these techniques capitalize on the actual psychological processes that students utilize in learning. All other things being equal, the more effectively instructional techniques take advantage of the actual learning process, the more efficiently a student will learn. If this assumption is correct, then research efforts directed at uncovering basic processes will help improve instruction by making it easier to capitalize on these processes. A further advantage of knowledge of basic psychological processes is that this knowledge should make remediation

---

a A theory must be falsifiable, that is, it must be clear what kind of data will confirm or deny it.
b A theory must be perfectly explicit, that is, all the terms and relations must have explicit definitions.
c A theory must be comprehensive, that is, it must include a description of the entire system it purports to explain.
d A theory must possess descriptive adequacy; it must describe all the facts accurately.
e A theory must be internally consistent; none of its parts may contradict one another.
For a more detailed discussion of theory see Schutz (1967) and Hempel (1952).

more efficient. Knowledge of basic processes allows researchers to pinpoint specific aspects of the process that are deficient in remedial readers. Reading teachers could use this information as a basis for remediation.

This is not to say that instruction cannot succeed without this basic knowledge. Quite obviously it often does. Knowledge of basic processes is offered here as only one way of improving instruction.

In the discussion that follows, seven major approaches to reading comprehension will be evaluated on the basis of the degree to which they have contributed to an understanding of the basic comprehension process. They are the skills approach, the measurement approach, the factor analytic approach, the correlational approach, the readability approach, the introspective approach, and the models approach.

Editor's Note: Dr. Simons reviews the seven approaches to reading comprehension identified in the preceding paragraph. He describes each approach, cites research related to it, and criticizes each in its failure to produce much information about the process of comprehension.

Conclusion: Approaches to Comprehension

The effort expended in the various approaches to comprehension have produced little knowledge of the reading comprehension process. As Spache (1962) points out, it is still not known:

> . . . (1) exactly what thinking processes operate in comprehension, (2) how may the reader's facility in each of these processes be measured, and (3) how can ability in these processes be improved in instruction? (page 63)

The accumulated knowledge of the comprehension does not go much beyond Thorndike's description in 1917.

In the next section some important reasons why the comprehension process has been resistant to explanation will be considered. These reasons will help decide the direction new work in comprehension should take.

Why the comprehension process has been resistant to explanation. In searching for the reason for the lack of success of past research efforts in comprehension, it would be unfair to place the blame on the poor methodology that this research has exhibited. It could thus be assumed that methodologically more sophisticated research would produce meaningful results. While it is true that many of the past studies, as in any field of research, have had severe methodological difficulties (Cleland, 1964), improving methodology alone will not produce major breakthroughs in knowledge.

The reason for the lack of progress in comprehension research goes much deeper than poor research methodology. The current lack of descriptions of the mental processes involved in reading comprehension render it very difficult to establish adequate behavioral criteria for successful comprehension. This in turn is due to comprehension being a covert mental process that along with other cognitive processes takes place without any overt behavior being produced.[2] Thus the behavior that is measured in research,—answers to questions on comprehension tests,—may be only indirectly if at all related to the comprehension process. Furthermore, it is difficult to distinguish, in anything but an arbitrary way, between behavior that reflects the comprehension process from behavior that reflects other psychological processes—such as motivation, memory, attitude, attention, and personality. To put the problem simply, it is almost impossible to conduct fruitful empirical research when there is a lack of knowledge of which behaviors provide relevant measures of the process under investigation.[3]

This problem is not unique to education. Kuhn (1962) writes that it is characteristic of the early stages of scientific development.

> In the absence of a paradigm [theory], all of the facts that could possibly pertain to the development of a given science are likely to seem equally relevant. As a result, early fact gathering is far more a nearly random activity than the one that subsequent scientific development makes familiar. (page 51)

That comprehension research is at this "early fact gathering" stage with the concomitant inability to separate relevant from irrelevant facts is evidenced by the proliferation of comprehension skills and tests to measure them and the inability to distinguish comprehension from other psychological processes. The problem is not that more facts are needed but that it is impossible at present to give a coherent explanation of the facts that already exist.

Linguistic theory and psycholinguistic research as a basis for comprehension research. A recent development in linguistic theory, transformational grammar (Chomsky, 1957, 1965) holds promise for opening a

---

[2] It is true that eye movements and pupil activity can be observed during comprehension. But these phenomena are difficult to interpret. Also, there are no doubt neurological changes that take place, but these are not easily monitored. Even when they can be monitored they also resist interpretation. The reason, as Fodor (1968) points out is that neurological explanations of behavior are dependent upon adequate psychological explanations that are lacking in the case of comprehension.

[3] The difficulty in selecting the appropriate behavior as a criterion for comprehension can be contrasted to the word recognition process in which there is a clear cut behavioral criterion for successful performance, that is, correct oral pronunciation. For this reason word recognition appears to be more amenable to empirical research at the present time.

new perspective on reading comprehension. Transformational grammar is a theory of the inherent structure of natural language. It is a formal description of the structural relations of sentences, the manner in which words in sentences are related to each other. It includes a description of the superficial structural relations (surface structure), or the manner in which sentences can be subdivided into groups of words. It also includes a description of the underlying structural relations of sentences (deep structure), that is, the logical subject and object or a sentence. And finally it includes a description of the manner by which surface and deep structure are related through transformations (see Jacobs and Rosenbaum, [1968], for a readable description of transformational grammar).

Reading comprehension involves understanding sentences and understanding sentences involves using the information about the structural relations of sentences as described by transformational grammar. Knowledge of structural relations is necessary for sentence comprehension because sentences are not merely strings of words, but strings of words related to each other in very specific ways.

The important structural relations for understanding sentences are given not only in the surface structure or the word order or form classes of the words, but also in the underlying or deep structure of sentences. And sentence comprehension cannot take place without the recovery of these underlying relationships.

For example, take the sentences:

1. John is eager to please.
2. John is easy to please.

In order to comprehend these sentences a reader must at least recover the underlying structural relations of these sentences. He must know that in 1 John is one who is doing the pleasing and the person pleased is unspecified, while in 2 the reader must know that it is John who is pleased and the one who is doing the pleasing is unspecified. This information is described by the deep structure in linguistic theory.

If a reader is to understand the sentence, "What was taken?" for example, he must be able to recover the following information that is contained in the deep structure.

(1) that something was taken
(2) that something was taken by someone (unspecified)
(3) that the person producing the sentence seeks information, (is asking a question)
(4) that the sentence refers to a past action
(5) that the person asking the question is more interested in what was taken than in who took it.

Thus a necessary condition for sentence comprehension, which is a prerequisite for the comprehension of larger units of discourse, is the recovery of deep structure. (Wardhaugh, 1969, chapter 5.)

Psycholinguists have investigated the psychological reality of the linguistic concept—deep structure. They have done this by showing that deep structure differences, when surface structure is held constant, are consistently reflected in recall, recognition, comprehension and learning of sentences (Bever, Mehler, and Carey, 1967; Blumenthal, 1967; Blumenthal and Boakes, 1967; Davidson and Dollinger, 1969; Levin and Wanat, 1967; Mehler and Carey, 1967). Two typical examples of these studies are described below.

Blumenthal (1967) compared subjects' recall of two types of sentences. Recall was aided by a prompt word taken from the sentence. Both types of sentences had the same surface structure but they differed in their deep structures. The first type was a standard passive, such as, Gloves were made by tailors. In the second type of sentence the by-phrase was replaced with a nonagent adverbial by-phrase: Gloves were made by hand. In the first type "tailors" is the deep structure logical subject of the whole sentence, for example, tailors made gloves. In the second sentence "hand" is a verb modifier and does not relate to the whole sentence in the deep structure. Blumenthal found that the first type of sentence was recalled more easily than the second type. He also found an interaction between prompt words and sentence types. When the initial noun was the prompt word, there were no differences in the ability of subjects to recall the two types of sentences. But when the final noun was the prompt word, the standard passive: Gloves were made by *tailors*, was more easily recalled than the second type: Gloves were made by *hand*. These results could be predicted by the differences in the deep structure relations in the sentences. In the first sentence, "tailors" is the deep structure subject of the whole sentence, while in the second sentence, "hand" is related only to a part of the sentence as an adverbial. Blumenthal and Boakes (1967) replicated this study with a different set of sentences.

Levin and Wanat (1967) measured Eye-Voice-Span (the amount that a subject's eyes are ahead of his voice when he is reading aloud) of a subject's reading passive sentences that had the same surface structure but different deep structures. Two types of passive sentences were used. One type was the standard passive: His brother was beaten up by the gang. In the other type the underlying subject of the sentence was deleted: His brother was beaten up by the park. They found a larger EVS for the first sentence type than for the second sentence type. Thus deep structure differences produce differences in EVS.

In other studies Bever, Mehler, and Carey (1967) found deep structure differences to be reflected in eye movements, while Davidson and Dollinger (1969) found that these differences are reflected in paired-associate learning. And Mehler and Carey (1967) found that deep structure differences are reflected in sentence recognition. These studies provide ample evidence for the psychological reality of deep structure.

On the basis of linguistic theory and the psycholinguistic research discussed above, it appears that a promising approach for reading researchers to begin viewing reading comprehension is to examine more closely children's ability to recover the deep structure of sentences, since it seems clear that one aspect of the reading comprehension process involves recovering the deep structure of sentences.

It should be noticed that taking the approach discussed above of basing reading comprehension on theory and in particular on linguistic theory constrains the research for the time being to investigations of the processes involved in the literal understanding of sentences. The constraint is necessary because linguistic and psycholinguistic theories have advanced only to the stage of dealing with the literal comprehension of sentences, and there is little, if any, theory that deals with anything beyond the sentence level. However, the literal interpretation of sentences is one good place for comprehension research to concentrate because most of the comprehension skills discussed earlier assume a literal interpretation as a prerequisite. And as Huey (1968) states, "Language begins with the sentence and this is the unit of language everywhere." (page 123)

Suggested methods of measuring skill in recovering deep structure. Skill in recovering the deep structure of sentences can be measured in a number of ways. Three of these are described below. They all take advantage of the fact that in linguistic theory sentences that are paraphrases of one another, under certain conditions, have the same deep structure.

In the first method a child is presented with three sentences, two of which are paraphrases of one another. The child is asked to choose the one sentence of the three which is not a paraphrase of the other two. Here are three examples.

(1) **a.* What the boy would like is for the girl to leave.
b. For the boy to leave is what the girl would like.
c. What the girl would like is for the boy to leave.

(2) *a.* He painted the red house.
**b.* He painted the house red.
c. He painted the house that was red.

(3) *a.* The girl asked the boy when to leave.
b. The girl asked the boy when she should leave.
**c.* The girl asked the boy when he should leave.

---

* The asterisk indicates the sentence with a deep structure different from the other two.

In each item there are two sentences that have the same deep structure but different surface structures. In example (1) *b* and *c* meet these conditions. The third sentence in this item, *a*, has a surface structure similar to one of the other two sentences, *c*, but it has a different deep structure and consequently a different meaning. The same relationships exist in the other two simple sentences.

Thus if a subject is to choose the correct answer, he must recover the deep structure of at least two of the sentences. An incorrect choice would indicate that the child has not been able to correctly recover the deep structure of at least two of the sentences. These items then provide a measure of children's skill at recovering the deep structure of sentences.[5]

Another way of measuring skill in recovering the deep structure is presented in the following examples. In these items the child would be asked to fill in the blanks to make the sentences have the same meaning.

(1) For the girl to leave is what the boy would like.
What the __________ would like is for the __________ to leave.

(2) He painted the house that was red.
He painted the __________ __________.

(3) The girl asked the boy when to leave.
The girl asked the boy when __________ should leave.

Here again subjects must recover the deep structure of the sentences to answer the items correctly. Of course precautions must be taken in the measuring procedures discussed so far to correct for guessing and other strategies that subjects might use to get the correct answers without recovering the deep structure. With careful test development procedures, these problems can be overcome.

A third and more direct measure of skill at recovering deep structure, that obviates some of the problems mentioned above, involves presenting written sentences to subjects and asking them to paraphrase orally or in writing. Their responses could be scored on the degree to which the paraphrases reveal that they have recovered the deep structure of the original sentences. This task, while providing the most direct measure of skill, has some problems. Objective scoring procedures would have to be developed and the test would be time consuming to score. However these problems are not insurmountable (Fodor, Garrett, and Bever, 1968).

One comment needs to be made about the concept of deep structure. The objection might be raised that the term deep structure is merely

---

[5] Simons (1970) has developed a test composed of items of this type and in testing it found it to be a reliable and valid measure of children's ability to recover deep structure.

another way of referring to the meaning of a sentence. In response to this it should be pointed out that deep structure is a precise technical term in linguistic theory while the word "meaning" is vague and undefined and allows numerous interpretations. Furthermore, in linguistic theory the deep structure of a sentence provides the basis for but is distinct from its semantics. The word meaning as it is commonly used covers both the deep structure and the semantics of a sentence plus its connotations, metaphorical interpretations, and such.

Directions for Future Research

The methods described above for measuring skill at recovering deep structure, plus other methods as they appear, must be fully developed and tested. The most sensitive and efficient measures should be applied at different grade levels to determine the developmental aspects of the skill. And, of course, group differences such as SES, I.Q., and sex should be studied in this skill.

Research should also be undertaken to investigate the strategies children use in recovering deep structure. These strategies will probably come from work in psycholinguistics. For example, Fodor, Garrett, and Bever (1968) have studied some promising strategies which suggest that the main verbs in sentences play a major role in the recovery of deep structure. These strategies can provide a starting point for investigations by reading researchers into the deficiencies in children's use of these strategies. These investigations can then in turn lead to diagnostic tests to pinpoint specific deficiencies in sentence comprehension and can finally lead to instructional procedures to remedy these deficiencies. It is impossible to predict what the form of the diagnostic tests and instructional procedures would take because the research is just beginning.

The new direction for reading-comprehension research discussed in this article deals with only one aspect of the reading comprehension process. There are still to be explained the comprehension of larger units of discourse and higher levels of comprehension that go beyond a literal interpretation. A complete understanding of the comprehension process must explain these aspects as well. The research is limited by the absence of a theory upon which to base it. As theories are developed, work on the larger aspects of comprehension can proceed.

In conclusion, linguistic theory and psycholinguistic research provide the beginnings of a theory of language comprehension that promises a new perspective on reading comprehension. The challenge for reading researchers is to become more theory oriented and more knowledgeable in linguistics and psycholinguistics and to stay abreast of the growing literature in the field. The reward will be an opportunity to go beyond

Thorndike's description and to obtain a deeper understanding of the reading comprehension process.

References

Bever, T. G., Mehler, J., and Carey, P. "What we look at when we read". *Perception and Psychophysics* 2 (1967): 213–218.

Blumenthal, A. L. "Prompted recall of sentences." *Journal of Verbal Learning and Verbal Behavior* 6 (1967): 203–206.

Blumenthal, A. L. and Boakes, R. "Prompted recall of sentences." *Journal of Verbal and Verbal Behavior* 6 (1967): 674–675.

Chomsky, N. *Syntactic structures*. The Hague: Mouton & Co., 1957.

Chomsky, N. *Aspects of the theory of syntax*. Cambridge, Mass.: M.I.T. Press, 1965.

Cleland, D. L. "Needed improvement in research design in reading." In J. A. Figurel (Ed.), *Improvement of reading through classroom practice*. Newark, Delaware: (1964): 244–249.

Davidson, R. E., and Dollinger, L. "Syntactic facilitation of paired associate learning; deep structure variations." *Journal of Educational Psychology* 60 (1969): 434–438.

Fodor, J. *Psychological Explanation: An Introduction to the Philosophy of Psychology*. New York: Random House, 1968.

Fodor, J. A., Garrett, M., and Bever, T. G. "Some syntactic determinants of sentential complexity, II: Verb structure." *Perception and Psychophysics* 3 (1968): 453–461.

Hempel, C. G. *Fundamentals of concept formation in empirical science*. Chicago: University of Chicago Press: 1952.

Huey, E. B. *The psychology and pedagogy of reading*. Macmillan: 1908 (Republished: Cambridge: M.I.T. Press, 1968).

Jacobs, R., and Rosenbaum, P. *English transformational grammar*. Waltham, Mass: Blaisdell, 1968.

Kuhn, T. S. *The structure of scientific revolutions*. Chicago: University of Chicago Press, 1962.

Levin, H., and Wanat, S. *The eye-voice-span: reading efficiency and syntactic predictability*. Unpublished manuscript. Cornell University, 1967.

Mehler, J. and Carey, P. "The role of surface and base structure in the perception of sentences." *Journal of Verbal Learning and Verbal Behavior* 6 (1967): 335–338.

Schutz, R. E. "Testing theories of reading instruction." In John Bormuth (Ed.), *Research Designs in Reading*. Newark, Delaware: International Reading Association (1967): 1–8.

Simons, H. *The relationship between aspects of linguistic performance and reading comprehension*. Unpublished doctoral dissertation. Harvard Graduate School of Education, 1970.

Spache, G. *Toward better reading*. Champaign, Illinois: Garrard, 1962.

Thorndike, E. L. "Reading as reasoning: a study of mistakes in paragraph reading." *Journal of Educational Psychology* VIII (1917): 323–332.

Wardhaugh, R. *Reading: a linguistic perspective*. New York: Harcourt, Brace and World, 1969.

Walt Wolfram's article is one of the most comprehensive treatments of the problem that I have seen.

He examines four alternatives: (1) retaining existing materials and teaching standard English prior to teaching reading; (2) retaining existing materials and accepting children's reading in their own dialect; (3) revising reading materials to eliminate features problematic for the nonstandard speaker; and (4) revising materials to include nonstandard dialect language features in reading material for children. Wolfram concludes that none of these alternatives has been proven to be the best and that more research on the whole topic is needed.

As with the earlier article by Simons, a great deal of the original copy of this article, including reports of research and arguments pro and con on the topic, had to be edited for reasons of space limitations. Reading the article in its original form is recommended for those interested in this subject matter.

Sociolinguistic Alternatives in Teaching Reading to Nonstandard Speakers

Walt Wolfram

Introduction

The lagging reading level of lower-class minority groups, particularly blacks, has now become a matter of national concern. In response to this national crisis, a number of alternative approaches have been suggested in order to neutralize the discrepancy between middle-class and lower-class minority group reading-achievement levels. Some of these programs have little relevance to the cultural and linguistic differences between social groups, such as programs that deal with the amount of time devoted to reading in the school curriculum or the reduction of discipline problems that interfere with productive time usage. Although these nonlinguistic factors may be legitimate concerns in themselves, the sociolinguist has nothing to contribute to these areas. Other suggested programs, however, attempt to deal directly with the details of language involved in reading. In these matters, sociolinguistic expertise may be helpful, for it is now generally acknowledged that there are a number of linguistic differences between the language of the basal reader and the lower-class black child's indigenous dialect.

Basic to this discussion of reading materials for speakers of a nonstandard dialect is the fact that the dialect variously called "Black English," "Negro Dialect" or "Negro Nonstandard English" is a fully formed linguistic system in its own right, with its own grammar and pronunciation rules; it cannot simply be dismissed as an unworthy approximation of standard English. Although this dialect shares many features of other English dialects, it is distinct because there are a number of pronunciation and grammatical features that are not shared by other English dialects (Fasold and Wolfram, 1970).

The purpose of this paper is to describe and evaluate current approaches to the reading problem of lower-class blacks that attempt to deal with the linguistic differences between the child's indigenous system and the language of the standard English reader. It should be clear from the beginning that there is no unitary "linguistic approach"—that mythical but marketable item that has become a token of prestige in language arts curricula. Rather, there are several alternatives that attempt to eliminate the possible effect that dialect differences may have in the acquisition of reading skills. There are no panacean solutions. The advantages and disadvantages of each alternative must honestly be faced if we are to arrive at a feasible solution—one which will ultimately result in the significant reduction of reading problems in ghetto schools. The fact that we have no infallible alternative should not, however, be taken to mean that all alternatives that attempt to deal with the discrepancy between the language of the primer and the indigenous language of the child are equal. As the different approaches are evaluated, it should be apparent that some can be more highly recommended than others.

Although there are idiosyncratic aspects of practically every reading program that has been proposed, the various alternatives can be roughly divided into two main groups, those that call for different methods in teaching reading with extant materials and those that call for the development of new types of reading materials.

The Retention of Extant Materials

If the linguistic diversity between the dialect of the lower-class black and the dialect of the reading materials is going to be neutralized without altering basic materials for lower-class black children, then two options are open; either the child's language patterns must be changed to conform to standard English patterns prior to the teaching of reading, or some accommodation to the dialect in the child's reading of the traditional type of reader must be made. The feasibility of these two alternatives is discussed below.

Teaching standard English prior to reading. To neutralize the difference between the "language of reading" and the language that the lower-class black child brings to school with him, it has sometimes been suggested that the teaching of standard English should precede the teaching of reading in our ghetto schools. Although this procedure may appear to be similar to the simultaneous teaching of reading and standard English that is often engaged in, it is essential not to confuse these procedures. When teachers "correct" children for dialect interference in reading as well as the authentic types of errors that occur in learning to read, the teaching of standard English is usually done in a haphazard and unsystematic way. Furthermore, legitimate dialect interference and reading problems arising from the incomplete mastery of the reading process are often not distinguished from each other. The approach suggested here, however, first concentrates on the systematic teaching of standard English before any reading is taught; when a child has acquired a productive control over standard English, the teacher may proceed to the teaching of reading. The teaching of reading begins with the assumption that the source for dialect interference has been eliminated. This is not to say that the child's indigenous dialect will be eradicated, only that he will have capacity in standard English as well as the vernacular.

Most school curricula call for the teaching of standard English eventually, but the program described here inevitably means that standard English will be taught at the initial stages of the child's experience, since the acquisition of reading is one of the earliest priorities of formal education. One might further suggest that since standard English will probably be taught anyway, it is most reasonable to teach it before the failure to learn it can inhibit reading development.

Editor's Note: The author discusses some conflicting assumptions about language that underlie the position that standard English should be taught prior to reading. These assumptions are: (1) the opinion (held by some) that the nonstandard language system is incomplete and deficient, and (2) that teaching standard English prior to reading is a means of acquiring basic reading skills of standard language.

He also identifies problems with this position; namely (1) that due largely to peer group influence, vernacular speech persists despite attempts at teaching standard English, (2) that excessive amounts of time would be needed, and (3) that the first grade may not be the best time to teach standard English.

Before we can endorse teaching standard English as a prerequisite for reading, we must have evidence that it can be extensively taught given the current sociocultural facts, and that it is most effectively taught at the initial stages of education. At this point, the sociocultural facts that inhibit the widespread acquisition of standard English even as a second dialect do not suggest this alternative as a reasonable solution.

Dialect reading of extant materials. The other alternative which retains traditional materials does not involve the teaching of standard English in any form. Rather, it involves the acceptance of dialect renderings of standard English reading materials. Goodman is probably the most explicit spokesman for this position when he states:

> No special materials need to be constructed but children must be permitted, actually encouraged, to read the way they speak. (1969, page 27)

The child is given the standard types of reading materials and simply asked to read them aloud in a dialect-appropriate manner. If a child can read the passage in such a way that it systematically differs from standard English where his indigenous dialect differs, he has successfully read the passage. For example, if a lower-class black child reads a standard sentence such as *Jane goes to Mary's house* as *Jane go to Mary house* he is considered to have read it properly, since third person singular *-s* and possessive *-s* suffixial absence are part of the lower-class black child's vernacular. It is held that by permitting the child to read the traditional materials in his own dialect, the teacher can focus on the essentials of the reading process and the child will not be confused about reading problems that may result from dialect interference and legitimate types of reading errors arising during the course of the acquisition of reading skills.

Editor's Note: This position assumes that the standard English contained in beginning reading material is comprehensible to the child. And even if this assumption were true, there is a question that some information loss may occur as a result of dialect differences even when basic comprehension exists.

Another factor is the teacher's knowledge of the sound-symbol relationships of the dialect that would be needed to determine which reading errors are due to reading problems and which are the result of dialect differences.

Although the above discussion may suggest several disadvantages, it does have one very practical advantage: it can be established much much immediately than some of the other alternatives. For example, it can be adopted while further experimentation with other alternatives which require more drastic curriculum reorganization is carried out. Indeed, the teacher who thoroughly acquaints himself with the description of the dialect features and is convinced of the legitimacy of the dialect as a highly developed language system is in a position to start initiating this alternative. (For a nontechnical description of the predominant features of the dialect, see Fasold and Wolfram, 1970.)

The Revision of Materials

A seemingly more drastic alternative to the reading problem for speakers of a nonstandard dialect involves the incorporation of new types of materials into the reading curriculum for lower-class black children. Basically, there are two approaches that have been proposed, one which involves the elimination of all features that might be unfamiliar to the nonstandard speaking child and one that involves the writing of new sets of materials designed specifically to represent the language and culture the child brings with him when he enters school.

The neutralization of dialect differences. One method of revising current materials for nonstandard dialect speakers would be to simply eliminate features that might predictably be problematic for the lower-class speaker because these features are not an integral part of his linguistic system. This alternative essentially follows the suggestion of Shuy that grammatical choices in beginning material should not provide extraneous data. Shuy observes:

> In the case of beginning reading materials for nonstandard speakers, the text should help the child by avoiding grammatical forms that are not realized by him in this spoken language (third singular verb inflections, for example). (Shuy 1969, page 125)

It should be noted that this alternative would not incorporate any nonstandard features present in the dialect but absent in standard English.[1] For example, the use of *be* to indicate distributive action in a sentence such as *He be here every day* would not be used, since this feature is unique to nonstandard black speech. Accommodation would be made only by excluding features in standard English that do not have isomorphic correspondences in the dialect. It capitalizes on the presumed similarities of large portions of the grammar of these dialects so that the possibility of grammatical interference is eliminated. This alternative would concentrate only on grammatical differences since differences in pronunciation would involve most of the words in the English language. It thus appears that this alternative would involve the neutralization of grammatical differences along with the acceptance of dialect pronunciations of reading materials, as was suggested in one of the previously discussed alternatives.

---

1. In the article by Shuy in which this procedure is suggested, this is only one of several types of changes that Shuy recommends for materials that are to be used by black dialect speakers.

Editor's Note: Basic to this alternative is the assumption that there is a common core between the standard and the nonstandard language systems. The author identifies very specific problems in eliminating nonstandard constructions from beginning reading materials.

Although several apparent disadvantages of this alternative have been described, this discussion must not be concluded before pointing out some potential advantages. For one, a modification of this method may eliminate some of the most salient features of standard English which might be unfamiliar to the lower-class black child who comes to the schoolroom. Also, it would not incorporate socially stigmatized features of language, eliminating the controvery that inevitably surrounds the codification of nonstandard patterns in reading materials. The types of changes that this alternative would require in materials could, in fact, be incorporated without necessarily being noticed by teachers who are using such materials.

Dialect readers. The final alternative dealing with linguistic aspects of the reading problem among lower-class blacks involves the use of readers that are written in the vernacular of the children. That is, every effort is made in the beginning materials to represent the cultural and linguistic content that is indigenous to the child. As a brief illustration of how such materials might differ from the conventional materials, Wolfram and Fasold have compared two versions of the same passage, one in standard English and one in the dialect of the children.

Standard English Version
"Look down here," said Suzy.
"I can see a girl in here.
That girl looks like me.
Come here and look, David.
Can you see that girl?"...

Black English
Susan say, "Hey you-all, look down here!
I can see a girl in here.
The girl, she look like me.
Come here and look, David!
Could you see the girl?"... (Wolfram and Fasold, 1969, page 147)

The second passage is a deliberate attempt to incorporate the features of the children's dialect into the basal readers. The absence of third person singular *-s* (for example, *Susan say, she look*), pronominal apposition (*That girl, she . . .*), *could* for *can* and *you-all* are direct efforts to accurately represent the indigenous dialect of the lower-class black child.

It should be noted that although dialect-specific grammatical features have been incorporated, the conventional orthographical system of English has been retained. The retention of conventional English orthography has been proposed for two reasons. As we mentioned earlier, the conventional spelling does adequately represent the phonological units of the dialect at a more abstract level, so that, for example, there is formal justification for representing word-final *f* in *toof* as *tooth* (cf. Fasold, 1969). From a sociological standpoint, extra-linguistic matters such as other printed material and official education also make this alternative most reasonable. For these reasons, most producers of dialect readers employ the conventional orthography. Stewart (1969, page 195), however, would make one major compromise in the direction of a literary-dialect orthography, namely, the indication, by an apostrophe, of those cases in which a word must take a prefix in order to become like its standard English equivalent. This generally involves unstressed initial syllables, such as *'cause* for *because*, *'round* for *around*, and *'posed to* for *supposed to*. This adaptation is based on the fact that "Negro-dialect speakers do not always know that a prefix is 'missing' from their version of a particular word" (Stewart, 1969, page 195).

Although it has sometimes been misunderstood by opponents of this alternative, the proposal of dialect readers does not advocate an eventual dualist reading system in American society. It is only proposed as an initial step in the adequate acquisition of reading skills. Once reading fluency has been attained in the dialect readers and the child is sufficiently confident in his ability to read, a transition from dialect to standard English readers is made. Stewart (1969) has illustrated the several stages of transition.

STAGE 1

Charles and Michael, they out playing.

Grammatically, sentences at this stage will be pure nonstandard Negro dialect. The vocabulary, also, will be controlled so that no words that are unfamiliar to the Negro-dialect-speaking child will appear. Thus, all linguistic aspects of text will be familiar to the beginning reader, and his full attention can be focused on learning to read the vocabulary. At this stage, no attempt should be made to teach standard-English pronunciations of the words, since the sentence in which they appear is not standard English.

STAGE 2

Charles and Michael, they are out playing.

At this stage, the most important grammatical features of standard English are introduced. In the example, there is one such feature—the copula. Apart from that, the vocabulary is held constant. Oral-language drills could profitably be used to teach person accord of the copula (*am*, *is*, *are*), and some standard-English pronunciations of the basic vocabulary might be taught.

STAGE 3

Charles and Michael are out playing.

Grammatically, the sentences at this stage are brought into full conformity with standard English by making the remaining grammatical and stylistic adjustments. In the example, the "double subject" of the nonstandard form is eliminated. Oral-language drills could be used to teach this and additional standard English pronunciations of the basic vocabulary could be taught. (Stewart, 1969, page 185)

The alternative that advocates the use of dialect readers seems to be based on three assumptions: (1) that there is sufficient mismatch between the child's system and the standard-English textbook to warrant distinct materials, (2) the psychological benefits from reading success will be stronger in the dialect than they might be if standard English materials were used, and (3) the success of vernacular teaching in bilingual situations recommends a similar principle for bidialectal situations.

Editor's Note: The author discusses each of the three assumptions identified in the above paragraph. First, the extent of the mismatch between beginning reading material and a child's language may be a problem for any child, whatever dialect (standard or nonstandard) he speaks. Second, while on the one hand there may be psychological support in using a language that is familiar to the child in beginning reading material, on the other hand many parents and community leaders see dialect readers as offensive and discriminating against the black child. Third, vernacular teaching has proven successful throughout the world, but there are questions about the validity of using this procedure for different dialects as well as languages.

Other things being equal, it would be expected that the reported success of teaching reading initially in the vernacular in other situations would recommend its usage for lower-class black children. But the fact that the sociopsychological factor we have discussed earlier may be sufficient to impede the acquisition of reading skills cannot be ignored. It should be noted in this regard, however, that in a number of bilingual situations where reading was initially taught in the vernacular, attitudes toward the indigenous language vis-a-vis the national language are quite comparable to the attitudes toward the nonstandard dialect of black children. That is, the vernacular is socially stigmatized both by the dominant class and those who actually use the stigmatized forms. Despite these attitudes, vernacular reading materials have been reported to be successful as a bridge to literacy in the national language.

Conclusion

It should be apparent from the above discussion that there is no magical potion for the reading ills of our ghetto schools. Whereas some of the alternatives seem to have more validity than others in terms of linguistic differences between standard English and lower-class black dialect, sociocultural or psychological factors may seriously impede the implementation of these alternatives. On the other hand, alternatives that do not face these sociocultural obstacles may not deal adequately with the linguistic differences.

But one should not mistake the attempt to honestly describe the problem areas of each alternative with the pessimistic conclusion that all is vanity. There are steps that can be taken immediately to remedy some of the sources for reading problems, and there are recommendations for curriculum overhaul that definitely deserve experimentation.

A first step can be the acceptance of dialect renderings of conventional reading materials. This may, at least, eliminate some of the child's reading problems that arise from the failure to differentiate authentic reading problems and legitimate dialect differences. The advantage of such an initial step lies in the fact that it can be implemented immediately; any reading teacher familiar with the phonological and grammatical structure of the dialect can employ such a procedure. But because the differences between the dialect and reading materials are considerably greater for the lower-class black child than his middle-class counterpart, this can be suggested only as an immediate stop-gap measure.

The magnitude of the reading problem suggests that experiments must be made with alternatives that may involve the potential changing of materials and curricula. For one, an experiment should be done on the effects of neutralizing potential problem areas for the nonstandard speaking child in beginning materials. Although complete neutralization may be impossible, one could make some modifications based on a criterion such as the avoidance of grammatical differences involving changes in order or *free* morphemes but not *bound* morphemes such as certain suffixial forms.

It also seems appropriate to recommend experimentation with dialect readers. It is not necessary to institute an extended program to incorporate dialect readers into all lower-class black schools, a project that might be a 5–10 year task—only experimentation with such materials so we can find out what potential they might hold for reading programs for lower-class blacks. Mere experimentation with such materials is however, controversial given the current sociopolitical feelings of the community. But what must be done is to convince the community, including administrators, community leaders, teachers, and parents, that such an alternative may hold promise for the acquisition of reading skills and to deny its experimentation may be to deny the child what should rightfully be his—the ability to read.

References

Fasold, R. W. "Orthography in reading materials for Black English-speaking children," in *Teaching Black Children to Read,* Washington, D.C.: Center for Applied Linguistics, 1969, pp. 68–91.

Fasold, R. W. and W. A. Wolfram. "Some linguistic features of Negro dialect." *Teaching standard English in the inner city.* Ralph W. Fasold and Roger W. Shuy (Eds.), Washington, D.C.: Center for Applied Linguistics, 1970, pp. 41–86.

Goodman, K. S. "Dialect barriers to reading comprehension," in *Teaching black children to read,* 1969, pp. 14–28.

Shuy, R. W. "A linguistic background for developing beginning reading materials for black children," in *Teaching black children to read,* 1969, pp. 117–37.

Stewart, W. A. "Negro dialect in the teaching of reading, in *Teaching black children to read,*" 1969, pp. 156–219.

Wolfram, W. A. and Fasold, R. W. "Toward reading materials for speakers of Black English: three linguistically appropriate passages," in *Teaching black children to read,* 1969, pp. 138–55.

Virginia F. Allen looks at the issue of teaching reading to nonstandard dialect speakers in somewhat conventional terms and from an instructional point of view. In her article she suggests some practical ideas on how to begin a reading lesson based on a group language-experience type of activity. She also looks at standard basic-decoding exercises as a way of building pupils' backgrounds in word analysis skills, and she identifies some intonational and structural features as a way of helping students learn to handle syntactically difficult sentences.

Reading the Language of Public Life

Virginia F. Allen

The term Public Language is not ideally satisfactory, but at least it is free from the evaluative connotations of "Standard" English. It directs attention away from distinctions of race or social class. Moreover, students find it a meaningful label for the set of grammatical conventions governing communications that are beamed at the general public, across ethnic and sociocultural lines.

Specific features of this grammatical system can be observed and described in a wide range of obviously public contexts outside the schoolmarm's domain: in wedding announcements, obituaries, telephone directories, cookbooks and appliance manuals—as well as in school textbooks. Quite probably, throughout the lifetime of our current students, most features now characteristic of this grammatical system will survive—features such as the *-s* inflection for verbs with third-person singular subjects, for instance, and the occurrence of *be* (vestigially, at least, as in *I'm* and *They're*) before the *-ing* form of a verb. Hence efficient reading of Public Language would seem to depend in part upon familiarity with that grammatical system, whether or not an individual chooses to use that system in his own speech.

When reading is a problem for intermediate grade students (or older ones) an obvious possible cause is the students' lack of experience in working from the *known* (their own language style) to the lesser-known (the written-down language of public life). One helpful way to deal with this cause of reading disability is to engineer a group-composition activity, starting with ideas expressed by the students in whatever way comes naturally. Once the points have been arrayed before the class on the chalkboard, they are then restyled by teacher and students collaboratively for the purpose of communicating to some segment of the public, and hence conforming to the conventions of public communication. Such an activity might go as follows:

Teacher: (at the chalkboard) Lincoln's Birthday is coming soon. Let's see what you remember about Abraham Lincoln. Who remembers one fact about him?
Sandra: Like freeing the slaves? (Teacher writes: 1. Freeing slaves)
Clarice: President of the United States. (Teacher writes: 2. Pres. of U.S.)
James: He born in a log cabin. (Teacher writes: 3. Born in log cabin)

After a few more contributions have been made, the teacher paves the way for rendering them into Public English by explaining: "The second graders are making some pictures for the display board in the hall. They need something about Lincoln for people to read along with the pictures. Now how can we put these facts you've mentioned into the right form for the display board?" Someone with clear handwriting is appointed to come to the chalkboard and write each sentence as soon as it has been composed by the class.

Teacher: Our first sentence will probably start with *Abraham Lincoln.* What should the rest of the sentence be?
Clarice: Abraham Lincoln was the President of the United State.
Teacher: Say it slowly enough for Gloria to write it . . . What word comes after United, class?
Class: States.
Teacher: What shall we do about fact number 1—freeing the slaves?
James: Abraham Lincoln was the President of the United States and he freed the slaves.
Teacher: Can anybody find a way to use *who* instead of *and* in that sentence Gloria just wrote?
Sandra: Abraham Lincoln was the President of the United States who freed the slaves. (Gloria writes the sentence.)
Teacher: Read it to us, Dan, and let's see how it sounds.

In the same fashion, other sentences are proposed, recast in "public" form, and then read aloud. When the entire piece has been composed, copies are made by the class, and the neatest copy is selected for the display board. Such an activity—a sort of elder brother to the Experience Chart—builds bridges between the students' everyday dialect and the kind of English found in printed materials.

Undoubtedly some reading disability is caused by the reader's lack of familiarity with Standard-English syntax and morphology. Some students might not understand the material even if they heard it instead of seeing it. Yet there is evidence to suggest that many Second-Dialect students comprehend *spoken* Standard English so readily that they can translate heard sentences into their own dialect, with lightning speed. When thirteen-year-old members of a street gang were asked to repeat certain sentences after a Standard model, says Labov[1], "they failed because they perceived only the meaning and not the superficial form." For instance, when instructed to repeat "Nobody ever sat at any of those desks, anyhow," David said: "Nobody never sat in none o' tho' desses anyhow." Labov found that David was "typical of many speakers who do not perceive the surface details of the utterance so much as the underlying semantic structure, which they unhesitatingly translate into the vernacular form." Apparently, then, reading comprehension depends on more than familiarity with Standard English syntactic and morphological features.

Roots of reading difficulty may extend as far back as the primary grades, when basic decoding skills were only haphazardly formed. If a student in any grade misreads material that he can understand in its *oral* form, the first thing to do is to find out how efficiently he can decode regularly spelled words. Nonsense words like the following would serve the purpose, printed on flash cards or on the chalkboard:

NUGG	FLENK	LOACHING
JEEB	HADGER	DAWP
KIPPY	TROON	MARPER

To spur efforts and attention, this assessment of decoding skills can take place within the context of a story, with a title like *Space Witch*, set in an alien world and developed orally by the teacher. At strategic points in the story (where the names of characters are introduced, for example, and where made-up names for objects and actions are encountered) the students decipher the printed words.

If this simple task proves at all difficult for any members of the class, the teacher's duty is clear: to give those students another chance to grasp the fundamental correspondences linking English sounds with the spelling patterns commonly used for representing them. Naturally primary-grade methods and materials designed for developing word-attack skills will not do for older students. In most cases the materials will need to be prepared by the teacher, moving from single words to simple sentences to brief paragraphs, all consisting mainly of regularly spelled words. (Irregularly spelled utility words such as *a*, *the*, *are* and *does* should be introduced into the materials gradually, and identified as "nonconformists.")

In addition to graded practice on materials designed to provide reliable bases for predicting how a given combination of letters will probably be pronounced, there is often a need for class discussion of the speech-writing relationship. Why does a certain chocolate manufacturer always print its name with an accent mark over the last *e*? Because otherwise people would pronounce it to rhyme with *wrestle* and *trestle*. Why?

---

[1] William Labov, "The Logic of Non-Standard English," in *Linguistic-Cultural Differences and American Education,* Alfred C. Aarons and others, eds., p. 70.

Because the combination *-le* is most commonly used to represent /əl/, not /liy/. At the end of what other words do we find the combination *-le*? What is the most common spelling for the /æ/ sound? for the /Σ/ sound? If we wanted to invent some names for new detergents and breakfast foods, some names people could pronounce easily just by looking at them in print, what might some names be?

It is good for students to become explicitly aware of the conventions that control ways in which spoken words are represented in print. It is good for their spelling, their writing and their reading, to notice which words are spelled as one would expect, and which are not. It is particularly instructive to compare the spelled forms of common *function* words with the ways in which those words sound in casual speech. For example, how would the /ən/ in the following be written in conventional spelling (the spelling used for the language of public life)?

down /ən/ out
down /ən/ alley
down /ən/ the farm
down /ən/ a minute
down /ən/ you're ready

If a student understands spoken utterances but has trouble reading the same material from a printed page, his difficulty may well spring from the discrepancy between the sound and the look of words and syllables which are unstressed in the stream of speech. The expert reader has somehow adjusted to this unsatisfactory aspect of English writing. For instance, he has learned to live with the fact that /əz/ may turn up written *is* (*Barnes /əz/ living*) or *has* (*Barnes /əz/ lived*) or *as* (*big /əz/ life*)—among other possibilities. The inexperienced reader may still be thrown off stride by words such as *is*, *as* and *has* when he meets them in print—not because the words themselves are unfamiliar, but because (in unstressed positions in sentences) they sound so different from the way they look.

We have noted that reading problems arise
—when lack of acquaintance with Standard English would place even *spoken* Standard sentences beyond the student's grasp.
—when lack of experience with the conventions of English writing prevent the student from recognizing even the words he actually knows.

Now to mention one more, which may prove an even more prevalent source of confusion and insecurity among poor readers. Often the student's reading disability stems from the fact that certain aids to comprehension which are provided by the voice in spoken sentences are not supplied at all in the writing system. Once in a classroom I saw the following sentence, written on the chalkboard:

Only by thinking do we make what we read our own.

Spoken aloud, this is not a very difficult sentence to understand. A speaker would call attention to *thinking* by saying it with extra volume and a rise in pitch. He would pause after *thinking*, to signal the end of a sentence sector. He would pause again after *make* (though the pause here would be briefer than the pause after *thinking*) and he would pronounce *read* and *own* quite loudly and deliberately. Through all these signals he would manage to convey the sense of a sentence which is far from easy to read—because the written sentence provides none of the stress-pitch-juncture signals supplied by the speaker.

Whenever the sentences to be read are relatively long, this kind of difficulty may be found—not, however, because length is in itself an obstacle to comprehension. Students themselves often write long sentences. Here is a fairly typical high school sentence:

> The wind is blowing hard and you hear strange noises and it makes you scared but you don't want to show it because people will laugh so you kid around and say, "Who's scared?"

Most sentences found in textbooks and other Public-Language media are actually shorter than this one. The difference is, of course, that professional writers avoid such obvious sector-markers as the ones this student has used: *and, but, because* and *so*, markers that cut the sentence into easily digestible chunks. Professional writers (that is, those who write for the public) are more inclined to use imbedded construction in their long sentences (clauses nested inside other clauses) and to depart from normal conversational word order for the sake of artistic effect, and to use participial constructions that look like predicate verbs but actually are not.

Such features of public prose would not trouble students unduly if the sentences could be *heard*, with the voice supplying cues by means of volume, pitch, and so on; but in print those signals are gone. What can be done to help students over this hurdle? First, students need a great deal of experience with listening to material read aloud by the teacher while following the printed version with their eyes. Second, students need to be *spared* the experience of reading aloud unfamiliar passages of public prose—and they particularly need to be saved from the damaging effects of hearing their classmates read aloud, since inexperienced readers almost inevitably distort the meaning of a sentence by misusing stress, pitch and juncture. Think, for example, what a *poor* reader might do to the following bit of advice by Russell Conwell, founder of Temple University, if suddenly pounced upon and told to read it aloud:

> Do what you can with what you have where you are today.

Suppose the student reader intones it as follows:

> Do what . . . you can with . . . what you . . . have
> where . . . you . . . are today.

It takes an old hand at reading public prose to splice together those disjointed fragments, deliberately ignoring the misleading pauses that obscure the syntactic units of which this sentence consists. Reading aloud should be done by the teacher, not by students.

A third way of helping students learn to handle syntactically difficult sentences is occasionally to print such a sentence on the chalkboard with spacing that makes the sectors of the sentence clear. The above precept, for instance, is much easier to read when spaced as follows:

Do what you can
with what you have
where you are today.

Advertisers (who know more about reading than most teachers do) take pains to convey their messages clearly by means of such spacing. It is a pity that textbook publishers have so seldom followed the lead of business and industry in this respect.

Finally, and this takes us back to the first classroom activity recommended in these remarks, the teacher can help the class *compose* sentences characteristic of the language of public life. Having themselves gone through the operations involved in transforming a pair of kernel sentences into one with an imbedded clause, the class is better prepared to recognize such a sentence in printed material, better prepared to replace mentally the "fences" that mark off the various "nested" elements in spoken English but are absent from print.

Of course other questions could be asked about students with reading problems. Is the subject matter content appealing enough to make the effort of reading seem worthwhile? Have the students had the kinds of life experiences that enable them to grasp the meaning of what they read? That these are valid questions no one would deny, yet they are less neglected than the questions I have been raising here. Since the Second-Dialect student's everyday speech is farther removed than other dialects from the language of public life, one may ask whether his reading problems cannot best be solved by classroom activities that focus his attention on features that characterize the kind of English customarily presented to the public eye. It may also be useful to ask to what extent the student has grasped the relationship between speech and writing in English, has developed decoding skills that enable him to recognize known words when he sees them, has adjusted to the many instances of mismatch between sounds and spellings, has learned to compensate for the absence in print of aids to comprehension that are supplied by the voice in speech. Such questions, with answers in terms of classroom activities, deserve special attention when teachers help students read the language of public life.

Ronald Wardhaugh's article is a concise, comprehensive, and up-to-date survey of the application of linguistics to the teaching of reading. He begins by citing research summaries of linguistics and reading. He then identifies some of the assumptions and theories that linguists bring to reading, highlighting the matter of phoneme-grapheme correspondences. He summarizes some of the theories of linguistics and looks at reading comprehension first from the transformationalist's view and then from a semantic base. Wardhaugh briefly identifies some of the work of linguists in the areas of poetry and of dialect study related to reading. He concludes by advancing three principles that "must be taken into account in any theory of reading which aims to produce . . . the kind of explanatory power that linguists themselves are now attempting to require of linguistic theory."

Wardhaugh's theory is, of course, presented more completely in his book, *Reading: A Linguistic Perspective* (New York: Harcourt, Brace, and Jovanovich, 1969).

Linguistics-Reading Dialogue

Ronald Wardhaugh

In recent years there has been considerable discussion of the relationship of linguistics to reading and of the possible application of the findings of linguistic research to the teaching of reading. Quite recently, several summaries of this discussion have appeared and certain conclusions have been drawn. In one such summary Carroll (1964), a psychologist with a long-standing interest in linguistics, criticizes reading researchers for their failure to incorporate linguistic findings into the procedures which they have chosen to examine in their research, and points out that though much reading research has been methodologically sound, it has been rather inconclusive because of its deficiencies in content. On the other hand, in another summary, Betts (1966) points out some of the relationships he perceives between reading and linguistics and criticizes linguists for dabbling in reading and for adopting a rather naive approach to the psychological and pedagogical problems in reading. In an attempt to summarize the whole reading-linguistics dialogue, Devine (1966) points out that although the dialogue has been characterized by statements of opinion rather than by statements of fact, it gives one good reason to be optimistic that the findings of linguistic research will prove to be of use to reading specialists.

Linguistics and Reading

The linguistics-reading dialogue so far has been one in which a particular view of linguistics has prevailed. In this view the main findings of linguistics that have application to the teaching of reading and to reading research may be summarized as follows:

a) language is speech and writing is a recodification of speech so that English graphemes and punctuation marks are representations, often imperfect, of phonemes and intonation patterns;
b) language is patterned, that is, grammatical;
c) language is spoken in dialects of which Standard English is one, albeit an important one; and
d) linguists prefer descriptions of linguistic data to prescription and to any kind of mentalistic introspection.

Although many linguists would agree with these statements, nevertheless they characterize but one part of current linguistic thought and omit the most significant concerns of linguists today. It should be noted too that even if they were comprehensive, current reading procedures lag sadly behind them and this linguistic lag itself deserves more than a passing comment.

Linguists agree that speech and writing may be considered to be different codes but insist that the speech code is in some way basic to the written code. Consequently, they insist that it is necessary always to make a clear differentiation between comments about the symbols of writing. However, in spite of the work of Bloomfield and Barnhart in *Let's Read* (1961) and of Fries in *Linguistics and Reading* (1963) even these very basic facts have not been taken into consideration in the majority of texts on reading. Fries, for example, insists on careful use of the terms *phonics*, *phonetics*, and *phonemics* and such careful use must be recognized as crucial if there is to be any really worthwhile discussion of these topics by reading specialists. However, except for what is on the whole a sound book by Cordts, *Phonics for the Reading Teacher* (1965), books on reading still continue to confuse statements about phonology with statements about orthography and to use the terms phonics, phonetics, and phonemics almost in free variation. A linguist cannot help but regard Heilman's *Phonics in Proper Perspective* (1964) as an example of just this type of confusion and wonder what kind of success such a perspective could possibly guarantee. Furthermore, a series of articles in *The Reading Teacher* by Clymer (1963), Bailey (1967), and Emans (1967) on phonic generalizations would have benefited from a much closer attention to linguistic data than any of the authors chose to give for here is a good example of the type of investigation of which Carroll speaks in which adequate methodology is dissipated on material that is often linguistically indefensible.

While this criticism of phonics is deserved, the linguists mentioned above, Bloomfield and Fries, are not above criticism for their views. Both overstress the importance of the phoneme-grapheme relationship and both oversimplify the process of reading. Learning to read means more than acquiring high-speed recognition responses to various letter patterns as Fries would have it. However, many of the teaching procedures he advocates, such as the use of contrast, the stress on vowels, the insistence on whole-word patterns, and the separation of reading and writing, seem to be excellent both linguistically and pedagogically.

Phoneme and Grapheme

Reading teachers and particularly reading researchers must make themselves aware of the phoneme-grapheme correspondence, the clear distinctions among phonics, phonetics and phonemics, and the difference between statements about speech and statements about writing. Fortunately, there is much linguistic research available on these topics. Current work in linguistics does, however, indicate that a word of caution is required on the subject of the phoneme. The majority of linguists have always viewed the phoneme as a convenient linguistic fiction, and a hard to define one at that, rather than as an absolute linguistic fact. Today many linguists manage to do without phonemes at all because such linguists believe that a distinct phonemic level is not required in describing a language. More important to them than the phonemic level is a level of representation that is sometimes called the morphophonemic. For example, instead of singling out the broad phonetic differences among the endings of *cats*, *dogs*, and *judges*, the [s], [z] and [ez], and calling these differences phonemic differences because of certain contrasts elsewhere in the language, as in *sip* and *zip*, such linguists point out that English plural formation is characterized by a morphophonemic sibilant, which is quite predictably realized in various phonetic shapes according to environment as [s], [z] or [ez]. This sibilant is therefore well represented by the English *s* spelling. Likewise, they stress the importance of what they call the morphophonemic connection in English between such pairs of words as *produce* and *production*, *nation* and *national*, and *long* and *longer*. In each case it seems that a phonemic spelling and an insistence on "traditional" phonemicization conceals rather than reveals the linguistic facts. It might even be said that English spelling in many cases is a good (or at least better than previously acknowledged) representation of the phonological facts of English. What this means for reading specialists is that there is reason to have serious doubts that a child beginning to read is well-served by a strict insistence on a one-to-one phoneme-grapheme correspondence when current linguistic research suggests first of all that the phoneme neither exists nor is always a particularly useful fiction and, secondly, that rules for pronouncing are dependent in part on grammatical and lexical information

That there is really nothing new in what has been said is readily apparent if one comes across an interesting paper by Edward Sapir (1963) which first appeared over thirty years ago entitled *The Psychological Reality of Phonemes.* Although Sapir claimed in this paper that phonemes have a psychological reality, a close examination of what he says shows that what he was talking about were morphophonemes rather than phonemes. He also seems to have been hinting at a distinction between linguistic facts, that is, linguistic reality, and linguistic data, that is, the observable characteristics of language, and this fact-data distinction is one which is extremely important in current linguistic thinking.

Linguistics: The Dialogue Within

From approximately 1930 to 1960 linguistic research was largely concerned with data, that is, with making observations of linguistic events and with procedures for classifying these observations. Out of this work came considerable development and clarification of such concepts as the phoneme, the morphome, and sentence pattern, the intonation contour, the linguistic level, the slot and its fillers, and so on. In fact this is exactly the kind of linguistic research that is referred to in most discussions of linguistics by reading experts. Lefevre's book, *Linguistics and the Teaching of Reading* (1964), is a good example of this type of linguistic endeavor and a good application of it to reading. However, it would not be unfair to say that there are severe shortcomings in this kind of linguistics and that linguistics surely has more to offer reading than Lefevre offers.

Classifications of collections of English utterances do not reveal a great deal about English. It seems fair to say that they do not, for example, account for a speaker's ability to relate some of the sentences to others within a corpus. They do not account for an ability to distinguish between sentences and nonsentences. They do not account for a speaker's feelings that some sentences are confused, or deviant, or ambiguous. They do not allow one in some principled way to predict possible English sentences that might occur in the future. And so on. A grammar accounting for the facts of English will be very different from the grammar presented by Lefevre and will not just present data. Instead, such a grammar will attempt to get behind the data and classifications of the data into the facts and into explanations of linguistic abilities.

Books and articles relating linguistics to reading have favored the data rather than the fact approach. For this reason they find it difficult to demonstrate an insightful and economical relationship between sound and symbol. Similarly, statements that writing is speech put down on paper are not as adequate as they should be. Raw speech is not language in any significant sense for the data of linguistic performance are not the facts of linguistic competence and the data of written performance are something else again. Speech performance is characterized by pauses, repetitions, syntactic shifts, and so on, whereas almost all the reading material presented to children is written in well-controlled sentences, a very different type of performance. The same basic competence apparently underlies performance in both speech and writing but the performances of speech and writing are not easily related to each other. The data are different, they are not easily convertible, and they are not at all convertible if a superficial view of linguistics is accepted.

It would be true to say that linguistics has not been the same since 1957, the year of the appearance of Noam Chomsky's *Syntactic Structures* (1957). In this book and since then (1965), Chomsky has put forward a theory of language which has revolutionized linguistics but which appears hardly to have touched the reading researcher. Perhaps this is not surprising for the theory is not easy to explain and any simple explanation is very likely to be distorted and misunderstood. The theory stresses the fact that a good explanatory grammar of a language requires a set of explicit syntactic rules that generate sentences of that language together with grammatical descriptions of the generated sentences and such a set of rules will reveal sentences to have deep structures on which semantic rules operate and surface representations that are mapped out by phonological rules. The phonological and graphemic surface features of sentences are automatic and superficial and contribute nothing to the understanding of sentences. Sentences may be understood correctly only if the listener or reader knows the deep underlying elements and only if he understands the deep relationships among these elements.

Comprehension: The Syntactic Basis

The importance of such a linguistic theory for an understanding of comprehension surely cannot be overestimated. Adequate comprehension of any sentence, spoken or written, requires more than just high-speed recognition, as for Fries, or left-to-right linear decoding, as in a stochastic model of the reading process, or recognition of surface patterns. In order to fully comprehend a sentence a listener, or reader, must be able to relate the correct deep structure to the surface structure of the sentence and to project a consistent semantic reading on the individual words. A reaction to the surface structure alone, that is, a recognition of individual sounds, letters, words or superficial syntactic patterns, is insufficient for comprehension, since comprehension requires that each sentence be given both syntactic and semantic interpretations in depth.

The following sentences offer illustrations, deliberately oversimplified for the purposes of the argument, of a few major syntactic problems that appear to be of interest in an understanding of comprehension.

1. The boy took the pen.
2. The pen was taken.
3. Who took the pen?
4. What did the boy take?
5. What was taken?

Sentence one requires the comprehender to assign a deep reading which will show that *The boy* is the deep subject of the sentence, *took the pen* the predicate, and *the pen* the deep object.

i The boy took the pen.

Sentence two differs from the first in that different elements and different relationships are present. The deep subject is an unspecified SOMEONE and the deep object is *the pen.*

ii SOMEONE took the pen (Passive).

This deep structure accounts for the fact that a correct interpretation of *The pen was taken* requires an understanding that an unspecified person did the taking and this unspecified person took the pen, *the pen* being the underlying or deep object of the sentence through the superficial or grammatical subject.

The deep structures of sentences three, four, and five may be represented as follows:

iii (Question) SOMEONE took the pen.
iv (Question) The boy took SOMETHING.
v (Question) SOMEONE took SOMETHING (Passive).

Still another group of sentences illustrates the need for the comprehender to understand exactly what is in the deep structure and what is not there.

6. The dog amazed the boy.
7. The boy was amazed by the dog.
8. The boy was amazed.
9. The dog's strength amazed the boy.
10. Who was amazed by the boy's strength?

These sentences have deep structures that may be represented as follows.

vi The dog amazed the boy.
vii The dog amazed the boy (Passive).
viii SOMENOUN amazed the boy (Passive).
ix SOMETHING [The dog was strong] amazed the boy.
x (Question) SOMETHING [the dog was strong] amazed SOMEONE (Passive).

In order to comprehend the above sentences it is necessary to be aware that an unspecified SOMENOUN is the deep subject "causing" the amazement in eight, that SOMETHING is "causing" the amazement in both nine and ten, and that this SOMETHING is the fact that *The dog was strong*, the only plausible interpretation of *the dog's strength.*

The type of analysis just illustrated could be carried much further into ambiguous sentences, complement structures, complex sentences, pronominal substitutions and various kinds of noun and verb classes. Here it serves the purpose of illustrating the interest that linguists are now taking in accounting for how sentences are understood, particularly in specifying what there must be in sentences and in speakers to make communication possible. A transformational-generative grammar offers an explicit characterization of the grammatical elements in sentences, a characterization which strives for completeness and that clearly distinguishes what is important about the underlying facts of language from what is involved in actual performance. The theory says nothing about performance, that is, about how a human being actually generates or interprets sentences. *It does say though that anyone who wants to understand how a human being does either such task must recognize the facts just presented and that anyone who does not cannot hope to discover anything very revealing about actual sentence production and interpretation. An adequate model of the comprehension process must also in some way encompass the linguistic facts just presented.*

Comprehension: The Semantic Basis

Interest in transformational-generative grammars has also fostered some intriguing work in semantics, particularly that of Katz and Fodor (1963). Katz and Fodor have proposed a semantic theory that relates closely to Chomsky's syntactic theory. How that theory might apply to basic language competency in reading may be characterized as follows. The comprehension of a sentence requires that that sentence be given a reading of its deep grammatical structure together with a reading of its semantic content. This latter reading requires that the lexical items, or words, in a sentence be interpreted in a manner consistent with each other and that inconsistent readings be rejected. The ability to give a consistent reading would imply that sentence production and interpretation requires in producers and interpreters some sense of a semantic norm and that this norm can be explicitly characterized.

Some illustrations, based on suggestions from Nida (1964), may serve to clarify these basic concepts.

11. The man sat in the chair.
12. The man died in the chair.

In sentence eleven a correct interpretation of the meaning of *chair* would be one that marked this occurrence of *chair* for such characteristics as "object," "human use" and perhaps "harmless." Sentence twelve might arouse a suspicion that a "harmless" rather than "harmful" distinction cannot be guaranteed because the verb *died* appears in the sentence. Sentence twelve is consequently more likely to pose an interpretation problem than sentence eleven. In sentences thirteen and fourteen the ambiguity of twelve is resolved. "Harmful" replaces "harmless" as a characteristic of *chair*.

13. He died in the electric chair.
14. He died in the chair for his crime.

Electric in thirteen and *for his crime* in fourteen require that *chair* be given a different reading from *chair* in eleven and illuminate some of the difficulties encountered in twelve. In sentences fifteen and sixteen a similar meaning for *chair* to that in eleven seems to be required.

15. He took the chair.
16. He accepted the chair.

However, the addition of *at the meeting* to fifteen would require a "role" rather than "object" characteristic for *chair* just as would the addition of *at the university* to sixteen. Furthermore, *chair* in fifteen would now require an additional "judicial" characteristic just as *chair* in sixteen would require an additional "academic" characteristic.

The Language of Poetry

A general ability to recognize the correct syntactic and semantic interpretations of sentences is also basic to any kind of specific ability to recognize that a particular sentence is incapable of a syntactic or semantic interpretation, that is, it is either ungrammatical or nonsensical. It is also basic to an ability to interpret deviant sentences, particularly the deviant sentences of figurative and poetic language. Sentences seventeen to twenty-one are examples of such sentences.

17. My dog passed away yesterday.
18. Salt is eating away my car's fenders.
19. All nature sleeps.
20. He sat in black despair.
21. The king was a lion in battle.

Normally only human beings pass away, only certain animates eat and sleep, only concrete things are capable of color, and lions are nonhumans whereas kings are human. These sentences deviate from the English norm but not far enough so that they cannot be given interpretations which relate them to that norm. Because such interpretations can be achieved the sentences can be understood and it is possible to account for the human-ness of *dog* in seventeen, the animism of *salt* in eighteen and *nature* in nineteen, the metaphoric blackness of *despair* in twenty and the animal attributes of *king* in twenty-one. Anyone with an interest in poetry can see how that interest and linguistic knowledge come together at this point. Linguists are indeed conducting research that is relevant to an understanding of poetic and literary style and some of this research is proving to be most revealing. Again the basic distinctions between competence and performance and between grammars accounting for facts and grammars accounting for data provide the insights.

The Dialect Problem

In writing about linguistics and reading it is appropriate to mention the dialect work that is being conducted in several large cities, for example by Labov in New York (1966), and by Steward in Washington, D.C. (1965), and by McDavid in Chicago (1965). These investigations are producing descriptions of the English spoken in such cities that will be invaluable for teachers of English and reading. The language of many children in these cities is very different from that of their teachers and of their textbooks. The dialect studies tell us what the main phonological and grammatical differences are and the findings suggest that teachers should clearly differentiate the teaching of the language habits of any kind of standard spoken English from the teaching of reading. It is possible to read standard written English in almost any dialect and a standard printed text can be associated with dialects that show considered phonological and grammatical variation from what might be considered the standard spoken dialect of a particular city or region. There are several reports in the literature of children reading the standard written forms in non-standard spoken forms that are the dialect equivalents of the standard forms only to be told that the readings are "incorrect" by the teachers. In each sentence the child understood what was on the page, understood it in fact so well that he gave the printed words the "correct" phonetic realizations in his own dialect and in each case the teacher revealed her confusion between teaching the child to read and teaching him to speak a different dialect. Likewise, the problem of teaching a child to say *with* and not *wif* or to distinguish *den* and *then* is in most cases a dialect problem not a reading problem and almost never is it a speech correction problem in the usual sense of that term. Again a little linguistic knowledge can go a long way in helping teachers to arrive at sensible attitudes and procedures in teaching spoken and written English to such children.

Concluding Observations

It will be apparent that no definition of reading has been offered in this paper but at least one has been rejected, reading as high-speed recognition. Reading is much more complicated a process than mere recognition and it is in no sense a passive process. It requires effort to get meaning from the printed page. It requires perceptual skills not required in oral communication, particularly, of course, visual skills. A written text is also a special type of linguistic performance; it is not just speech written down. In addition, most of us read and comprehend far faster than we can listen and comprehend and this fact must be explained somewhere in a theory of reading that incorporates the view of language advanced here. However, no matter what definition of reading is finally agreed to certain basic linguistic principles must be recognized in such a definition.

The first principle is that a clear understanding of any kind of language use can be based only on discovering answers to the questions of what language is and how language works. Transformational-generative theory gives clues to the answers to these questions. The second principle is that there is an important distinction between competence and performance. In teaching, the concern is with the former for it is competence that allows one to produce and understand new sentences. Performance, on the other hand, is but a record of those particular sentences that were produced along with all the imperfections that occurred in their production. Performance acts, of course, at the same time as a kind of screen through which we must investigate all competence. The final principle is that most if not all language behavior is rule-governed behavior and this fact must be taken into account if one is to seek to reinforce or change existing behavior. These three principles must be taken into account in any theory of reading that aims to provide reading teachers and reading researchers with the kind of explanatory power that linguists themselves are now attempting to require of linguistic theory.

References

Bailey, Mildred H. "The utility of phonic generalizations in grades one through six." *The Reading Teacher* 20 (1967): 413–418.

Betts, E. A. "Linguistics and reading." *Education* 86 (1966): 454–458.

Bloomfield, L., and Barnhart, C. L. *Let's read.* Detroit: Wayne State University Press, 1961.

Carroll, J. B. "The analysis of reading instruction: perspectives from psychology and linguistics." In *Theories of learning and instruction, n. s. s. e. 63rd yearbook, part I,* E. R. Hilgard (Ed.) Chicago: University of Chicago Press, 1964.

Chomsky, N. *Syntactic Structures.* The Hague: Mouton, 1957.

———. *Aspects of the theory of syntax.* Cambridge, Mass.: M.I.T. Press, 1965.

Clymer, T. "The utility of phonics generalizations in the primary grades." *The Reading Teacher* 16 (1963) 252–258.
Cordts, Anna D. *Phonics for the reading teacher.* New York: Holt, Rinehart & Winston, 1965.
Devine, T. G. "Linguistic research and the teaching of reading." *Journal of Reading,* 9 (1966): 273–277.
Emans, R. "The usefulness of phonic generalizations above the primary grades." *The Reading Teacher* 20 (1967): 419–425.
Fries, C. C. *Linguistics and reading.* New York: Holt, Rinehart & Winston, 1963.
Heilman, A. W. *Phonics in proper perspective.* Columbus, Ohio: Charles E. Merrill, 1964.
Katz, J. J. and Fodor, J. A. "The structure of a semantic theory." *Language* 39 (1963): 170–210.
Labov, W. *The social stratification of English in New York City.* Washington, D.C.: Center for Applied Linguistics, 1966.
Lefevre, C. A. *Linguistics and the teaching of reading.* New York: McGraw-Hill, 1964.
McDavid, R. I., Jr. "Social dialects: cause or symptom of social maladjustment." In *Social dialects and language learning,* Roger W. Shuy (ed.) Champaign, Illinois: National Council of Teachers of English, 1965.
Nida, E. A. *Toward a science of translating.* Leiden, Netherlands: E. J. Brill, 1964.
Sapir, E. "The psychological reality of phonemes." In *Selected Writings of Edward Sapir.* D. G. Mandelbaum (Ed.) Berkeley and Los Angeles: University of California Press, 1963.
Stewart, W. A. "Urban Negro speech: socio-linguistic factors affecting English teach ing." In *Social dialects and language learning.* Roger W. Shuy (Ed.) Champaign, Illinois: National Council of Teachers of English, 1965.

Daisy M Jones' article is a practical look at what various branches of linguistics have to offer the reading teacher.

After sketching a background of what linguistics is and what a linguist does, Jones points out where linguistics can be applied in the areas of words and meanings in reading (see table, page 294). Looking first at historical or geographical linguistics, she gives examples of how these areas can lead to a greater understanding of words and also how they can aid in comprehension through an understanding of English sentence patterns.

Turning to descriptive or structural linguistics, Jones examines phonology, morphology, and other aspects of linguistics to show how they can contribute to the improvement of children's word-attack skills. Finally, she examines the place and function of sentence patterns as an aid to comprehension. The conclusion is a brief examination of the different roles of the linguist and the teacher, and what the former can contribute to the latter.

Implications of Linguistics for the Teaching of Reading

Daisy M. Jones

We have been hearing a lot about linguistics. Many people, both professionals and laymen, are looking for a method, a technique, a recipe, a panacea—something that will guarantee that, if applied in the right amounts at the right time, will lead to perfect results every time. But it is not quite that simple. There are a number of reasons why this is so. English is not consistent enough to guarantee uniform stimulus-response patterns. Learners are not like automobiles coming off the assembly line. They don't all respond in the same way. Each learner is a custom job, and it is the responsibility of the teacher to help him learn in his unique way.

Let us then look at linguistics and the work of the linguists to see what they have to offer. We begin with orientation in terms of definitions. *Linguistics* as a study is a branch of anthropology. *Anthropology* is defined as the science that deals with the origins, development, races, customs, and beliefs of mankind. In as much as language is a part of the development and one of the customs of mankind, it is then a branch of anthropology. A *linguist* is one skilled in, or a student of, languages; one who studies the history and structure of language. *Linguistics* pertains to the study and comparison of languages, the science of language, its origin and growth, and the likenesses and differences among languages.

How does all this relate to the teaching of reading and the other language arts to the child in the elementary school? This treatise is not designed to add new information to the subject. It is not even written by one who lays claim to being a linguist. It is an attempt to interpret the various positions of linguists in the light of classroom teaching. It is hoped that it will help the teacher of reading to gain perspective on the subject and see where her work fits into the total linguistic picture.

First, let us consider what linguistics is *not*. It is not a method or a technique. It is not a tool. Then what is it? It is an organized body of knowledge relating to the tools we use in communication. It is something a teacher should know, though it is not necessarily something she will teach to the children at the lower-elementary level.

If you have been confused in your interpretation of linguistics, it is probably because you have read different authorities who were talking about different facets of the subject. As you applied your own generalizations, perhaps they didn't seem to fit. Let's look at an organizational pattern that may help you to see what the linguist is talking about.

Historical and geographical implications of linguistics may be applied either to word patterns or to meaning patterns. Descriptive or structural implications of linguistics may be applied either to word patterns or meaning patterns. The historical linguist is attempting to trace the history and origin of the language. He may also be trying to isolate certain linguistic patterns in geographical settings. The structural linguist is attempting to describe the language as is exists now. He, too, may be dealing with word patterns. He also deals with meaning-bearing patterns that include more than the isolated word. This description may extend to the phrase, the sentence, or sometimes even the whole group of sentences that are needed to give complete meaning.

Historical or Geographical Study of Word Patterns

Look at the upper left-hand column of the diagram. The area of emphasis is historical and geographical. The pattern is based on words. The historical and geographical implications of word patterns are interesting and worth knowing, and the truly professional teacher should be informed. It is doubtful if much of the material will be taught to the elementary-school child as an organized body of knowledge, though some of it may be challenging to a few superior students. It should, however, be part of "the stock in trade" for the professional educator who is attempting to teach children to read. A thorough understanding of this phase of linguistics will help the teacher to recognize patterns in the language, to understand difficulties encountered by the learner, and to make judgments about what to teach to whom and when.

Some examples of the historical and geographical emphasis on word patterns may help to clarify this point of view.

LINGUISTICS—AREAS OF EMPHASIS

Pattern	Historical or Geographical	Descriptive or Structural
Word-Patterns	Word origins Derivations New words New meanings Coined words Colloquialisms	Phonemes Morphemes Sound-symbol relationships Word structure— roots affixes inflections Semantics
Meaning-Patterns	Influences of other languages Structure of English Sentence patterns Word order Regional speech	Syntax Sentence parts Punctuation Figures of speech Paragraphs Meaning patterns— pitch stress juncture

(1) Word origins from other languages are abundant in English. "*Pend*" from the Latin meaning "to hang" is evident in such words as pendant, independent, suspend, depend, and pending. The Latin root *"porto"* meaning "to carry" is evident in such words as portable, import, transport, export, and many others. The dictionary points out word derivations from Old English, Old French, Anglo Saxon, Latin, and Greek, and others.

(2) New words enter our language to meet new needs. If you were to look in a dictionary bearing a copyright date of 1900, you probably would not find such words as astronaut, aquanaut, refrigerator, helicopter, and a host of others.

(3) New meanings for familiar words occur frequently. The child who thinks of a *range* as a stove will get a different concept when he sees the word in such expressions as "on the open range," or "the mountain range." Similar experiences will be met with such words as *diamond* (a gem, a baseball field, a geometric shape), *spring* (a flexible piece of steel, a source of water, a season of the year), *square* (a square deal, a square box, a "square" person).

(4) Coined words are constantly entering our language to meet new situations; for example a *scuba* diver is one who uses a Self-Contained Underwater Breathing Apparatus. The words pasteurize and mesmerize come from the names of persons who contributed to the development of those processes.

(5) Then there are colloquialisms—words that take on different meanings in different geographical settings. To people in some parts of the country *poke* means to punch, to others it means a sack for carrying something. To some, *reckon* means to calculate, to others it means "I suppose so." Examples could be added endlessly. Every student of language has his own favorite illustrations.

Historical or Geographical Study of Meaning-Bearing Patterns

Now look at the lower left-hand column of the diagram. The area of emphasis is still historical and geographical, but the pattern is based on sentences or meanings. Historically, languages have developed to meet the needs of the times. Geographically, they have developed to meet the needs of the people in a given place. A study of this development of language leads to a study of the means of communication of thought. Out of this grows the study of the sentence patterns that have evolved in different languages and in different regions.

Some examples of the historical and geographical emphasis on sentences and meaning-bearing patterns will further clarify this point. English has borrowed much of its structure from other languages. The following sentences illustrate some of the more common sentence patterns that children are familiar with long before they start the learning-to-read process:

Boys run.
Boys are noisy.
Boys run fast.
Dogs are animals.
Boys like dogs.
Boys teach dogs tricks.
Boys teach dogs clever tricks.
Boys teach dogs clever tricks quickly.

These are only some of the simple sentences. Many children use compound and complex sentences with subordinate clauses, relative pronouns, prepositional phrases, and even participles, with ease, although they have not learned to identify or name them.

The sentence pattern in English usually has the modifier preceding the substantive it modifies, for example, "the clever dog," and the modifier following the verb it modifies, for example, "Dogs learn quickly." Some of these patterns are reversible without distorting the meaning and some are not; for example you might say, "Dogs quickly learn" but you would not say, "the dog clever." Sentence patterns and word order vary from one language to another. In Latin the verb comes last. Many of the amusing expressions, for example, "He went the stairs up," that result from confusion of one language pattern with another are explainable if one understands the patterns of the various languages.

Regional speech is accounted for by localization of cultural groups in certain geographical areas. This explains the speech characteristics of the Pennsylvania Dutch, the western colloquialisms, and the dialects peculiar to certain sections of the country. Historical influence has given our language some special qualities also. Pioneer expressions and figures of speech have added color to the meaning of language, for example, "soft soap," "slick as a greased pig," "sharp as a tack," and "black as coal." Most modern children have never seen soft soap, have not experienced the pioneer frolic of catching a greased pig, may never have used a carpet tack for its original purpose, and might not even be familiar with coal, therefore, these expressions must be explained if they are to have meaning when they occur in literature. Many other examples could be added from the familiar language of the logging camps, military life, the gold rush days, and World Wars I and II. How many children today know what we mean by a four flusher, a GI or a doughboy?

Descriptive Study of Structure of Word Patterns

Next, let us turn our attention to the upper right-hand column of the diagram. Here the area of emphasis changes to structural linguistics or a description of the language as it is at present. The pattern at this point is based on word structure. The descriptive or structural phases of linguistics deal with the language as the child is now using it as a tool of communication both in the expressive phases that include speaking and writing, and in the impressive phases that include listening and reading.

Much of the research done in recent years, and many of the proposed beginning reading programs on the market, are centered around word patterns. A study of phonemes includes the isolated sounds and the letters that represent them, for example, *p*, *t*, *d*, *m*, *l*, and so on. A study of morphemes includes a unit of structure, the pronounceable parts of words such as the *am* in ham, or the *our* in sour.* The emphasis is on a regular pattern of sound-symbol relationships, such as the *t* in time, butter, dot; or the *a* in cat, sand, bag, man.

Further applications of descriptive and structural linguistics lead to a study of word patterns. It is well to note at this point that letters do

---

**Editor's Note:* This is not to say that these elements are morphemes (or meaning-bearing parts) of these particular words.

not make sounds. Not all of them even represent sounds. Vowels represent many and varied formations of the resonance chamber producing open sounds; for example, consider the shape of the oral cavity in forming the *o* in hot, home, some, for, son, or. Each is different. Consider the *a* in cat, cake, call, star, about, said, was. Again each is different.

Consonants are divided into two groups depending on whether or not they can be prolonged. Plosives, such as *b*, *p*, *d*, *t*, *k*, and so forth, must be released by a vowel. They represent only a position of the vocal organs. Continuants such as *m*, *n*, *l*, *s*, *r*, and so forth, can be prolonged, and may be sounded separately, but for what purpose?

Syllabication divides words into pronounceable parts. This may aid in spelling and sometimes in analysis for meaning, but it is of questionable value in reading for meaning. Accent varies with the word pattern and the meaning. Compare this list—visit, habit, travel, label, shovel, signal, neighbor—with this list—control, patrol, regret, decide, equip, accept. Mispronunciation often results from the application of rules of syllabication and accent where they do not apply. One may have formed the habit of placing the accent on the next to the last syllable in words with three or more syllables such as inter*lop*er, auto*ma*tic, indi*ca*tion, and invi*ta*tion, then when he applies the same principle to the word *determiner* he comes up with det-er-*min*-er instead of de*ter*miner. In the same manner, when one changes the noun *beau*ty to the adjective *beau*tiful, he keeps the accent on the first syllable, but in changing the noun *rem*edy to the adjective form he does not keep the accent of the first syllable which would give *rem*-e-di-al, but instead moves the accent to the second syllable and gets re-*me*-dial.

This phase of linguistics also involves word structure based on roots, affixes, and inflections. Sometimes the study of word structure moves beyond mere word recognition based on symbol representation and incorporates the semantics involved in the various meanings of such words as fast, run, rose, fly, lie, fall, game, green, and many others. Add to this the variations caused by homonyms and heteronyms that depend on recognition of spelling and sometimes origin for both pronunciation and meaning.

A method of reading that stops with recognition of words assumes that the pupils will assemble the words into meaningful relationships. Bright children from highly literate environments may learn to read this way, but the ones who are linguistically deprived may progress no farther than the mechanical process of associating sound with symbol. Mere recognition of words is not reading. Reading is finding out what the sentences mean. In many present day situations too great an emphasis has been placed on words and their pronunciation. What really matters is the function of the words in the utterance of sounds that express ideas. Some linguists think that it makes no difference whether words are meaningful or of the nonsense variety. Others seem to be of the opinion that children ought to read meaningful words from the beginning. Some say that from the start all reading activity should be based on meaning of the whole sentence.

Descriptive Study of Structure of Meaning-Bearing Patterns

Finally, examine the lower right hand column of the diagram. Here we continue the emphasis on descriptive or structural linguistics but the pattern is now based on meanings. After all, it is the getting of meaning that reading is all about. And by the same token, it is the expression of ideas that language is all about. Meanings are expressed, not necessarily by single words but by larger syntactical units made up of phrases, and often whole sentences. We need to teach larger segments of sound in order to maintain meaning in its entirety. Many children who seem deficient in reading at higher-grade levels are really deficient in general-language ability. This justifies time and effort spent in the development of oral language prior to and along with the use of language in the reading situation. Beginning reading should be couched in the spoken-language form that is familiar to the child. Reading stories to children and talking with them helps them to become familiar with the language patterns they will encounter in reading.

Lefevre proposes attention to larger structural patterns. He refers to this as a syntactic-semantic approach. For this the teacher needs a knowledge of the structural system of English, not necessarily in order to relay it to the child, but in order to know what, how, and when to point out organizational patterns that exist in the child's language. This is what Lefevre calls the "meaning-bearing pattern."[1]

In order to get full meaning from the printed page a child needs to learn to interpret the sentence in its entirety and in its relation to the rest of the sentences in the total setting. This involves the syntax of the sentence itself; that is, the construction or use of a word in a phrase, or clause, or even in the whole sentence; the arrangement of words in the sentence and the grammar dealing with this. It also involves the interpretation based on punctuation, figures of speech, total paragraphs, and meaning patterns as revealed by change in pitch, stress, and juncture in oral speech.

Consider the alteration of meaning as influenced by omission or addition of sentence parts, and by the placement of punctuation. Notice what the addition of the final phrase does to the meaning of the following:

---

[1] Lefevre, Carl A. "A Comprehensive Linguistic Approach to Reading." *Elementary English,* (October 1965): pp 651–659.

The girl wanted the dress.
The girl wanted the dress to be discarded.

In one case she wanted the dress; in the other case she did not want it.

Consider the different points of stress in reading the sentence:

He hit him

in answer to the following questions: Who hit him? What did he do to him? Whom did he hit?

Notice the difference in stress in reading the sentence:

He is an elevator operator

when answering the following questions: Is he a telephone operator? Is he an elevator repairman?

In Matthew 26:27 we read, "Drink ye all of it." Does that mean for all of you to drink of it, or for you to drink all that is in the cup? Try reading it aloud each way.

Consider what punctuation can do to meaning, and consequently to the inflection of the voice in interpreting print. Read these two sentences:

You went to the mountains.
You went to the mountains?

Unless the reader is aware of the terminal punctuation mark and its implication for meaning as well as vocal inflection, he may see no difference.

Read these pairs of sentences noting the effect of the punctuation marks.

Woman without her man is a raving maniac. (Woman is the maniac.)
Woman, without her, man is a raving maniac. (Man is the maniac.)
This bears watching. (You are doing the watching.)
This bear's watching. (The bear is doing the watching.)
Let me call you sweetheart.
Let me call you, sweetheart.

Sometimes vocalization is identical but the difference in meaning is represented by the spelling of the words or the spacing. Consider these examples:

The consecrated cross I'd bear.
The consecrated cross-eyed bear.
I scream.
Ice cream.
Greene House, greenhouse, and green house.
The sun's rays meet.
The sons raise meat.

Sometimes words are identical and you have to decide on both pronunciation and meaning from context. For example:

These garments are 89 centers.
We plan to work in 89 centers.

Then consider these:

in a *minute*, and a *minute* speck
Real *live* bears *live* in the park.
You may *present* the *present*.

Sometimes one word can serve several functions in the same sentence. This headline appeared in a newspaper:

Police police police picnic.

The first *police* is the subject, the second is the verb, and the third is an adjective modifying the word picnic.

Sometimes the change of just one word will change the meaning and even the grammatical structure of an entire sentence. Consider these:

The body's calcium needs are balanced daily.
The body's calcium needs to be balanced daily.

In the first sentence the word *calcium* modifies the word needs and in the second sentence it is a noun and is used as the subject of the sentence. In the first sentence the word *needs* is the subject of the sentence and in the second it is the verb.

And who isn't familiar with the informal language of conversation as contrasted with the more formal language seen in print? Witness: hafto, didja, kinda, whadja, wuza goin', and so on. One girl said to another, "Squp." It was obvious what she meant when the two turned and started up the stairway. Then there is the question, "Jeet yet?" and its answer, "No. Jew?"

Words or sentences or even paragraphs are islands in the sea of meanings. We need to teach the total relationships for real meanings.

This story illustrates the principle that knowing the words does not necessarily prove that the meaning is clear:

A lobbyist was opposing a large appropriation for a state college. He sent the following letter to the legislators:

Dear Congressmen:

Before you cast your vote on Senate Bill No. C—192–a, please give careful consideration to the following facts gleaned from the campus. You should know that up at the state college the men and women students use the same curriculum. The boys and girls often matriculate together. A young lady student cannot get an advanced degree until she shows her thesis to the male professors.

Signed: Bill Smith, Lobbyist
for Economy in Government

Note: Senate Bill No. C–192–a was defeated 187 to 3.

Summary and Conclusions

The linguist is a student of language and its structure.
The educator is a student of human growth and development and the resulting learning patterns.

Each has something to contribute to the other. The linguist needs to know more about how learning takes place, and the educator needs to know more about how the language is structured before either can presume to prescribe the work of the other.

Both the linguists and the educators tend to agree that taking words apart and analyzing them has advantages over a synthesizing of the parts into words, and that the ultimate goal of reading should be the use of words in meaningful settings.

Linguists and educators tend to disagree on the initial emphasis especially in reading. The linguist would organize the program around the structure of the language and attempt to help the child adapt his learning techniques and sequences to a logical order. The educator would organize the program around the developmental steps in the child's growth and attempt to help him discover and organize his understandings about the structural patterns observable in his language.

The good teacher should understand thoroughly the linguistic structure of the language she is using as a medium of teaching. This seems to be one of the serious lacks in the education of today's teachers. The good teacher should understand the learning patterns, levels, and sequences in child development and therefore be prepared to help the learner progress along parallel lines developing concurrently such concomitant learnings as concepts on which reading is based, familiarity with both the aural and the visual stimuli, acquaintance with sentence patterns, awareness of word structure, and generalizations about frequently recurring and useful patterns. In this way she may lead the learner to independence in both the mechanics of reading and the acquiring of meaning.

The teacher who understands both the learner and the language is in a position to introduce one to the other in a mutually beneficial setting.

William West addresses himself to the practical question of values of linguistics in high school reading, but most of what he has to say applies to the elementary grades as well.

After a brief and delightful introduction, West identifies and explains "eight definite contributions that linguistics can make to high school English and reading"; namely, it provides: intrinsically interesting material, a language-learning method, a scientific approach, a basis for remedial help, insight into the melody of language, a source for vocabulary development, tools for increasing precision in complex thinking, and finally a basis for insight into literature.

Values of Linguistics in High School Reading

William W. West

Introduction

I recently visited a used car lot and went through the time-honored ritual of kicking the tires, slamming the doors, sniffing the carburetor, and twisting the steering wheel of a miserable old clunker that seemed to promise cheap second-car transportation. None of these hallowed operations, however, "sold" me on the vehicle. But then as I sat in the driver's seat, inhaled deeply and caught the "new car smell," I fairly vaulted from the cockpit and shouted, "I'll take it."

Imagine my consternation when I picked the car up to see a familiar drop out, a former student, squirting into other clunkers bottled "new car odors" from an aerosol spray can.

A similar situation exists in educational publishing today, and teachers who are not impressed with new covers, kodachrome pictures, and gratuitous changes in old texts leap delightedly for the order blank at the least whiff of "linguistics." And in some cases the linguistic content and the linguistic procedures are as fundamental—and as ephemeral—as the new car smell in my wife's current calamity. If we are to avoid the pitfalls of the bandwagon and the frustrations of calamitous delay, we ought to know what values linguistics has for high school reading. In my opinion, the values of linguistics for high school programs are much slighter than for elementary programs. Nonetheless, I can think of eight definite contributions linguistics can make to high school English and reading:

1. It provides intrinsically interesting material.
2. It suggests a method of language learning.

3. It brings the scientific method to the study of language.
4. It structures a way of developing awareness of phoneme-grapheme correspondence in remedial students.
5. It provides insights into the melody of the language students can use in oral reading, in reading for meaning, and in punctuating.
6. It refines our approach to the development of word families and the increasing of vocabulary.
7. It gives us tools for increasing precision in complex thinking.
8. It suggests insights into literature.

But even with these eight values of linguistics listed, it is well to remind readers of Emmett Betts' 1964 warning: "At the present time there is no substantial evidence that the study of either descriptive grammar or generative grammar increases the pupils' ability to write or to read."[1] Now, almost five years later we must still preface a discussion of each of these values with an identical warning: "At the present time there is no *substantial* evidence . . ." But note that the stress on the word substantial is "phonemic" here—that is, it changes the meaning ever so slightly: there is beginning to be evidence, but it is not yet substantial.

1. Intrinsically interesting material. The first value of linguistics is that it provides intrinsically interesting material. What student can fail to be fascinated by such subjects as the way language changes? They love such information as the fact that an Elizabethan girl was complimented to be called homely (home-loving, domestic), that the seventeenth century criticism of St. Paul's cathedral as "awful, atmospheric, and artificial" really meant "awe-inspiring, mood-inducing, and built with great artifice or craftsmanship," that decimate once meant to "kill every tenth man of a captured army." They are fascinated, too, by discussions of the possible origins of language—even though these discussions can lead to no definite conclusions. Did language come from spontaneous animal cries (the *bow-wow* theory), from emotional exclamations (the *pooh-pooh* theory), from the imitation of natural sounds (the *ding dong* theory), from the use of sound to coordinate group efforts (the *yo-he-ho* theory), from sounds naturally associated with bodily movement (the *hi!* theory), or from the simplest sound combinations (the *ga* theory). They are fascinated by the varying geographical, social, and occupational dialects; by the various kinds of changes that occur in words; by the kinds of new words that develop; by the foreign words that enter English, and so on almost without end.

It is easy to entertain students with this kind of information, and a certain amount of such entertainment is valuable in stimulating an interest in and continuing observation of language, but Kreidler warned ". . . on variety, style, social or geographic dialects, or historic periods, the textbook writer can quickly exhaust the information which the linguist has provided."[2] I'm not sure that either the teacher or writer will exhaust the material, but he may continue past the point of interest and into the valley of diminishing returns.

2. Language-learning method. A second value of linguistics is that it suggests a method of language learning. Recent researches by Roger Brown and Ursula Bellugi, among others, show that students learn language by using language. Brown and Bellugi report that during the early stages of language development, children use three basic methods of learning language: (1) They imitate language they have heard, systematically reducing the length of sentences and retaining the important meaning-carrying "telegram-style" words; (2) The child uses language which may vary somewhat from the adult norm, and the parent imitates his speech, but expands and corrects it; and (3) The child "induces" the underlying structure of the language by finding analogous patterns: thus, *hop*, *hopped*, *hopped* becomes—mistakenly—*go*, *goed*, *goed*.[3]

It becomes apparent that language develops as children use language; as John Dixon summarizes ". . . language is learnt (sic) in operation, not by dummy runs."[4] My own theory as to the reason that the so-called "general American television announcer dialect" has not invaded and leveled the delightful variant regional dialects of our country is that children do not learn this dialect because they don't produce it! At the risk of alienating reading teachers, I will suggest that one thing linguistics suggests for reading programs is more *production* of language—oral and written—before reading.

3. Scientific study of language. A third value of linguistics for high school reading programs is that it brings the application of the scientific method of language. Indeed, if one reads some authorities (notably Postman and Weingartner[5]) he may come to believe that this is the major contribution and value of linguistics. The scientific method involves: (1) stating a problem or question in "researchable" terms; (2) collecting and organizing data; (3) proposing a hypothesis or a solution; (4) evaluating the solution or hypothesis; (5) stating (and acting upon) the accepted solution or hypothesis.

Modern man uses this scientific method to a greater or less degree in many areas of his life; why should he not, then, apply it to the study of his language? By having students propose researchable questions and follow through on them, we teach the scientific method, we learn the actual facts of the language, and we communicate information and linguistic attitudes likely to remain long after deductive learnings are forgotten. What are some researchable questions? Here are some that have been asked recently: What is the relative "verb density" of two different writers (that is, the proportion of verbs to other words) and what is the effect on their style? What proportion of the sentences of good, modern expository writers begin with something other than the subject noun cluster? What is the status in your community of "who-whom," of "can-may," of "like as a conjunction," and so on. Many of these "researches" can be connected with reading and literature.

4. Remedial help. A fourth value of linguistics is in what it says to us for teaching remedial students phoneme-grapheme correspondence. Like many other linguistic insights, this is more pertinent to instruction in the elementary school. Theoretically at least, our students should have developed their recognition of phoneme-grapheme correspondence. Actually, we have some poor readers and poor spellers who might be helped through a linguistic approach. The basic problem with the learning of which letters and letter patterns represent what sounds is that traditional reading and spelling books teach students the most common words first—the words most frequently used. *And the words most frequently used are the ones most likely to be irregular in spelling.*

To illustrate, the spoken language has slowly changed from what it was when English spelling was "fixed," and the words most frequently used have not only had more opportunity to change in sound, but also there is more resistance to changing their spelling so it fits the current pronunciation. If someone were to initiate the spelling of *ufemizm* in place of *euphemism*, few people would object both because they would probably not even see the word from one year to the next and because they just wouldn't care. But change the spelling of *have* to *hav* and see the complaints you engender!

This is the problem of the child learning to read and to spell. We teach him a regular pattern such as *a-consonant-e* as in *wave*, *save*, *cave*, and so on, but before he has "set" this pattern in his mind, we show him *may*, *weigh*, *they*, *steak*, *wait*, and several other common words. It is as though on the blackboard we wrote a-consonant-e for the "long a" sound and then directly on top of it wrote each of the other spellings. The effect of the additional spellings is to interfere with the original pattern so the child forgets his most important graphemes.

Somewhere I read that because of the fact that there are about 200 spellings of English for the forty-odd sounds of English the word *circumference* could theoretically be spelled in 396,000,000 different ways. Dubious, I took the spellings for each sound in *circumference* as listed in the front of the Thorndike-Barnhart Junior Dictionary—and I discovered that the mathematically possible combinations totaled over two billion! It's no wonder Johnny can't spell or read.

This information is of little value to the secondary teacher, but if an occasional student is so retarded as to be having problems with phoneme-grapheme correspondence, begin him with groups of words that represent the regular-spelling patterns: The short vowel sound, as in lad, beg, rid, lot, but:

vowel-consonant	vowel-consonant-consonant
tab	mast
fed	elk
it	think
cot	odd
sup	stunt

The long vowel sound, as in rate, scene, hike, hope, fume:

vowel-consonant-vowel	vowel-consonant-e	vowel-vowel
hoping	hope	moat
hating	hate	wait

Exceptions? Of course, there are exceptions—thousands of them, and they must be taught eventually. But don't teach them until the student has learned the regular patterns to the point of saturation—so the new learnings won't erase the old. To use the example of Robert Allen of Teacher's College, Columbia, don't teach the spelling of *have*. As a pattern it leads nowhere. It really should be pronounced as in *wave*. So teach wave *instead* because it leads to rave, crave, save, shave, and dozens of other words. The most completely-worked-out volume for teaching these patterns is that of Ralph M. Williams (*Phonetic Spelling for College Students*, New York: Oxford University Press, 1960). Despite the title, it's pretty much a linguistics approach.

5. The melody of language. A fifth value of linguistics for high school reading programs is that it helps students realize consciously the melody of the language and the importance of the melody in sending and receiving meaning. To ignore all the fine points of intonation at this time, it is enough to emphasize that the pauses, the stresses, and the pitch level are phonemic in English—that is, they make a difference in meaning. By having students listen to good oral readings, perhaps recorded, by having them mark passages for oral reading, by having them read orally and chorally material they have prepared, and by having them attend to their own oral reading and its connection both with meaning and with punctuation, some little insight into meaning-bearing units may be acquired. The meaning-bearing units are the clusters of words that must be read together—phrases, clauses, complete subjects, and so on—if meaning is to be communicated.

A very slight contribution to reading from this aspect of linguistics might be the recognition that English has four degrees of stress (three stressed and one unstressed) rather than the two recognized in traditional scansion of poetry. Try taking an ancient nursery rhyme and working it out in the Italian-French iambic pattern: it will look pretty irregular:

/ ∪ / ∪ / /
Sing a song of sixpence,
∪ / ∪ / ∪ /
A pocket full of rye;
/ ∪ / ∪ / /
Four and twenty blackbirds
/ / ∪ /
Baked in a pie.
/ ∪ / ∪ / ∪
When the pie was opened,
∪ / ∪ / ∪ /
The birds began to sing;
/ ∪ / ∪ / ∪ /
Wasn't that a dainty dish
∪ / ∪ / ∪ /
To set before the king?

I don't know to whom I am indebted for the insight that traditional scansion doesn't work with old-English poetry. The early-English poets counted only the very heavy primary stresses, so if you mark those only, you get the regular two beats per line, regardless of the number of unstressed syllables: sing six/- pock- rye/ four black-/ Baked pie, and so forth. When working on scansion of English poems and the regular feet seem sadly irregular, try counting only the primary accents. And, of course, call attention to Gerard Manley Hopkins' deliberately archaic "sprung rhyme" which used this insight in the late nineteenth century.

6. Vocabulary development. The sixth value of linguistics in high school reading is that it aids in the building of word families and in increasing vocabulary. Reading teachers have traditionally done a great deal in this area, putting together roots, bases, stems, prefixes and suffixes to show word families. Linguistics has really little additional to say in this area—discounting the jargon—except *Keep it up!*

7. A tool of precision. The seventh value of linguistics for high school reading is that it provides tools for increasing precision in complex thinking. Recent studies of the language and dialect of the underprivileged show that an utterance in this social group is likely to cut off thought rather than to invite it. A disgruntled worker might announce, "The man don't care about us, ain't that right?" And this tag question invites a chorus of "Yeah." End of thought. In a middle-class situation, a worker might make the same statement in his own dialect: "The boss is kind of teed-off today, isn't he?" But the intonation of the final phrase—a true question, rather than an agreement-getter—would invite such responses as "He seems okay to me." "I haven't had any trouble." "Oh, you mean because he slammed his door . . ." and so on. The nature of the statement invites disagreement, questioning, analysis, and concretization. In short, it invites refinement and correction.

There is, admittedly, a strong difference of opinion among linguists as to the best way to stimulate the refinement of language that bespeaks precise thought. One school opts for direct study of the language structures. Another demands that situations challenging thought and speech be set up. A third suggests a compromise with challenging situations followed by analysis of structures. Without question, the transformational grammarians offer more insights than any other group into the way language can be used in communicating refined thought, but teachers and writers have a long way to go in developing techniques for using these insights without drowning students in structure, terminology, and symbolism.

8. A medium of insight. Finally, linguistics can help students in a high school reading program as they use its insights to puzzle out structure and meaning; for example: "These two lines have parallel structure; they must have somehow parallel meanings." "In this phrase in ordinary speech someone would use a noun; why did Cummings use an adverb?" "The predominant phoneme clusters in this passage are sibilants; what is their effect?" "These two lines don't scan regularly; what happens if we look only at the primary stresses?" "That line doesn't make sense; suppose we try to rearrange it into a regular sentence pattern?"

Perhaps a final observation from a linguist on what the task of teaching English and the language arts really consists of is appropriate at this point. Dr. Peter Rosenbaum, the research linguist of the IBM Corporation's computer-assisted-instruction team, says that the teaching of English is "the designing of environments which demand the creative use of language." In short, even as a linguist, Rosenbaum recognizes that challenging students, stimulating them, even irritating and frustrating them until they *must* use language to read, write, listen, speak, and think, results in the greatest improvement in linguistic ability. Rosenbaum does not rule out a direct attack on language, but he puts it into perspective. And this, too, is an insight from linguistics.

Bibliography

1. Betts, E. "A New Era: Reading and Linguistics," *Education* 84 (May 1964): p. 518.
2. Kreidler, Charles W. "The Influence of Linguistics in School Grammar," *The Linguistic Reporter* 8 (December 1966): pp. 1–4.

3. Brown, Roger, and Bellugi, Ursula. "Three Processes in the Child's Acquisition of Syntax," *Harvard Educational Review* 34 (Spring 1964): pp. 133–152.
4. Dixon, John. *Growth through English Reading.* (England): Association for the Teaching of English. (1967): p. 13.
5. Postman, Neil, and Weingartner, Charles. *Linguistics: A Revolution in Teaching,* New York: Holt, Rinehart & Winston, 1967.

Postscript

You don't have to use the *Merrill Linguistic Series*, the *Bloomfield-Barnhart Let's Read*, or any other series of linguistic readers currently on the market in order to apply linguistic principles in your reading class. Certainly, a background of linguistics will help you do a better job in the event that you are ever handed such readers and expected to use them. But even without a formal published linguistic program, your own knowledge of linguistics will enable you to see new vistas in reading and will likely suggest ways that you can put linguistics to work to improve your reading instruction.

Sight Words

Teaching sight words (words that a child can recognize instantly on sight) has long been an early step in reading programs. But which words should be included in the list of sight words to be taught? Many lists have been compiled (the best known is the Dolch list), but a survey of basal-reading series shows that they do not completely agree on which words or how many words children ought to learn by sight.

Fries' distinction between form and function words (presented in this book on pages 214–215 in the section on structural grammar) suggests to me the importance of teaching function words as sight words. Exactly how many of these function words there are is a moot point, differing according to what words one considers as function words. Francis says they number about 154; Lefevre says there are about 300. Exact numbers notwithstanding, we do know that function words make up a relatively small and stable list of the total number of words in our language and that they include pronouns, auxiliary verbs, conjunctions, articles, prepositions, and other "minor" word classes. Despite their relatively small number, these words make up from 30 percent to 50 percent of all running words in our reading material. They are often phonetically irregular and difficult to pin a lexical meaning on (how do you define *about* or *because*), but since they are used so often, you can be sure that many if not most of these words are already part of your pupils' speaking vocabularies.

A simple example will illustrate how form and function words work in our language. In the sentence The *dog chased* the *cat* down the *street*, the form words are italicized. Half of the words in the sentence are function words, half are form words. Deleting the function words, we have *dog . . . chased . . . cat . . . street*. This sequence of words produces a mental image (it may be up the street or across the street or around the street, but at least we can envision a feline and a canine on a street).

Deleting the form words, however, we have *The . . . the . . . down the,* which makes no sense at all. From this example, it is obvious that function words can't be the only words taught in the beginning stages of reading but, because of their high frequency in reading material at all levels, they ought to be taught as words to be recognized instantly.

Try this kind of form-function analysis on your own classroom reading materials. Which words are used over and over?

I've used this type of activity while working with older remedial readers and adult functional illiterates who profess "I can't read anything." Taking a newspaper (either a daily or a school newspaper such as *Know Your World*), I've had the learner underline or circle every word he can already recognize. Usually he circles common function words, that occur so frequently he soon discovers that he can, in fact, read quite a few words in a running text.

The degree to which a word is phonetically regular also suggests teaching it as a sight word. Some words in English are so phonetically irregular that analyzing them is an exercise in futility. I once asked a group of students whether they would teach the word *chalet* (a word that I took from an early story in a second-grade basal) by means of decoding or sight. A few answers ran something like this: "Decoding. First, I would teach the sound for *ch* and then tell the pupils that this is an exception to the rule because of its French origin. Then I would teach the 'long vowel at the end of an open syllable rule' and explain that the first vowel in *chalet* is an exception to this rule. Next I would write the syllable *let* on the board and tell the children that although this syllable is usually pronounced /let/ in English, it is pronounced /ley/ in this case because of the French origin of the word." It would have been better to avoid the rules and exceptions and teach the word as a sight word at the outset. While historical or comparative linguistics can be useful in helping to explain the background and phonetic irregularities of some English words, linguists offers little in the way of helping children decode these words on a letter-sound correspondence basis.

Phonics

Phonics is defined as the application of phonetics in teaching reading. It has been used both as the major focus and basis of beginning reading instruction and as an integral part of the reading-skills program.

Many reading teachers are puzzled about the difference between linguistics and phonics aproaches and don't quite understand Bloomfield's criticism of the phonic method. The *-ap*, *-ip*, *-op* patterns remind them of the old phonics word families of the "grunt and groan" days. While there are inescapable similarities in both approaches, the difference between linguistics and phonics rests in their different orientations, the different ways they approach language. The phonics teacher sees words basically as written words and talks about "the sounds of letters." The linguist, on the other hand, sees speech as the first form of language. Thus, rather than teaching the sound of a letter, the linguist begins with the assumption that the child already knows the sound and then shows children which letters are used to represent this sound. While they approach the topic from different directions, the result is in some cases the same: an emphasis on sound-symbol relationships often using phonetically regular words.

Because of this similarity, we often find such standard phonics activities as following verbal directions, listening to stories read aloud, identifying familiar sounds, building a large speaking vocabulary, discriminating between different shapes and letter forms, associating beginning sounds with pictured objects, matching sounds, establishing left-to-right directionality, identifying rhyming words, categorizing and classifying words and objects, reproducing sequences of sounds, and learning the alphabet, classified as *psycholinguistic activities*. Some of the terminology changes too; for example, the old *auditory discrimination* of phonics becomes the *auditory association* of linguistics.

Developing an awareness of the child's sound features in his own speech—his pronunciation of consonants, vowels, and the existence of syllables—gives a linguistic base to your phonics instruction. Maybe (and I know this is debatable) a first step in phonics instruction ought to be teaching children the concept of a phoneme as a basic indivisible speech sound and then have them identify phonemes in their own speech. By changing a simple sound in a word, they can create their own minimal pairs.

What linguistics offers that phonics often doesn't is precision and exactitude. As a result of thorough linguistic analysis, we can now identify precisely which sound-symbol relationships are regular, which are not, and under what conditions the sounds and symbols of our language match in various ways. Books such as *Letters and Sounds: A Manual for Reading Instruction* by Robert E. Schell (Englewood Cliffs, N.J.: Prentice Hall, 1972), a recent publication containing a comprehensive inventory of sound and letter relationships in American English, should prove useful to teachers, whatever approach they use.

Structural Analysis

Structural analysis, the unlocking of words through the use of meaningful structural units within the word, is another skill that is part of any reading program. Here's where a knowledge of morphology can be useful in building reading power. Some applications of morphology to building vocabulary have been suggested earlier (page 99).

Beginning with basic features such as inflectional endings (can your pupils hear, read, and understand the difference between *girl* and *girls*), structural analysis builds on a knowledge of roots, prefixes, suffixes, and compound words as clues in word attack.

How many prefixes can your pupils recognize in print? How many suffixes? Do they know the common roots of English words? Can they apply this knowledge in unlocking the meaning of new words they meet in their reading?

Recognizing and decoding compound words is also part of structural analysis. Your students need to know that both parts of a compound word must contribute to the meaning of the new word. For example, the *car* in *carport* or *carfare* is not the same as the *car* in *carpet*, *carrot*, or *carbon*. (This is where some children run into problems in "finding little words in big ones.")

Take the word *like*. How many new words can your class build by adding preflxes and suffixes? (*unlike, likely, unlikely, likable, likeness, likes,* and so on.) Numerous exercises and activities can be (and have been) designed to develop these skills.

Comprehension

"Words, words, words, I'm so sick of words!" That's what Liza Dolittle said in *My Fair Lady,* and I'm sure she was expressing the sentiments of many school children and their reading teachers. In reading and in language instruction, our focus has long been on words—lists of sight words, words that pupils know, new words in a story. Yet we know that knowing the meaning of each individual word does not guarantee comprehension. Words are only stepping stones to meaning. How many times have you been faced with a passage to translate on a foreign language exam, where you knew the meaning of each word, yet couldn't make any more sense out of the passage than "The blue-beaded grasshopper climbed under the holy fence to get a haircut."

Linguistics focuses attention on language patterns in sentences as the key to comprehension, the ability not only to know the words but also to understand the relationship of one word to the others. Words need to be seen in terms of the whole passage in order for understanding to take place.

How closely do the sentence patterns in your class reading material correspond to the sentences your pupils use in their everyday speech? Having children translate the reading into their own words, an activity long used by many reading teachers, is a good test of comprehension. Then they can reveal whether or not they have grasped the deep structure of the sentence.

You may want to use the ideas suggested by Simons in his article as a means of testing your children's comprehension. Here's where a knowledge of new grammar can help in the reading process.

At the upper levels, a knowledge of semantics will help your students in reading between the lines.

Language patterns put a new dimension on another basic reading skill, *context clues.* In the application of context clues, the reader uses the sense of the sentence or clues in the passage surrounding an unfamiliar word to determine the meaning (and sometimes the pronunciation) of that word. For example, the meaning and pronunciation of *content* is determined by the use of the word(s) in the sentences *He was content to stay home* and *The content of this book is very interesting.* In materials designed for reading instruction, authors usually provide passages in which a pupil can learn to apply this skill. In subject-area reading material, students need to more skillful in figuring out new words by using context clues.

Oral Reading

In oral reading pitch, stress, and juncture come to the fore. For years, we have been telling children to read as if they were speaking, and then giving them sentences to read like "Father said, 'Oh, Oh. Here is Spot.' " If kids really were to read this sentence as they would say it, they would probably read, "Dad said, 'Hey, here's Spot.' "

Intonation puts expression into oral reading; that is, the printed symbols are translated into spoken sounds with the normal melody present in our speech. Examples of various interpretations of oral expressions that were changed by changing the pitch, stress and juncture were presented earlier. The same kind of activity can be carried on using written expressions. Make a list of short expressions such as

Have some tea.
How brave you are.
It will rain tomorrow.
You learned to drive today?

Let pupils read these expressions with various interpretations. For example, *Have some tea* can be read as a command or an invitation, *How brave you are* can be read admiringly or sarcastically, and so on. Students can do this type of activity in pairs.

Extend the list to include longer sentences. For example

After eating my pet my friend and I were tired.
For your birthday I'll send candy and nuts to you sweetheart.

In the first sentence, *my pet* could either have been eaten or have been tired after having eaten, depending on how you read it. The kind interpretation of the second sentence would include "... candy and nuts . . ." A more unkind rendition would be ". . . candy / and nuts to you . . ." (It's difficult to write about intonation because the medium in which it operates (speech) is missing in the printed text.) In the different interpretations of the second sentence, notice how the whole tone of the final word (sweetheart) changes from the kind to the unkind. Exercises such as these will show students the role that pitch, stress, and juncture play in oral reading.

One of my very favorite sentences to illustrate this point is *Woman without her man is a raving maniac.* In this sentence, it would appear that the woman is a raving maniac without her man. But in reading it *Woman—without her, man is a raving maniac,* it is the man who is a raving maniac without woman. Even though the words are the same in both instances, the intonation completely reverses the meaning.

Developing pupils' oral reading skills in a linguistic or any other kind of reading program suggests the use of plays. Unlike most other forms of literature, plays were written to be spoken aloud and thus are particularly appropriate for developing oral reading skills.

Pitch, stress, and juncture constitute the suprasegmental phoneme system in English and, like the regular segmental phonemes, they are represented in writing by graphemes. For the suprasegmental phoneme system, the graphemes are puntuation marks: the period representing falling terminal juncture; the question mark usually representing rising terminal juncture; the comma, colon, and dash representing sustained terminal juncture; and so on. As in the case of all sound-symbol relationships, the correspondence is rather imperfect, but it is necessary for students to learn these correspondences as they exist.

When using lists of sentences and expressions similar to the ones suggested above, you may want to leave out the punctuation marks and let the students punctuate according to the way they read the items. Underlining can be used to indicate words with particularly heavy stress. Learning to use punctuation is usually a regular part of language instruction at all grade levels, and whenever it is taught, its function as representing speech features should never be overlooked.

Pitch, stress, and juncture are not limited in their application to oral reading alone. While reading silently, the reader must sense the intonation and melody in his mind's eye in order to comprehend what he reads.

Literature

A number of ways in which linguistics has influenced the teaching of literature have already been identified. The importance of reading literature aloud—particularly poetry—cannot be overestimated. Studying the language of literature can lead students to insights as to how literary artists use their language. But beware: over-analysis can kill interest altogether. I'm just getting over my hatred of daffodils because of grade school assignments that forced me to dissect William Wordsworth's poem about those lovely flowers. Direct experience, rather than literary criticism, ought to be the chief aim of working with literature, at least in the early years.

Analysis of the sound and rhythm patterns of prose and poetry might be good preparation for choral-speaking activities. Remember what Lefevre has to say about the four-stress system of English in this respect. Depending on the level of your class and your own background and knowledge in such matters, you might want to look at various authors' use of dialect in their writing (Bobby Burns, Mark Twain, Charles Dickens, and others) or the use of language in literature during different periods (the Elizabethan era versus the Victorian or some other period).

Dialect

No matter which regional or social-class dialect the children in your class speak, a good starting point might be for you to analyze the sound system they use. On an individual basis, have each one pronounce a list of words such as *pan, pen, pin, pond,* and *pun; pave, peet, pine, phone,* and *prune.* You might want to include nonsense syllables as Allen suggested. What are the variations between your language and that of your pupils in the beginning, middle, and ending sounds of words? What are the phonetic caution points that you should be aware of in teaching reading?

Dialectologists identify grammatical areas where nonstandard dialects differ from standard English. Some examples are: the use of *ain't;* dropping or changing the standard form of the verb *to be* (as in *He be going.*); variant verb features (*brang* for *brought*); dropping the suffixes marking the past tense or third person singular of verbs, or the plural and possessive forms of nouns; pronoun forms and the like. Wolfram's article may help you identify some of these grammatical conflict points to be aware of in teaching reading.

A thorough analysis of the phonological and syntactical features of the dialect of the children you teach (available in a publication such as *The Linguistic Atlas*) might prove helpful in suggesting points of emphasis or adjustments you need to make in teaching reading.

Spelling

A linguistically-based spelling program groups words according to their patterns of sound-symbol correspondence. Once a pattern has been introduced to (and learned by) your class—the letter combination *oa* as in *boat, goat,* and *road,* for example—other words that correspond to this pattern ought to be presented. You could make a class dictionary or have your pupils keep spelling notebooks in which words are grouped according to their sound-symbol patterns.

The nature of our alphabetic writing system could also be an interesting and worthwhile subject for discussion. Your children have probably enjoyed some experience with picture puzzles and rebus writing that could be extended to the classroom. We sometimes use logograms (symbols for frequently recurring words) in our writing; for example, $4 + 3 = 7$ represents Four and (plus) three is (equals) seven. Write a short rebus puzzle on the board, such as I C U or I AM Y Y U U IT. (I am too wise to use it.) The inclusion of pictures will increase possibilities:

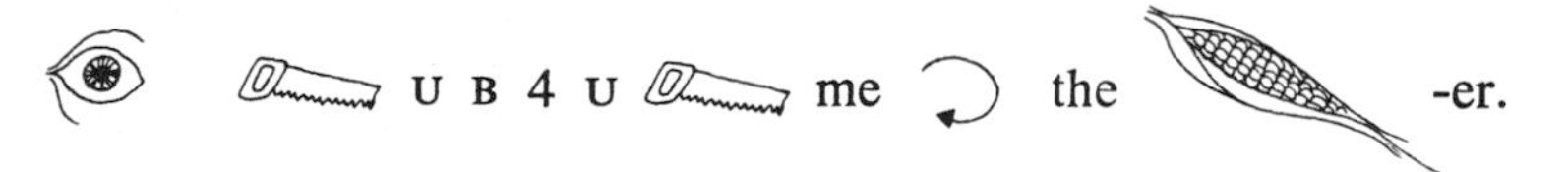

(I saw you before you saw me around the corner.) Let pupils make up their own rebus puzzles for others to decode.

After this type of activity, children may be able to discuss the advantages and limitations of this kind of writing in contrast to our own alphabetic writing system.

A study of the history and development of the alphabet might be an interesting class project, or an individual assignment for capable students who are interested.

Conclusion

Because learning to read is a language process, virtually anything we do under the banner of reading instruction might be classified as a linguistic activity and can be justified on linguistic grounds. For example, in a study cited earlier (page 7), Carol Chomsky found that there was a strong correlation between a number of reading-exposure measures and language development in terms of acquisition of certain syntactic structures. In other words, the more a child is exposed to reading (either being read to or reading on his own) the more adult syntactical patterns he can be expected to know and use. Of course, reading specialists have been recommending the practice of reading aloud to children and good teachers have been following this practice for years, without being conscious of the direct contribution that they were making to a child's acquisition of complex syntactic structures. What linguistics does, then, is to allow us to add a new dimension, or to reinforce positive practices that we have been using all along.

The linguistics revolution is still going on. You can be sure that linguists will keep coming up with new theories—not only in reading but in other areas of language instruction as well—and that teachers will be expected to present these new theories to students or to use the theories to improve their language instruction. This has always been, and will continue to be, an exciting and challenging task. Good luck in it!

One More Step

Questions and activities for further learning.

1. Using the material presented in the articles by Bloomfield, Fries, LeFevre, Simons, Wardhaugh, and others, develop a synthesis that might be legitimately called *the linguistic approach to reading.* Don't forget readiness factors, evaluation, instructional techniques, and materials.
2. Select a primer or first reader from a conventional meaning-oriented basal reading series and compare it with a book from a linguistic series intended for the same grade level. What similarities and differences are apparent between the two?
3. In what specific ways can a knowledge of linguistics contribute to better phonics teaching in the classroom?
4. Take a look at a standardized reading test currently in use and determine the means used to measure reading comprehension. Try applying Simons' theory of measuring comprehension with the material contained in this test.
5. Wolfram proposes four alternatives to teaching reading to speakers of nonstandard English; Allen also gives some suggestions. In which of Wolfram's alternatives would Allen's ideas be particularly appropriate? Which of the alternatives and suggestions do you favor? Why?

The Final Step

It has been said that there is no part of the language arts curriculum that can be left untouched by linguistics. Now that you have read the book, think of the applications and implications that linguistics has for your language-arts teaching. Don't forget dramatics, storytelling, choral speaking, discussion, and all the other areas of language instruction.

The text of this book was composed on Lintotype in 10-point Times Roman and the heads in Helvetica Bold by Holmes Typography, Inc. of San Jose, California. Display heads and article titles in Univers Demi-Bold were set by Spartan Typographers, Oakland, California.

Printing and binding were done by The George Banta Company of Menasha, Wisconsin.

Sponsoring Editor: *Karl J. Schmidt*
Project Editor: *Toni Marshall*
Designer: *Joseph di Chiarro*

3456/54321